Essential Psychiatry

Essential Psychiatry

John Sheahan
SRN RMN RNT

Tutor, Institute of Advanced Nursing Education, Royal College of Nursing and National Council of Nurses of the United Kingdom.

MTP**PRESS LIMITED·LANCASTER·ENGLAND**
International Medical Publishers

Published by
MTP Press Limited
Falcon House
Lancaster, England.

ISBN: 0-85200 052-9

Printed by UPS (Blackburn), Northgate,
Blackburn.

Contents

Contents

1

Introduction

1.0 Introduction

As a nurse you are going to be caring for other people, many of whom may be very ill and distressed. Some may have lost their ability to reason, whilst others may never have had this facility. This has a number of effects. For example, it may give rise to personal fears, anxieties and bewilderment, or to aggression and destructiveness. It causes social upsets within the family, at work and in society. Coupled with this are the economic effects, first to the individual and secondly to the community.

From the nurse's point of view, all these aspects are important but there are two aspects which are of particular importance. In order to do your job well you will need a lot of knowledge and this will mean much study. You will, after a time, look upon increasing your knowledge as a pleasure to be enjoyed and not as a chore to be endured. This love of knowledge, or more precisely, love of wisdom is called *Philosophy*. During your professional career you will be forming relationships with other people. Your relationships are going to be different, in one important respect, from ordinary relationships, because of the mental state of those with whom you will relate. Impaired mental function puts the other person at a disadvantage. Due to your position as a nurse you will know a great deal about those in your care. You will need some guiding principles to keep your conduct on a sound professional basis and these are provided by that branch of philosophy called *Ethics*.

1.1 Philosophy

Philosophy is defined as the love of wisdom, and the study of philosophy concentrates on providing fundamental explanations for everything that happens about us. The sciences, such as chemistry, physics and biology, provide explanations of how and why things work. These explanations are based on facts derived by experiment. The explanations thus offered are limited by the experimental methods of each science and at best are only part of the total picture. The task of philosophy is to give an all-embracing picture of the world around us.

Philosophy tries to provide explanations for abstract concepts such as truth, goodness, beauty, the nature of reality and the existence of God. Many great men have contributed to the subject and a few of these will be mentioned in case you would like to read some of their works. The most notable philosophers of early times were Plato (428–348 B.C.) and Aristotle (384–322). St. Thomas Aquinas (1225–1274) and René Descartes (1596–1650) were notable philosophers of later times. In more recent times, among the names frequently mentioned are those of Benedict de Spinoza (1632–1677), John Locke (1632–1704), David Hume (1711–1776) and Immanuel Kant (1724–1804).

A Specialist has been defined as one who knows more and more about less and less. Much of learning today is concerned with examining particular topics in detail and in depth. One of the values of philosophy is that is has an integrating influence on the whole world of learning. Secondly it helps to put things in perspective. It also helps man to be thoughtful and reflective and not a slave to his emotions and this, as we shall see later, is important in mental health. We frequently say of a person who remains cool, calm and collected when disaster or tragedy befalls, that he was philosophical about it or that he behaved philosophically. Philosophy develops man's capacity to think, to reach objective decisions and at the same time frees him from prejudice.

1.2 Ethics

Ethics is sometimes called the philosophy of conduct or moral philosophy. It comes from the Greek word ethos which means custom, usage, habit and includes characteristics such as disposition, temper and character. Philosophy helps man to be more reflective and thoughtful and ethics, which is a branch of philosophy, helps man to be more reasonable, for the aim of ethics is to instruct reason so that it can make the correct judgements about the morality, the right or wrong, of human acts. Ethics supplies principles for man's moral guidance.

1.3 Ethical aspects of nursing

Scientific knowledge and technical skill is more advanced than ever before, yet the ethical considerations become increasingly complex. Take abortion for example. In skilled hands this is a technically safe operation, but when the law relating to abortion was recently changed, the main arguments were about the ethical aspects. In fact a conscience clause was included for the benefit of those who strongly objected to this operation on ethical grounds.

There is the question of terminal illnesses and the use of drugs to control pain. Some believe that drugs should be freely given to provide freedom from pain, whilst others maintain that this is wrong if the drugs have the effect of shortening life. It is possible to keep the victims of serious accidents alive for a long time with the aid of technical apparatus. There comes a time when it is obvious that the person will not recover and the question of withdrawing the help of the apparatus arises. This poses a profoundly difficult ethical problem, for there are some who will maintain that every effort must be made to maintain life, whilst others would argue of the futility of prolonging a vegetable-like existence.

The transplant of organs from one person to another is a major technical achievement, but again, the main arguments have centred round the ethical considerations. In the case of heart and liver transplants there is the problem of deciding when the donor is dead. Then there is the question of putting the inconvenience of a major operation on a seriously ill person, when the advantages to be gained are known to be limited.

In the field of psychiatry, the question of brain surgery arises. The operation of leucotomy can bring relief from distressing symptoms, but sometimes the side effects can be as incapacitating as the original disease. Should the operation of leucotomy be done? Then there is the question of behaviour therapy. Is it right to use methods which cause the person to be sick or to feel discomfort due to the passage of an electric current? There is an ethical principle which says that the end does not justify the means. Likewise there is a practice of rendering people unconscious by the use of electricity in electro-convulsive therapy. These are forms of treatment which continually raise ethical questions.

There is a major ethical discussion in progress about whether the lives of people suffering from distressing diseases should be ended and there have been unsuccessful attempts to introduce legislation to make euthanasia lawful. Euthanasia means a gentle and easy death, but it is now taken to mean legalized or mercy killing and is unacceptable to the medical and nursing professions.

1.4 Code of ethics

A nurse has many responsibilities and among these are those to the the sick, the doctor and other professional colleagues, the nursing profession and last but not least her own conscience. She will therefore need guidance to meet these responsibilities and this has been provided in the International Council of Nurses 'Code of Ethics'. Representatives from forty-six countries adopted the code at Sao Paulo, Brazil in July 1953. The code, which was revised in 1963, is as follows:

1. The fundamental responsibility of the nurse is threefold; to conserve life, to alleviate suffering and to promote health.

Comment: It will be seen that the practice of euthanasia would be incompatible with these principles.

2. The nurse shall maintain at all times the highest standards of nursing care and of professional conduct.

Comment: To give less than one's best would be unacceptable.

3. The nurse must not only be well prepared to practise but shall maintain knowledge and skill at a consistently high level.

Comment: Nurses, like people in other professions, become perpetual students. In order to keep up to date professional magazines should be read regularly and copies of textbooks should be kept up to date.

4. The religious beliefs of a patient should be respected.

Comment: This is always important, but particularly so now for people move freely about the world.

5. Nurses hold in confidence all personal information entrusted to them.

Comment: It helps some people to be able to confide in others in times of difficulty. In hospital a nurse is often told personal details and she reads others in the person's medical history.

6. Nurses recognize not only the responsibilities but the limitations of their professional functions; do not recommend or give medical treatment without medical orders except in emergencies, and report such action to a physician as soon as possible.

Comment: Nurses tend to be consulted by a variety of people on an even greater variety of problems. Nurse training does not provide training in the diagnosis of illness, therefore, it must be recommended that medical advice is sought.

7. The nurse is under an obligation to carry out the physician's orders intelligently and loyally and to refuse to participate in unethical procedures.

Comment: A physician accepts overall responsibility for those in his care and is therefore entitled to co-operation and loyalty. At the same time the nurse is the keeper of her own conscience.

8. The nurse sustains confidence in the physician and other members

of the health team; incompetence or unethical conduct of associates should be exposed but only to the proper authority.

Comment: When there is unethical conduct by colleagues, this poses a difficult problem which must be faced. There may be legal repercussions and all nurses would be well advised to belong to a professional organization which would advise.

9. The nurse is entitled to just remuneration and accepts only such compensation the contract, actual or implied, provides.

Comment: This means that a nurse does not accept gifts from those in her care, for gifts may be given in the hope of gaining preferential treatment and this would be unacceptable. At other times gifts may be given as a tip and this is also unacceptable to a professional person.

10. Nurses do not permit their names to be used in connection with the advertisement of products or with any other forms of self advertisement.

Comment: If advertising were allowed there would be a danger that professional interests would take second place to commercial ones.

11. The nurse co-operates with and maintains harmonious relationships with members of other professions and with nursing colleagues.

Comment: Team work is the keynote of modern medical and nursing care and of course good relationships are essential for this.

12. The nurse adheres to standards of personal ethics which reflect credit upon the profession.

Comment: Unless the nurse's personal conduct is of a high standard, it is unlikely that she will aspire to high professional standards.

13. In personal conduct, nurses should not knowingly disregard the accepted pattern of behaviour of the community in which they live and work.

Comment: This would apply to nurses who travelled abroad and found themselves working among people of a different culture.

14. The nurse participates and shares responsibility with other citizens and other professions in promoting efforts to meet the health needs of the public—local, state, national and international.

Comment: Disease knows no boundaries, therefore the efforts to control disease and to promote health must not be in any way insular.

1.5 Personal aspects of illness

The history of psychiatry shows that the lot of the mentally ill has never been a happy one. They have at times been thought to be possessed of devils and thus outcasts from society; their problems have been misunderstood or ignored.

It is against this background that the personal aspects of mental illness must be considered, for though society now has a more enlightened approach, it must be remembered that attitudes change very slowly. From your own experiences you will have observed that people discuss mental illness in a different tone. Euphemisms may be used and people may try so hard to say the right thing that their approach is guarded.

The mentally ill person has a double obstacle to overcome. He has to overcome the effects of his illness and he has to come to terms with an often unhelpful and sometimes even hostile society.

The effects of specific disorders can be quite crippling. Fear and anxiety can be so great as to make life a nightmare, when it is impossible to make a decision. Disorders affecting intelligence result in perplexity, bewilderment and confusion. In thought disorders, the world around us is misinterpreted and instead of normal percepts, those formed are of a distorted and frightening nature. These distorted percepts torment the person so that his behaviour is often seriously affected. When the mood is affected as in depression, joy and happiness vanishes and all that remains is unrelieved gloom. At times this gloom may be so great and the outlook on life may appear so futile, that the person cannot see any solution but to end life by his own hand.

We shall develop the effects of these disorders when they are considered in detail later, but at this early stage it is important to attempt to understand what it is like to be mentally ill, for if your help is to be effective it must be based on a sound understanding of the sick person's dilemma.

1.6 Social aspects of illness

The family is the basic unit of society and most people have family ties, though some choose to cut these ties. There is the immediate family which consists of husband and wife and children. In addition there is the so called extended family, that is, grandparents, uncles, aunts, cousins and in-laws. Illness causes disruption of this family unit. Near relatives may lose sleep, miss work or more seriously have their own health affected through caring for the sick member. The sick person, particularly in the case of illness of long duration, loses normal social contacts and becomes socially isolated.

When the person is ready to return to work again, there is the problem of working a full working day when one has been out of the habit. In some cases illness means a loss of job and the person has to begin to look for a job and then has the problem of settling down in a new setting. In the case of the mentally ill, there is an additional problem in that many employers are unwilling to employ them. Without adequate support in the early days, the demoralizing effect of being unable to get a job is enough to cause a relapse of the illness.

Mental illness affects people at all levels of society from the professor to the cleaner, but there tends to be a greater number at the lower levels. This is explained by the fact that some people at the higher levels when affected by illness tend to drift down the social scale. A university graduate, because of mental illness, may be doing a menial job and living in slum surroundings. This is known as 'social drift' and increases the incidence of mental illness at the lower social levels.

A poor environment with poor housing and a high population density can be a source of mental stress. People living in such environments are often unskilled and are those likely to find themselves unemployed when work is scarce. Such people frequently have large families which adds to the economic strain. Slum conditions, unemployment, large families and consequent shortage of money leads to crime. If the father is sent to prison for criminal activities, the mother is likely to have to go to work or to increase the existing level of work. This means that the parental supervision of the children will be inadequate and truancy and delinquency may follow. Thus the die is cast for another generation of deviants.

1.7 Economic aspects of illness

It is the duty of every nation to provide facilities for the care of the sick. In this country this is done through the National Health Service. The nation spends over £1,800 million per annum on this service and this represents about five per cent of the national income or five new pence in the pound. The National Health Service provides 454,000 hospital beds for the care of the sick and nearly half of these, actually forty-seven per cent are occupied by the mentally ill. The cost of maintaining these beds is in excess of £180 million a year. This represents a considerable expenditure but it is not the whole story. During 1970 over ten million working days were lost through strikes, but the number lost through illness was 300 million or 30 times greater. About 25 million of the illnesses were psychiatric. But this is not all, for there are over 250,000 accidents in industry each year. We shall look at accident proneness again when we consider the mental mechanisms and we shall see that there is a psychological element.

It will be seen that illness has economic effects on the individual, though these have been greatly eased by providing a free health service which is backed up with sickness, injury, unemployment and social security payments. The effects at a national level are also great. There is the loss of productivity which means that delivery dates cannot always be met and this sometimes means a loss of export orders which are vital for the country's economic survival. Coupled with the loss of productivity is the cost of injury and social security benefits. It is estimated that the cost of accidents alone is over £220 million a year.

1.8 Summary

There are many facets to caring for others including a basic philosophy and ethics. It is important to be able to think deeply and to reflect on the problems of the day. It is equally important to have reasonable conduct in relation to others and the principles governing this are supplied by ethics. They are personal, social and economic aspects to illness and this adds to the complexity of the study of human problems, but these many dimensions also ensure a greater range of interests and thus a greater challenge.

2

Mental processes

2.0 Introduction

It has been said that the art of the physician is based not only on clinical experience but on a systematic understanding of the functions and structure of the human body. These sentiments equally apply to a nurse or any other helper concerned with the mentally ill. It is recognized that when help is given to a sick person, the whole person should be considered from the physical, social and psychological aspects. This will be borne in mind throughout this book, but to include all aspects in detail would result in a very heavy book. The approach then will be mainly a psychological one. In keeping with the opening of this chapter we shall now consider the nervous system and the mind in some detail.

2.1 The beginning

If cells of the human species are examined they are seen to contain 23 pairs of yellow bodies (chromosomes). If these cells are further examined they are seen to be composed of tiny bead-like structures called genes. On even closer examination, the nuclei within each cell are found to contain two types of acid, ribonucleic acid (R.N.A.) and deoxyribonucleic acid (D.N.A.) This latter acid, D.N.A. is said to be the chemical basis of life. The cells increase in number by each cell dividing and giving two daughter cells, which in turn gives rise to two more and so on. This process is called mitosis and it ensures that each of the daughter cells have exactly the same number of chromosomes, genes and the same quantity of nucleic acids as the parent cell. There is an exception to this as far as the germ or reproductive cells are concerned. They undergo a special type of division which is called meiosis (Fig. 2.1). This results in a halving of the number of chromosomes, genes and nucleic acids in each cell. A male germ cell is called a spermatozoon and the female one is called an ovum. At fertilization a spermatozoon enters the ovum and fertilizes it. There is a pooling of genetic material and the chromosome complement is restored to the full number. Thus as offspring resulting from fertilization has inherited half of its characteristics from the genes of its father and half from its mother. The quality of these genes is of fundamental importance and abnormalities result in a variety of disorders. Precisely how important is the quality of these genes, has not yet been satisfactorily determined, as at the moment it is the subject of much debate which is revolving around intelligence. Sir Cyril Burt, an English psychologist, who is concerned with the factors which influence intelligence, has come to the conclusion that genetic factors make a ninety per cent contribution to the development of this function. In America, Professor Jensen of California has concluded that the figure of eighty per cent is more correct in this respect. Another worker in America, F. S. Fehr has come up with the answer that intelligence is only thirty-eight per cent inherited. We cannot but conclude that whilst inheritance is important we cannot say so with precision as yet. We shall return to genetic influences and genetic disorders later, but at the moment we shall consider the development of the new individual.

2.2 Development (embryology)

When two germ cells, a spermatozoon and an ovum also called gametes, fuse together, fertilization is said to take place and results in the production of a zygote. Fertilization usually takes place in the uterine tubes although it can occur elsewhere. The zygote undergoes a process called cleavage. This is the term given to repeated mitosis which takes place following fertilization. It produces a small mass of cells called the blastula. By the time the blastula reaches the uterus it consists of a considerable number of cells. It is now called a blastocyst and becomes implanted in the wall of the uterus. Following implantation, membranes develop and the life-line to the mother is established. This is the beginning of the embryo stage which lasts about eight weeks after which time it is recognizably human. From now on the embryo is referred to as the foetus. As we shall see, intense development takes place during the embryonic period and a study of these activities is called embryology. We shall consider these activities in relation to the nervous system only.

Up to the blastocyst stage all the cells are alike. Once implantation of the blastocyst takes place, groups of cells begin to acquire characteristics. This process is known as differentiation. The first stage of this process is not too specific as it gives rise to three different types of tissue only. These are the ectoderm, the mesoderm and the endoderm. These three basic tissues further differentiate to give rise to all the tissues and organs in the fully grown body. The ectoderm gives rise to the nervous system which first appears as a neural groove at about two and a half weeks. At three and a half weeks the groove becomes more pronounced and looks like a tube. At four weeks the neural tube is closed and the three primary vesicles of the brain are represented (Fig. 2.0). At this stage nerves and ganglia can be

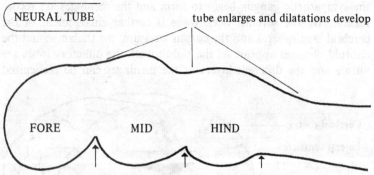

Fig.2.0. Diagram to show neural tube.

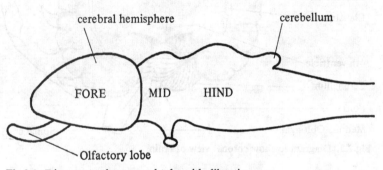

Fig.2.1. Diagram to show neural tube with dilatations.

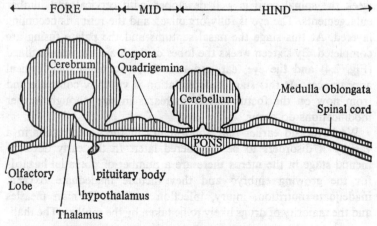

Fig.2.2. Diagram to show further development of dilatations.

seen to be forming. At five weeks there are five brain vesicles and the cerebral hemispheres begin to bulge and the nerves and ganglia are more obvious. In the sixth week nerve plexuses are present, the sympathetic ganglia begin to form and the meninges are recognizable. By the seventh week there is further enlargement of the cerebral hemispheres and the corpus striatum, the thalamus and the choroid plexuses appear. At the eighth week the olfactory lobes are visible and the different layers of the meninges can be recognized

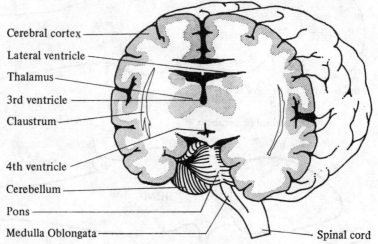

Cerebral cortex
Lateral ventricle
Thalamus
3rd ventricle
Claustrum
4th ventricle
Cerebellum
Pons
Medulla Oblongata
Spinal cord

Fig.2.3. Diagram to show coronal view of brain.

and the brain attains its general structural features. By the tenth week the spinal cord is well developed with cervical and lumbar enlargements. The eye is fully organized and the retina is becoming layered. At this stage the nasal septums and the palate fusing are completed. By sixteen weeks the lobes of the brain are well outlined (Fig. 2.4) and the eye, ear and nose have acquired their typical appearances. At this stage differentiation is virtually complete and from now on the foetus mainly increases in size, though further modifications do occur.

We have said earlier that abnormality of the genes results in a variety of disorders to be considered later. In the early developmental stage in the uterus there are a number of potential hazards for the growing embryo and they include inadequate oxygen, inadequate nutrition, injury, infection such as German measles and the majority of drugs likely to be taken by the mother. The thali-

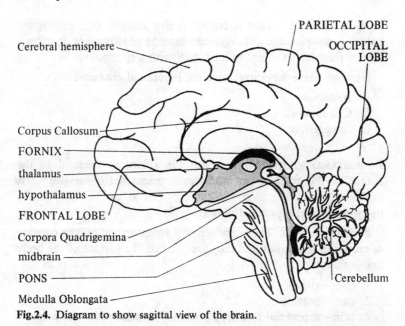

Fig.2.4. Diagram to show sagittal view of the brain.

domide tragedy is an example of how a drug taken by the mother during pregnancy can have disastrous effects on the embryo. Like the genetic influences, the development hazards will be considered more fully when we come to consider mental illness.

2.3 The developed nervous system

From our brief account of growth within the uterus, we have seen that the development of the nervous system begins very early and is considerably advanced by the end of three months. Some further development does take place, but the main feature is that the foetus increases in size during the last six months in the uterus. At birth the infant has a complete, though not very efficient, nervous system. The feeling or sensory side is fairly efficient as the infant is aware of discomforts and can make these known. At first vision is uniocular, that is the child sees out of each eye independently. The ability to focus both eyes on an object does not come until the infant is six weeks old. The infant is deaf at birth and only loud noises are appreciated. The perception of fine sounds does not come until later. Motor activity, the ability to do things, is limited to aimless thrashing of the limbs at birth and skills such as walking are not possible until the infant is ten or twelve months old. Intelligible speech is not possible until eighteen months or two years. It takes a similar time for an infant to feed itself with a spoon.

Nervous tissue has three principal functional characteristics:

A. Irritability.
B. Conduction.
C. Integration.

A. IRRITABILITY. Irritability means the ability to respond to the stimuli in the environment and this is essential for survival. It is achieved by sense organs which are placed at various sites in the body and are grouped as follows:

a. *Exteroceptors.* These are sensory receptors or organs capable of receiving sensations and they are sited on the surface of the body and include:

1. eyes—vision.
2. ears—hearing.
3. skin—superficial and deep sensation, temperature and pain.
4. nose—smell.
5. tongue—taste.

These are the five senses or the special senses.

b. *Proprioceptors.* (*L. proprius*, one's own; *capere*, to receive). Like the exteroceptors, the proprioceptors are sense organs but they are sited in the skeletal muscles, the tendons and joints, the lungs, heart and abdominal viscera. They receive stimuli which arise within the body itself.

c. *Interoceptors.* Similarly the interoceptors are sense organs and these are sited in mucous membrane of the respiratory and alimentary tracts. Though removed from direct influence by the external environment, these receptors nevertheless, are stimulated by agencies originating outside the body such as air and food.

It can be seen that the entire body is supplied with sense organs and whatever the nature of the stimulus, there is in the healthy person, a means to receive. But receiving the information is not sufficient. It must be transmitted so that action may be taken. It would be no use if the sense organs in the nose were stimulated by a high concentration of coal-gas in the environment, or those in the skin by an unusually high or low temperature if the information were not passed on. The person could be either gassed or burned or suffer from frostbite. This brings us to the second functional characteristic of nervous tissue, which is conduction.

B. CONDUCTION. Conduction is the job of the nerve fibres. When a sense organ of any kind is stimulated an impulse is said to be set up. An impulse (*L. impellere*, to drive before) means a sudden force or thrust. The term message is sometimes used instead of impulse. Impulses from the sense organs are transmitted along the nerve fibres to the spinal cord and in the spinal cord they are again transmitted along fibres to the appropriate centre in the brain. These are called *sensory* nerve fibres. In the brain the incoming information is analysed and action is taken. The frontal lobe of the brain initiates this action and creates impulses which are transmitted in nerve fibres which leave the brain and these are called *motor* fibres. The sensory or incoming fibres and the motor or outgoing ones are quite specific in action and allow only a one-way transmission of impulses. No interchange of roles is possible. Nerve impulses travel along the nerve fibres at high speed, at approximately the same speed as a racing car, yet there are emergencies when this speed is not fast enough and the route to the brain is not followed. The sensory impulses go to the spinal cord only, and in emergency this can initiate motor action. This is a *reflex action* and is the mechanism used to achieve the very quick response which results when a hot object is touched or when one stands on a sharp object.

Failure of the sense organs is potentially dangerous because an individual is unaware of hazards in the environment. It follows that transmission failures have similar circumstances. The transmitting fibres can be damaged by injury or disease processes. Syphilis of the spinal cord for example, damages the sensory fibres, particularly those to the proprioceptors. The result is that the person is unaware of the position of his feet in relation to the ground and develops a stamping gait. It might be useful to think of the nervous system as the manager of the muscular system. When there is a nerve supply to a muscle (innervation) muscular activity is possible, and conversely, when the nerve supply is deficient or absent then the resultant muscular activity is also deficient or absent. Some of the motor fibres are damaged when a haemorrhage occurs in the brain, as occurs in the condition commonly called 'stroke'. The limbs affected are stiff and fine movements are no longer possible. This is called a *spastic* paralysis. If the entire motor nerve supply to a limb is cut off muscular activity will cease and this is called a *flaccid* paralysis.

C. INTEGRATION. This is a vital function and is carried out by the nerve cells. It has been estimated that an average person has over 10,000,000,000 nerve cells and ninety per cent of these are found in the brain and are often called *Betz* cells, the remainder are in the spinal cord. As we have seen there are sense organs all over the body and as we are seeing, hearing, feeling, smelling and tasting for most of the time, the brain is continually bombarded with a variety of sensory stimuli. The brain in turn has to initiate the appropriate responses in reply to these stimuli. All this means a considerable amount of activity. As there is so much happening and if chaos is not to result, there must be very careful control over events. This control function is called integration. This is achieved by the action of the inhibitory and facilitatory mechanisms. In front of the motor area of the brain lies the suppressor band and this contains inhibitory fibres. As their name suggests such fibres inhibit some motor impulses. Conversely fibres arise in the area of the hypothalamus which facilitate the passage of motor impulses and these are called facilitation fibres. It is the balance between these opposing influences that makes integration possible. We have seen that an infant's movements are poorly integrated and this lasts for some time. Anyone who has, for example, seen the handwriting of five, six or seven year olds will observe that it is usually clumsy, big and shaky. As the young person gets older the writing becomes more uniform; this is due to improved muscular co-ordination and integration. It is true that some people are exceptionally clumsy and drop and break objects at an alarming rate. There are diseases which damage the nerve cells such as Huntington's chorea and Parkinson's disease which seriously affect the integration function of the nervous system and result in involuntary, purposeless movements. In the case of Huntington's chorea the movements may be so strong and frequent that a person is unable to attend to personal details such as washing, dressing and eating.

2.4 The organization of the nervous system

We have seen that the principal functions of the nervous system are perceiving stimuli (irritability), transmission of the impulses set up by these stimuli (conduction) and analysing the stimuli, establishing an order of priorities and ensuring smooth, efficient purposeful and co-ordinated muscular movements (integration). It is now time to have a close look at the organisation of the system concerned with these vital functions. The basic unit of the nervous system is the nerve cell or neurone. Each neurone has two parts, a cell body and an axon. When small pieces (sections) of cell bodies are examined using a microscope, they have a greyish hue. It is for this reason that collections of neurones are referred to as grey matter. If a nerve fibre (the axon) is similarly examined, it is white in appearance and is thus called white matter.

We have already said that an average person has about 10,000,000,000 neurones and ninety per cent of these are in the brain. For this reason the grey matter or cortex of the brain is a convoluted structure. This allows more cells to fit in a small space. The cell body contains the nucleus of the cell and this controls the metabolism of the whole unit. As the majority of the cell bodies are in the brain, this is the reason why an injury or haemorrhage in this area has such widespread results. The majority of the cells in the body have the power of regeneration or healing. Most of us have scars on the surface of our bodies to prove this. Neurones are so specialized in nature that they have no such powers. We are given one set and if we abuse or ill-use these, then the resultant functions will be permanently impaired. The impairment of function is proportional to the number of cells lost.

Radiating from the cell body are branches called dendrites. These dendrites transmit impulses towards the cell body and synapse with, and receive impulses from axons of other nerve cells. Stimulation of one neurone by another takes place at the synapse. (*L. Synapse*, 1 clasp). A synapse is formed by the axon of one neurone and the cell body or a dendrite of another. There is no physical contact at the synapses, and at such gaps the nervous impulse is transmitted through a chemical medium. The chemicals at these points are either of an excitory or an inhibitory nature. Each cell body, unless it is a sensory cell, has synapses with several nerve fibres. An impulse, when it reaches a synapse, has to stimulate the next neurone if it is to produce any further effect. This stimulation takes a little time and it is referred to as synaptic delay. Such stimulation may fail to occur if the impulse arrives from the wrong direction. As we mentioned earlier, this transmission of impulses is a one-way process and the synapses are responsible for this. It is necessary to have repeated stimuli in order to achieve action and this is called *summation*, which is the additive effect of several stimuli. Summation can be explained as follows: Suppose a neurone has synapses with the nerve fibres of neurones A, B, C. If impulses arrive separately from A, B, and C, they may fail to produce an impulse in the neurone, but if all three arrive simultaneously, stimulation is much more likely to occur. This increased responsiveness on the part of the neurone due to the effect of summation is called *facilitation*.

The main fibre leaving the cell body of the neurone is the axon. These may vary in length from a few microns up to 90 cm. long. The sciatic nerve has a long axon; it may be up to 90 cm. long in a tall adult. The function of the axons is to transmit the nervous impulses and in common with conducting cables, most of the axons are insulated. This insulation is provided by the presence of myelin. Such nerves are called myelinated or medullated. Fibres which lack a myelin sheath are called unmyelinated or non-medullated; their axons are bounded merely by the usual plasma-membrane of all cells. The myelinated fibres are surrounded with Schwann cells and these produce the fatty-like material called myelin. The myelin forms a sheath which completely envelops the fibre except at regularly spaced intervals. These intervals are called nodes. Sometimes the myelin is destroyed by disease processes and impaired function results usually in the form of paralysis. The best known of such diseases is disseminated sclerosis sometimes referred to as multiple sclerosis. All the post-ganglionic fibres of the automonic nervous system are non-myelinated. (We shall consider the autonomic part of the nervous system later). There are also a number of non-myelinated fibres in the dorsal nerve roots of the central nervous system.

In the case of motor nerve fibres, these give rise to small fibres called fibrils at their end-points where they join muscles. These end-points terminate just short of the motor end-plate in the muscles. There is no physical contact between the muscles and the nerves. The final passage of the nerve impulse is through a chemical medium across a synaptic connective tissue interval by means of chemical transmitters, in this instance called acetylcholine. In the case of the post-ganglionic fibres of the sympathetic part of the autonomic nervous system, the chemical transmitter is noradrenaline.

The Nervous system is organised from:

A. *Neurones*. These are specialised in irritability, conduction and integration. These are further subdivided according to function. The motor neurones (Fig. 2.5) transmit impulses from the brain and spinal cord to the effector organs (muscles and glands). Association neurones transmit impulses between neurones and sensory neurones (Fig. 2.6) transmit impulses from the environment to the spinal cord and brain.

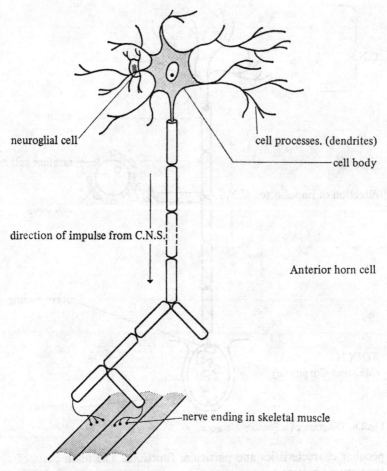

neuroglial cell

cell processes. (dendrites)

cell body

direction of impulse from C.N.S.

Anterior horn cell

nerve ending in skeletal muscle

Fig.2.5. Diagram of a Motor Neurone.

B. *Accessory or supporting cells.* These are non-receptive and non-conducting. These include the neuroglia in the central nervous system (glia = glue, nerve glue). This glue-like material is found supporting the neurones in the brain and spinal cord. They also include the Schwann cells which have already been mentioned, and the satellite cells in the ganglia of the peripheral nervous system. A ganglion is a small mass of nervous tissue containing, in the main, numerous cell bodies. These are found in the spinal and cranial nerve roots and in connection with the autonomic nervous system.

The nervous tissue is organised into a system of the body with

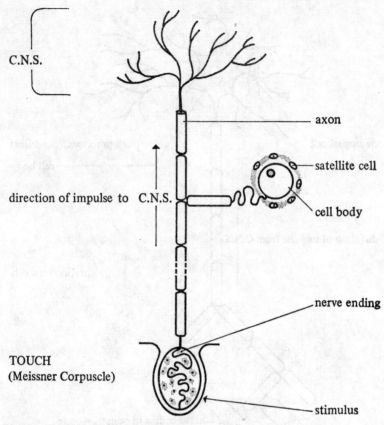

C.N.S.

axon

satellite cell

direction of impulse to   C.N.S.

cell body

nerve ending

TOUCH
(Meissner Corpuscle)

stimulus

Fig.2.6. Diagram of a Sensory Neurone.

peculiar characteristics and particular functions. The main parts of
the nervous system are:

A. The central nervous system which includes the brain and spinal
   cord.
B. The peripheral nervous system which includes the motor and
   sensory nerves outside the spinal cord.
C. The autonomic nervous system which controls a variety of
   functions within the body without our being aware of it.
   This in turn is composed of two parts, the parasympathetic
   and the sympathetic.

2.5 The brain

The brain is an extremely delicate and sensitive organ. Unlike other organs in the body there is no connective tissue or 'packing' material to protect it, apart from the neuroglia already mentioned. The organ is housed in a strong bony case, the skull, which provides a good deal of protection. The various areas of the brain are given the name of the bones which cover them; these are frontal, temporal, parietal and occipital.

The brain has two cerebral hemispheres. These hemispheres are connected at the centre by a structure called the corpus callosum. This is an arched mass of white matter, made up of transverse fibres which connects the roofs of the lateral hemispheres as well as the cerebral hemispheres. When a section is cut through the brain it is seen to comprise of a narrow convoluted area of grey matter (cell bodies) on the outside and a white area (nerve fibres) on the inside. In the centre there is a system of channels which are enlarged at certain points. The enlargements are the ventricles containing a fluid-like cushion for the delicate organ, and the channels connect the ventricles to allow for the free circulation of this fluid. Surrounding the ventricles on each side are collections of grey matter and these are collectively called the basal ganglia.

2.6 The nerves

In order to keep in touch with all parts of the body, there is a comprehensive communication system. It consists of twelve pairs of cranial nerves which keep the brain informed of what is happening around the head and neck, so that it may take appropriate action. These include the nerves concerned with sight, hearing, smell, taste, touch and temperature. Some of these are sensory nerves, some are motor nerves and some are mixed with branches carrying out sensory and motor functions. The thirty-one pairs of spinal nerves carry out a similar function for the rest of the body.

2.7 Localization of brain function

We have said earlier that nerve impulses are transmitted to special centres in the brain. Here they are interpreted and action is taken. We shall now consider the localizing of function within the brain. The cerebrum contains the higher centres and controls learned and conscious behaviour. The higher centres usually accredited to the frontal lobes, enable us to conform to the conventions imposed on us by society and makes sophisticated behaviour possible. These centres

are subject to a variety of influences. For example if the blood supply
is inadequate, confusion and changes in behaviour occur, as happens
in elderly people. Drugs and poisons affect these centres and result
in changes of behaviour. One of the explanations of drug taking is
that the drugs allow an escape from the pressures of society. Alcohol
is seen to do this. A person who has drunk alcohol is said to be less
inhibited and is therefore more sociable. Alcohol serves a function in
society as a social lubricant and enables people to mix better, but
continued excesses have disastrous consequences. The motor area is
contained in the frontal lobe where motor action is initiated and it is
also the centre for skilled acts. When head injuries involving the
frontal lobe occur, the range of functions of this part of the brain
become very apparent. The person has little or no control over
behaviour and flies into a temper at the slightest provocation. There
is no hesitation about using foul language and concentration and
attention are non-existent depending on the degree of the injury.
Judgement and reason are impaired, skilled acts are not possible
and a formerly skilled person becomes clumsy. The speech centre is
found in the left side of the frontal lobe. This has a practical bearing
in diseases of the nervous system. Each side of the brain controls
opposite sides of the body. If a person has a haemorrhage or 'stroke'
affecting the left side of the brain the speech area may be affected and
the right side of the body is partially paralysed. The frontal lobe plays
a major role in the integration of the functions of the nervous
system and hence the clumsy movements when the area is affected
by injury.

The parietal lobe contains the sensory centre. All sensory stimuli
from the body are transmitted to this area where they are interpreted.
The centre for hearing is in the temporal lobe and that for vision in
the occipital lobe. There are large uncharted areas in the cerebral
hemispheres, that is, they have not been ascribed any functions.
It has been suggested that these areas are responsible for mental
processes such as intelligence, memory, judgement, imagination
and thought. These are functions associated with the mind and we
shall return to them again when we come to consider the mind.

2.8 The basal ganglia

If we move away from the cerebral cortex, the next areas of grey
matter we meet are the basal ganglia (Fig. 2.7). These consist of the
globus pallidus, the caudate nucleus, the putamen, the substantia-

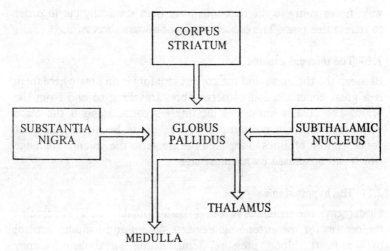

Fig.2.7. Diagram to show relationships of basal ganglia.

nigra and the subthalamic nucleus. The caudate nucleus and the putamen constitute the corpus striatum. The nerve pathway from the corpus striatum to the globus pallidus carries inhibitory fibres from the suppressor areas of the cerebral cortex (already mentioned) and the caudate nucleus. These fibres run down to the reticular formation in the medulla. The facilitatory fibres from the cerebral cortex run through the putamen to the globus pallidus and then to the thalamus. From the thalamus they run to the reticular formation in the midbrain.

The basal ganglia are concerned with modifying and co-ordinating voluntary movement of the skeletal muscles. Disease of this area results in Parkinson's disease as we mentioned earlier and involuntary muscle movement results. The movements of the hands and fingers are characteristic and are described as pill-rolling. Some of the drugs used in the treatment of mental illness affect the basal ganglia, chloropromazine is an example, and we hear of drug-induced Parkinsonism.

2.9 The thalamus

Close to the basal ganglia and just below the lateral ventricles is found an egg-shaped structure called the thalamus. This is an important relay centre for sensory fibres on their way to the cerebral cortex. It is thought that crude sensation and pain may be felt here. In cases where there is severe pain which is not relieved in the usual way, fibres going to the thalamus have been surgically cut in order to relieve this pain. The procedure is not always successful.

2.10 The internal capsule

Between the thalamus and the corpus striatum is an area where there is a great concentration of nerve fibres travelling to and from the brain. The area is known as the internal capsule and is the place where the haemorrhages causing 'strokes' occur. Because of the great concentration of fibres in the area the greater is the potential damage which can be caused by haemorrhage.

2.11 The hypothalamus

Underneath the thalamus is found the hypothalamus. This contains the centres for the autonomic nervous system and includes control of the heart, blood pressure, temperature, metabolism, kidney function and it is thought to influence sleep. It affects sleep by its effect on kidney function. At night less urine is produced and so the person is not disturbed to empty the bladder. Less urine is produced because there is a higher concentration of the anti-diuretic hormone which is responsible for preventing loss of water from the kidneys. The production of this hormone is under the influence of the hypothalamus.

2.12 The brain stem

At the base of the cerebrum is the brain stem. This includes all the structures in this area excluding the cerebral hemispheres and the cerebellum and is composed of the midbrain, the pons and the medulla oblongata. The twelve pairs of cranial nerves originate from this area.

The midbrain receives impulses from the eye and the ear and serves as a centre for visual and auditory reflexes. The grey matter contains the cell bodies of the third and fourth cranial nerves and the red nucleus.

The white matter of the midbrain carries fibres linking the red nucleus with the cerebral cortex, thalamus, cerebellum and the basal ganglia. It also contains ascending sensory and descending motor fibres.

Continuous with the midbrain is the pons (*L. Pons*, bridge). The pons acts as a bridge between the brain stem and the cerebellum and relays impulses to and from the cerebellum and the cerebral cortex. The grey matter gives rise to the nuclei of the fifth, and sixth cranial nerves and the motor division of the seventh.

The lowermost part of the brain stem is the medulla oblongata. This extends from the lower border of the pons to a plane corresponding with upper border of the first vertebra (the atlas). Nerve fibres when arranged together in bundles are called tracts. The motor tract known as the pyramidal tract, because it looks something like a pyramid in appearance at this point, crosses over in the medulla. This accounts for the statement made earlier that the body is supplied with nerves from the cerebral hemisphere of the opposite side. The cross-over is technically referred to as the decussation of the pyramids. About ninety per cent of the motor nerve fibres cross-over and the remainder pass through uncrossed. The medulla oblongata contains the nuclei of part of the seventh, eighth, ninth, tenth, eleventh and twelfth cranial nerves as well as the gracile and cuneate nuclei. It also contains sensory fibres. The cardiac, respiratory and digestive centres are found in the medulla.

2.13 The red nucleus

There is a mass of grey matter in the upper part of the midbrain called the red nucleus. This is an important cell-station of the extra-pyramidal tract. It has connections with the thalamus and the basal ganglia above and with the cerebellum below and gives rise to two descending spinal nerve tracts; the rubro-reticular and the rubro-spinal.

2.14 The reticular formation

Also in the brain stem is found a scattered collection of intermingled grey and white matter called the reticular formation. This formation is considered as part of the extrapyramidal system. When we considered the basal ganglia we saw that fibres from these structures went to the reticular formation and that these fibres were either of a facilitatory or an inhibitory nature. The reticular formation thus plays an important part in the integrating function of the nervous system. It has been found that if part of the reticular function is destroyed, a deep sleep and insensibility to sensory impulses results. Therefore it seems that this diffuse structure is responsible for keeping us awake. It has been suggested that the slight kick people give when dropping off to sleep is due to the reticular formation giving up its functions resulting in involuntary muscular movement.

2.15 The cerebellum

Posterior to the brain stem at the level of the pons, the medulla oblongata and encompassing the fourth ventricle, is the cerebellum. Like the brain it has two hemispheres and these are called the cerebellar hemispheres. It is composed of masses of grey matter, the cerebellar nuclei, and white matter. The centres for balances and equilibrium are sited in the cerebellum. It plays an important part in the co-ordination of nervous function and disease of this organ results in *ataxia* and irregular muscular contraction due to the lack of integration of movement and posture. The cerebellum is well connected to the remainder of the nervous system. On the motor side we have already mentioned its connections with the red nucleus, from whence the rubro-spinal and the rubro-reticular tracts arise. On the sensory side two tracts, the anterior and the posterior spino-cerebellar tract go to the cerebellum, via the superior and inferior commissures which attach the organ to the brain stem.

The cerebral cortex initiates purposeful movements. During such movements the proprioceptors are continually supplying information to the cerebellum about the changing positions of muscles and joints. The cerebellum is then responsible for collating the information and for sending out impulses to bring about co-ordinated movements of different muscle groups.

2.16 Blood supply to brain

All cells in the body require energy if they are to do their jobs. The energy in the form of nutrients, carbohydrates, fats and protein, and the oxygen needed to release the energy from the nutrients are conveyed by the bloodstream. Nerve cells have a high energy requirement and are very sensitive to any lowering of supplies. Take the example of the fit young guardsman who has to stand on parade for a long period of time. Because he has to stand upright and keep still, the blood supply, and thus the energy supply to the brain is reduced. The result is that the guardsman faints. This is a protective mechanism because it is much easier for the heart to get blood to the brain when the person is lying flat.

The brain has a good blood supply for it is supplied by four arteries which arrive by different routes (Fig. 2.8). In front there are the two internal carotid arteries which are branches of the common carotids. At the back, the vertebral arteries travel in the bodies of cervical vertebrae. At the base of the brain the two vertebral arteries form

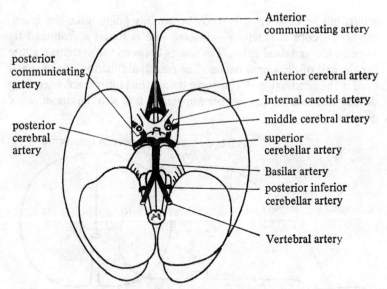

Fig.2.8. Diagram to show circulation of blood in brain.

the single basilar artery. This later divides to give rise to the two posterior cerebral arteries. Each posterior cerebral artery gives rise to a posterior communicating artery. The function of these communication arteries is to link the posterior cerebral artery, which is on either side at the back, to the internal carotid artery, which is on either side at the front. Both internal carotid arteries are joined by the anterior communicating artery. It will be seen that blood vessels form a circle which is known as the circulus arteriosus cerebri. Formerly, under the old anatomical terminology, this circle of arteries was known as the circle of Willis.

2.17 The spinal cord

The spinal cord, like the brain, is composed of grey matter and white matter, but the distribution of each is different. In the brain the grey matter is on the outside but in the case of the spinal cord it gives an H shaped formation on the inside. The H is surrounded with white matter which forms the motor and sensory tracts and also gives origin to the spinal nerves (thirty-one pairs).

The spinal cord extends from the medulla oblongata above, which is at the level of the atlas vertebra, to the level of the lower end of the first lumbar vertebra below. This is the arrangement in an adult, but in children it extends below this point. Like the brain, the spinal cord is carefully protected and is found surrounded by bone in the vertebral canal. The spaces between the vertebrae allow for the exit of the spinal nerves. The principal function of the spinal cord is the conduction of the nerve tracts, the motor tracts travelling downwards and the sensory ones upwards. It is also the site of reflex action.

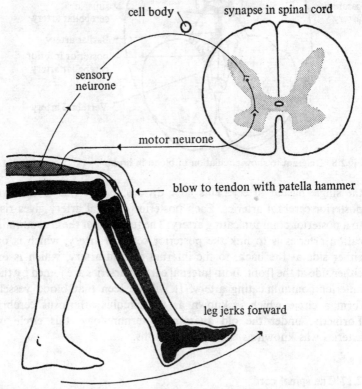

Fig.2.9. Diagram to show reflex arc.

2.18 Reflex action

Reflex action is an emergency action taken to protect the person from some injury or other, and its main value is the speed with which it is carried out. The following are the components necessary for a reflex action: A sensory stimulus is necessary to start the action and this may be pain, touch, pressure or extremes of temperature. There must be a sensory receptor and a sensory pathway. The sensory pathway travels via the posterior root ganglia to the posterior horn of the spinal cord. In the grey matter of the spinal cord there are connector neurones which connect with the motor neurones fibre. This leaves the anterior horn of the spinal cord and goes to the effector organ which may either be a muscle or a gland. In the case of a muscle immediate contraction results, removing the person from danger (Fig. 2.9). If any of the components are missing reflex action is not possible. If there is a disease process in the posterior horn of the cord as happens in the condition known as syringomyelia (*syringo*— syringe) which results in syringe-like holes, then the person is unaware of temperature and pain stimuli. It is possible for such a person to become badly burned without being aware of it.

If the anterior horn or the peripheral nerve fibres are damaged, no muscular contraction is possible and a flaccid paralysis and muscle wasting results. Poliomyelitis, which fortunately is now rare, affected the anterior horns and thus produced muscle wasting and a flaccid paralysis. Even more important to life, muscles of respiration were involved and resulted in the sufferer having to remain in an iron lung for life.

2.19 The nerve pathways in spinal cord

The motor pathways (Fig. 2.10) are composed of four distinct elements:

A. *The pyramidal tract*, supplied by the upper motor neurones, Betz cells, from the motor cortex of one cerebral hemisphere to the lower motor neurones of the other side of the body.

B. *The extrapyramidal tract*, which consists of a composite group of neurones, with their cell bodies in the basal ganglia of the hemi-

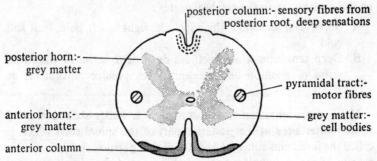

Fig.2.10. Diagram to show nerve pathways of spinal cord.

sphere and in the brain stem and their axons distributed to the lower
motor neurones.

C. *The cerebellar motor tracts*, chiefly consisting of fibres which
run from the cerebellum to the cells of the extrapyramidal system
in the basal ganglia and brain stem.

D. *The lower motor neurones*, comprising all nerve cells which
supply skeletal muscle; that is, the cells of the anterior horns of grey
matter in the spinal cord.

The effect of disease on the motor pathways depends on its site.
In the case of a 'stroke' already mentioned, it is the upper motor
neurones that are involved and the result is a spastic paralysis because the muscles are still getting some nerve supply. In the case of
lower motor neurone lesions, it is the neurones in the anterior horns
that are involved. Disease at this point or beyond, poliomyelitis
already mentioned, is an example, means that the muscles receive
no innervation whatever and are completely inert (flaccid paralysis).
The lower motor neurones and fibres are sometimes called the motor
units and the pathway along the fibres is called the final common
pathway, because in addition to innervation from the pyramidal,
extrapyramidal and cerebellar tracts, it also carries innervation from
the autonomic part of the nervous system (to be mentioned later).
In fact the final common pathway provides a route which is shared
by all the possible sources of innervation to the organ.

The sensory pathways transmit impulses from the sense organs to
the brain via the thalamus. The posterior root of each spinal nerve is
composed of fibres which enter the cord. Of the fibres entering the
cord many are conducting impulses which never reach consciousness;
for instance, the ingoing fibres of the spinal reflexes of the spino-
cerebellar pathways. Two principal types of sensation are transmitted
by these pathways to the cerebral cortex:

A. Superficial sensation which includes light touch, pain, heat and
cold.
B. Deep sensation which includes deep pain, sense of vibration,
sense of position and recognition of passive movements at
joints.

Much deep sensation is transmitted in a wedge-shaped area of
white matter sited at the posterior part of the spinal cord which is
called the fasciculus cuneatus and its adjoining structure the fasciculus
gracilis. Sensory impulses to the thalamus are transmitted along the

lateral and anterior spinothalamic tracts and those to the cerebellum by the posterior and anterior spinocerebellar tracts.

We have mentioned earlier that the majority of the motor pathways cross over in the medulla oblongata. The sensory fibres also cross over. Those conveyed in the fasciculus gracilus and the fasciculus cuneatus, like the motor pathways, cross over at the medulla oblongata whilst those of the spinothalamic tracts cross over almost as soon as they enter the spinal cord. The fibres of the spinocerebellar tracts pass up on the same side of the spinal cord.

Although they have been mentioned, the cranial or the spinal nerves have not been described yet. These are important and will be considered later in an applied fashion when the examination of the nervous system is considered. From the point of view of the central nervous system the next thing to be considered is the coverings of the brain and spinal cord. These coverings are called the meninges.

2.20 The meninges

We have already said that the nervous tissue is very specialized and therefore it is also delicate. The brain and spinal cord are encased in bony structures which give protection: the skull and the vertebral column. The meninges provide further protection. There are three layers, the dura mater, the arachnoid mater and the pia mater (Fig. 2.11). The dura mater is the tough outermost layer. This in turn has two layers of its own. The outer or endosteal layer which is in contact with the inner surface of the skull bones and the innermost or meningeal layer. The dura mater is a tough, inelastic membrane which has a number of folds. The falx cerebri (*falx*—sickle shaped) is found between the two cerebral hemispheres. The tentorum cerebelli (*tendo*—to stretch) is a tent-like fold which separates the occipital lobes of the brain from the cerebellum. Like the falx cerebri, the tentorun cerebelli separates both cerebellar hemispheres.

The arachnoid mater is a fine membrane connected to the pia mater by threads through which the cerebrospinal fluid percolates. This cerebrospinal fluid will be considered later. The arachnoid space has a number of enlargements along its course and these are called cisterns. These are the cerebellomedullary cistern behind the medulla oblongata, the pontine cistern anterior to the pons, the lateral cistern located at the lateral fissures of the temporal lobes and the cistern of the great cerebral vein between the corpus collosum and the cerebellum.

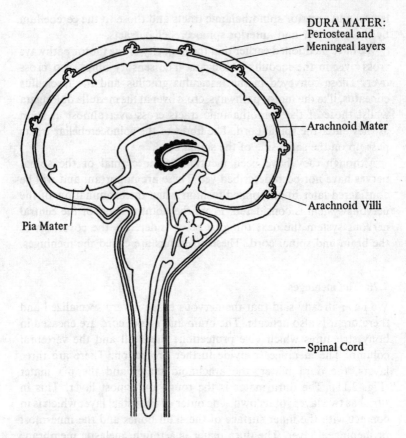

Fig.2.11. Diagram to show meninges.

Haemorrhage sometimes occurs into the subarachnoid space and this is called a subarachnoid haemorrhage. Between the dura mater and the arachnoid mater is a non-communicating space called the subdural space. The cerebral veins crossing this space have little support and are therefore vulnerable. Haemorrhage into this space is called subdural haemorrhage and because it is a non-communicating space the blood cannot escape, therefore intense pressure builds up.

The pia mater is the innermost covering of the brain. It is a very fine membrane which follows every convolution of the brain and has a very rich blood supply. Because of its good blood supply and because the causative organisms are blood-borne, the pia mater is the covering first involved in meningitis.

2.21 The cerebrospinal fluid

The cerebrospinal fluid circulating in the subarachnoid space (Fig. 2.12) is similar to blood plasma but it does not clot. It is a watery alkaline fluid and contains salts such as sodium chloride, glucose, waste products such as urea and creatine and a few lymphocytes.

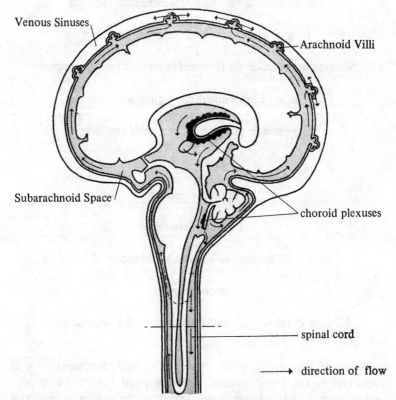

Fig.2.12. Diagram to show circulation of cerebrospinal fluid.

It has a specific gravity range from 1·005 to 1·008 and exerts a pressure in the range of 80–120 millimetres cerebrospinal fluid. The total volume of this fluid circulating at any time is about 125–150 ml. and quantity produced in 24 hours is about 500 ml.

This fluid is produced by the choroid plexus which are found principally in the left and right lateral ventricles. These plexus function somewhat like the glomerulus of the kidney. At the end of this process only the plasma-like fluid from the blood passes into the subarachnoid space. The circulation of cerebrospinal fluid can be illustrated as follows:

Cerebrospinal fluid produced in lateral ventricles
↓
Third ventricle via the interventricular foramen
↓
Fourth ventricle via the cerebral aqueduct
↓
Subarachnoid space via foramen in roof of fourth ventricle
↓
Cerebromedullary cistern
↓
Foramen in lateral part of fourth ventricle
↓
Pontine cistern
↓
Superior cistern
↓
From the cisterns
↓
Circulate in subarachnoid space
↓
Arachnoid villi
↓
Various dural sinuses and thus back to the circulation.

Some of the cerebrospinal fluid is absorbed, but most of it is returned to the blood stream. Cereberospinal fluid is being continually produced and continually lost from the system. Samples of this fluid are removed for diagnostic purposes and we shall consider this later in the section on investigations.

The cerebrospinal fluid has three functions:

A. It provides a protective covering for the delicate tissue it surrounds.
B. Alteration in volume can compensate for changes in the amount of blood in the skull and thus keeps the total volume of the cranial contents constant.
C. It allows for an exchange of metabolic substances.

2.22 The autonomic nervous system

The skeletal muscles are under voluntary contol and receive their nerve supply from the central nervous system. There is much muscular activity in the body which it not controlled voluntarily. The muscles involved are the visceral muscles and these are supplied by the automonic nervous system. This part of the nervous system controls the heart and secreting glands as well. Visceral muscle is found in the digestive tract, the air passages, the bladder, blood vessels and in the eye.

We saw earlier that in the case of skeletal muscle, innervation was by a single set of fibres carried in the final common pathway. Skeletal muscle has thus one nerve supply. The position of visceral muscle is different; it has a double nerve supply. One nerve is excitatory and causes the visceral muscle to contract. The other fibre is inhibitory and causes the muscle fibre to relax. This means that the autonomic nervous system has two divisions. These are the sympathetic part (Fig. 2.13a) and the parasympathetic part (Fig. 2.13b).

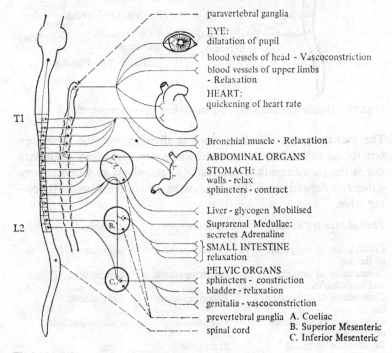

paravertebral ganglia

EYE:
dilatation of pupil

blood vessels of head - Vascoconstriction
blood vessels of upper limbs
- Relaxation

HEART:
quickening of heart rate

T1

Bronchial muscle - Relaxation

ABDOMINAL ORGANS
STOMACH:
walls - relax
sphincters - contract

Liver - glycogen Mobilised

L2

Suprarenal Medullae:
secretes Adrenaline

SMALL INTESTINE
relaxation

PELVIC ORGANS
sphincters - constriction
bladder - relaxation

genitalia - vascoconstriction

prevertebral ganglia A. Coeliac
spinal cord   B. Superior Mesenteric
                       C. Inferior Mesenteric

Fig.2.13a. Diagram of autonomic nervous system (Sympathetic)

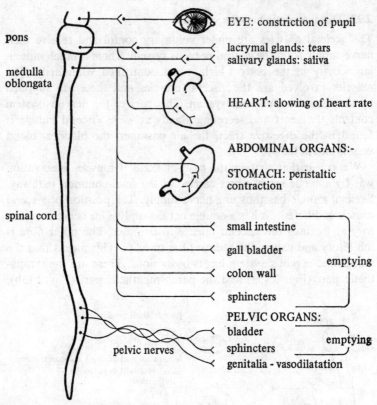

Fig.2.13b. Diagram of autonomic nervous system (Parasympathetic).

The excitatory nerve belongs to one division and the inhibitory one to the other, but the sympathetic is not exclusively excitatory nor is the parasympathetic exclusively inhibitory; each can assume either role depending on their location as we can see from the following table.

Visceral Muscle Causing	Excitatory Nerve	Inhibitory Nerve
Constriction of the pupil of the eye	Parasympathetic	Sympathetic
Constriction of bronchi and bronchioles	Parasympathetic	Sympathetic
Contraction of alimentary tract	Parasympathetic	Sympathetic
Contraction of sphincters of alimentary tract	Sympathetic	Parasympathetic
Constriction of blood vessels	Sympathetic	None

The anatomical origins of the two parts of the autonomic nervous system are different. The parasympathetic part leaves the central nervous system from two places or outflows as follows:

A. *The cranial outflow.* This arises from the brain stem within the cranium and involves some of the cranial nerves. The most important of these is the tenth nerve or the vagus nerve. It is widely distributed and supplies the contents of the thorax including the heart and the bronchi and the bronchioles, and most of the abdominal organs with parasympathetic innervation.

B. *The sacral outflow.* This arises from the region of the spinal cord at the level of the second, third and fourth sacral vertebrae. The two outflows together are referred to as the craniosacral outflow.

The sympathetic nerve fibres leave the central nervous system between the first thoracic and the second lumbar vertebrae. This is called the *thoracolumbar outflow.*

Just as the anatomical origins of the parasympathetic and the sympathetic nervous systems are different, so are the arrangements of the nerve fibres. In the case of the parasympathetic part, the preganglionic part of the nerve fibre is very long and the postganglionic fibre is short. The opposite is the case for the sympathetic part. There is uniformly short preganglionic fibre. The ganglia are arranged a short distance from the spinal cord and form a chain known as the paravertebral chain extending the length of the sympathetic outflow. The postganglionic fibres are sometimes very long.

Like the nerve fibres of the central nervous system, the fibres of the autonomic nervous system do not touch the effector organ: the final transmission of the nerve impulse is through a chemical medium. In the case of the parasympathetic part the transmitter is acetycholine, just as in the central nervous system Parasympathetic nerve fibres are called cholinergic. At the terminals of the sympathetic part, the transmitter released is noradrenaline and such nerves are said to be adrenergic. Noradrenaline is a precursor of the hormone adrenaline and is also produced by the supra-renal glands of the endocrine system. The noradrenaline circulating the bloodstream augments that produced at the sympathetic nerve endings. Adrenaline is the hormone of fear and fright and this has the function of preparing the body for these emergencies.

The functioning of the autonomic nervous system gives us many examples of how states of mind can effect the body. The simple condition of blushing is a reaction in the skin brought about by something embarrassing experienced by the subject. We shall consider these reactions more fully later when we consider conditions where the mind is thought to have a major influence over the matter; such conditions are said to be psychosomatic.

2.23 The mind

So far we have considered the structure and the function of the nervous system and we have accounted for a number of vital functions. There are however some which are left to be described and these must be attributed to the mind. 'He read each wound each weakness clear. And struck his finger on the place, and said: Thou ailest here and here'—(1822–88—Matthew Arnold). Such precision is not possible with the mind.

Some psychologists dislike the use of the word 'mind' because it implies that there is a special non-visible and non-spatial organ responsible for thinking and deciding. Others have suggested that the word 'mind' is a noun like 'arm' or 'leg' and while it does not stand for a physical object of any sort, it is a shorthand way of referring to certain functions of one part of the body, namely the brain. The mind is that which manifests itself in thought, feeling, purpose, desire, memory and so on. That which lies behind experience and behaviour.

The thoughts, feelings and drives which make up mental life are products of the function of the brain. In considering the mental processes it was therefore right to concentrate on the brain and nervous system because the working of the mind depends on the working of this system. Take a simple example. If a person goes blind a part of the nervous system is damaged and there are mental consequences. Likewise if a person goes deaf there is a reaction to the failure of this part of the nervous system, usually a degree of suspicion that people are talking about the subject. When there is a great degree of suspicion it is technically called paranoia. Damage or injury to the brain itself is shown in disorders of consciousness and impaired function. It can result in the impairment of language function resulting in *aphasia*, inability to recognize common objects *agnosia* and inability to perform simple movements *apraxia*. A local anaesthetic gives local loss of consciousness for a particular area. Yet a person can be totally paralysed and be conscious. Therefore consciousness does not depend on the ability to move limbs. Consciousness is relating to "experience" and has two dimensions, clarity and content. These are important dimensions and we shall return to them again later as we consider mental illness.

Experience is described as all 'information' about the external world which the brain has received through the sense organs and then converts into something which is described as 'mental'. The manner of conversion is not known. The spontaneous outcome of mental activity of the brain is also 'experience'. We have seen earlier that not all nervous impulses reach the brain and that their transmission is well co-ordinated giving rise to integrated function. The same principle applies to the mind. Only a fraction of information gives rise to awareness at any time and some of it never does. It can therefore be assumed that there is a system of filters which regulates the part of experience of which we become aware.

2.24 Levels of consciousness

There are three levels of consciousness which can be represented as follows:

a. *The conscious mind.* The conscious mind is that part of the mind which is aware of the environment and it has two components:

a. The focal area. This is the area involved when attention or concentration is focused on a single task, say, reading a book, writing a letter or solving a mathematical problem.

b. The peripheral area. This is the area where information is received but not given much attention. For example whilst reading or doing one of the tasks above, traffic may be passing noisily on the road outside, a train may be rumbling in the distance or an aircraft may be hovering overhead. Unless these stimuli are very intense they do not generally interfere with the job in hand, and are thus kept in the periphery of consciousness.

b. *The subconscious mind.* The subconscious mind is that part of the mind which stores past experience, which can be recalled and these are of two sorts:

a. Recent memories.

b. More distant but very vivid memories. This is said to be a biological safety device.

c. *The unconscious mind.* The unconscious mind is that part of the mind which contains past experiences which are not easily recalled. Information reaching the mind is never lost, but some of it is very difficult if not impossible to recover. Sometimes unpleasant material which may affect behaviour is stored in the unconscious mind and the techniques of psychoanalysis are designed to uncover and to help the person to come to terms with such material.

2.25 Structure of the mind

Psychology has been defined as the study of the mind, but we have said that the term 'mind' is a shorthand term for the functioning of the brain. The functioning of the brain results in behaviour, therefore psychology is concerned with a study of this behaviour.

We can refer to the 'structure' of the mind in the same way that we refer to the structure of a story, or of a play or of a piece of music, in that it has parts which are related to a whole. Behaviour is produced by a combination of experiences and drives. The nature of these drives, which used to be called instincts and still are by some, need to be explained.

2.26 Drives

Drives are said to be inborn energy forces which influence behaviour. They are responsible for unlearned patterns of behaviour and have been used to explain why migratory birds fly many thousands of miles to lay their eggs and hatch their young, and similar behaviour in a variety of other animals.

Some of the drives (instincts) will now be mentioned and these are:

 a. Drives concerning the self and these are concerned with such things as food-seeking, curiosity, aggression and escape.
 b. Drives concerning the herd. If these drives are to be fulfilled, social co-operation is necessary and some sacrifice of the 'self' drives must be made. Submission to the pattern of herd behaviour is necessary.
 c. The sex drives are directed primarily to ensuring the continuance of the species, and involve not only courtship and sex relations but also ensure parental care. In this way the young of the species are covered for a critical time in their lives.

These drives may be affected in a number of ways. Expression of the drive is followed by the achievement of the goal. Repression may occur, that is, the crushing of the expressed drive. In some cases frustration may result and also perversion. When the drive is used to a wrong end this is perversion and this often happens with the sex drive. Sublimation may also occur. This is the direction of a drive to a new and more socially acceptable goal.

2.27 Emotion

There is another dimension to behaviour and this is *emotion*. One of the inherited part of man's make-up is his tendency in certain situations to produce patterns of response which are called emotions. An emotion is something which has the effect of moving, stirring or agitating and when someone is upset we frequently say that the person was moved. Fear, anger, joy and surprise are examples of emotions, but the one most commonly seen and felt is that involving affect or feeling. As well as feeling the emotion also contributes an impulse to behaviour. Emotions are the interactions between a drive and the incoming experiences. They act as a bridge between the physical world explained by physiology and the mental world described by psychology. An emotion, then, has a physical and a mental side. The mental side consists of perceiving, feeling and doing. Take an example. A gas main explodes. The person hears (perceives), feels frightened (feeling) and takes shelter (doing). The physical side of an emotion consists of changes in viscera and skeletal muscles. These are often widespread and involve the co-ordinated activity of the central and autonomic nervous systems. The involvement of the autonomic nervous system in psychosomatic conditions has already been mentioned.

Emotions are driving forces serving intelligent variable behaviour, just as the inborn drives serve the need of unlearned behaviour.

2.28 Temperament

There is yet another dimension affecting behaviour and this is *temperament*. This has been the subject of study for a very long time. Aristotle, for example, based temperament on four physiological considerations:

a. Blood (Sanguine). The sanguine temperament was characterized by superficial emotions and inconsistent behaviour.

b. Phlegm (Phlegmatic). The phlegmatic temperament was accompanied by slowness of thought and movement.

c. Yellow bile (Choleric). The choleric temperament showed depth and stability of emotion and inflexibility of purpose.

d. Blackbile (melancholic). The melancholic or nervous temperament was characterized by rapidity of thoughts and movements.

We sometimes hear a person is 'emotional' if the person is subject to emotional outbursts. Likewise we hear of people being temperamental and both patterns of behaviour seem similar. In fact temperament is the general character of man's emotional reactions and there is a certain consistency in the emotional reactions of any individual.

One may show lasting loves or hates, another may show emotion in expression.

Temperamental differences are partly inborn and partly environmental. The inborn part is determined by the existing drives, physiological balance and the endocrine secretions. Environmental factors which act by changing the activity of the autonomic nervous system or the endocrine glands. Stimulation of the thyroid gland, for example, excites the emotional system and corresponds with the sanguine temperament of Aristotle.

2.29 Personality

All the factors we have mentioned and some not yet mentioned, combine to make the personality. Definitions of personality are usually inadequate because the term personality involves so much. It includes physical and mental characteristics such as height, weight, colour of hair, clothes, voice, interests, intelligence, abilities, attitudes and so on, but has been defined as the whole of the integrated characteristics of the individual. Temperament and character are but two aspects of personality. *Character* is defined as the integration of habits, sentiments and ideals which renders an individual's actions stable and predictable and involves honesty, loyalty and truthfulness.

2.30 Motives

As we mentioned above there are a number of factors which contribute to the personality which have not yet been mentioned and these will be considered now and the first are motives. A motive is a feeling-doing factor which operates in determining the direction of an individual behaviour towards an end or goal. It may be conscious or it may be unconscious. When there is an act of any kind a motive is sought, as in crime. Very often there is no conscious motive, therefore it must be assumed that there was an unconscious one. Motives are responsible for people taking up medicine, nursing, art, music, games, teaching, voluntary work and so on. Motives are very important when it comes to study. If a student is well motivated and of course intelligent, then studying will not be looked upon as a chore. When there is a conscious awareness of groups of motives acting towards a particular goal, this is *interest*. If a task is to be done well there must be interest. One sees a gardener, a car owner or a stamp collector spend many hours deeply absorbed attending to his object of interest and without the hope or the wish for any financial reward. On the other hand there are employees in factories where the work is of a repetitive nature who are well paid, but have little or no interest. This results in poor workmanship, boredom, a high incidence of casual sickness, in other words low morale. When selecting people for study or work it is therefore important to ensure that they are well motivated and interested.

2.31 Sentiments

When there are emotional dispositions centring on one part of an individual's make-up, this is called a sentiment. This can be expressed as follows:

$$\text{Ideas} + \text{feeling} = \text{sentiment}.$$

Sentiments which favour an idea engender love and conversely those which are against it engender hate. Indifference occurs where there is a lack of sentiment towards an idea. Sentiments can of course be changed and St. Paul provides an example. At first he hated and persecuted Christ. Later on the hate turned to love and he became a trusted disciple. Racial and generation differences modify behaviour and motives.

Moral sentiments, that is, those sentiments concerned with the right and wrong of an act or conduct, have essential qualities such as truth, fairness and beauty.

Sentiments usually develop around people to whom the individual is close. For example parents and teachers. They may be transferred to other persons showing the same qualities, such as classmates or to a whole nation resulting in patriotism. Sometimes sentiments are not well developed and in the case of a child may result in apathy towards knowledge and a lack of imagination. Such a child may play truant from school, become involved in stealing and similar anti-social behaviour and before long is on the road to delinquency.

Sentiments need to be expressed and if for any reason this is not possible an abnormal *complex* results. This holding back of sentiments may be conscious at first. If a person is prevented from being self assertive, frustration occurs and an inferiority complex develops. There is however a safety valve in the form of dreams which is the natural way of dispersing pent-up energy forces.

2.32 Habits

Habits are a factor which also contribute to the personality. A habit is an automatic response to specific situations, acquired normally as a result of repetition and learning. Strictly speaking habits apply only to motor responses, but the term is often applied more widely to include habits of thought which are also referred to as attitudes. Habits are useful and aid efficiency by allowing certain actions to be carried out quickly without having to think out each stage. Some habits such as drug taking can be a disadvantage. This is the inability to refrain from taking a particular drug when it is not medically necessary and may even be detrimental to the individual's health.

2.33 Attitudes

Attitudes, which have been more or less replaced by sentiments by some, have been defined as a morbid state of an individual towards a value. Love of money, desire for fame, hatred of foreigners and respect for authority are examples. Attitudes are very important from the point of view of learning. If the attitude is a positive one, learning is more likely to be successful. Attitudes are also important from the point of view of mental illness. If the public are to accept people fully with mental illness in the same way as people with physical illnesses are accepted, the questions of attitudes arise. Unfavourable attitudes must be changed before full acceptance can be achieved. Attitudes are of paramount importance in race relations. Attitudes are a more or less permanent state of readiness of mental organization. They predispose an individual to react in a characteristic way to any object or situation and can be helpful to the individual and others, as a guideline to expected behaviour. When attitudes are of an anti-social nature they can be stumbling blocks with far reaching effects. They are then called *prejudice*.

2.34 Traits

The term personality is an all embracing one. It has so many dimensions that it is difficult to include them all simultaneously in any form of measurement. Personality factors tend to be measured separately and these separately measurable elements are called traits. These include things like introversion (inward looking) extroversion (outward looking), dominance, perseverance, egoism (more concerned with self), altruism (more concerned with other people) and so on. We shall mention some of the methods used when we consider personality tests.

2.35 Conscience

There is another factor which affects behaviour and this is conscience. This is usually considered above the mind and used to be referred to as the super-ego (above the self). Conscience is the individual's system of accepted moral principles or principles of conduct and we have already mentioned this when we considered ethics. The constraints of conscience apply when the act is contemplated which threatens or violates the person's principles. There are emotional and intellectual aspects to conscience and its overall effect is a beneficial modification of behaviour. Conscience can also cause a person to be out of step with society. Take the example of those who object to war on grounds of conscience. They are not kindly looked upon by society and in times of war suffer because of their pacifism.

2.36 Development of the mind

There are a number of needs which must be supplied if the mind is to develop properly. We have seen earlier that every person has a number of inborn drives. It follows then that there are a number of needs, if these drives are to be satisfied and these fall into two groups:

A. PHYSICAL We have already mentioned that we should think of the whole individual and not just the physical, mental or social aspects in isolation because physical needs have psychological consequences and conversely. The physical needs are those for food, water, shelter against extremes of light, wet, wind, heat and cold, and sex.

B. PSYCHOLOGICAL. These are the fundamental needs for mental health and happiness and include:

a. *Security*
1. Protection from danger as in the case of children and sick people.
2. Financial. This means regular employment, without the fear of unemployment and includes adequate pension provision for retirement.
3. Social. We have a need to be in an environment in which we are socially secure and have friends. This applies to school, office or factory work, or to retirement. Social security means being

accepted by the group, being permitted to make some contribution such as to accept advice, humour, hospitality or opinions. It is important for the individual to know that the group accepts and respects his individuality and self respect.

b. *Affection*. This involves friendliness, understanding and the giving of assistance. Affection is important for mental health and everyone needs it in some form in their environment.

c. *Independence*. In the case of a child this means freedom from the aprons strings and may show itself at about eight to ten months and is strongly present at the two year stage. Stemming from independence is the need for responsiblity and this is essential for mental growth. People who are irresponsible usually have had little opportunity to exercise responsibility.

d. *Development of initiative*. The opportunity to observe, criticize, to ask questions, to do and make and to explore is essential for mental growth of children. An alert environment is essential for the mental health of all ages at work, in the home and in hospital. The lack of a stimulating environment results in monotony—in illness this can lead to apathy and regression, particularly for the aged. At work it can have similar effects to poor motivation, that is, poor workmanship, no job satisfaction, high casual sickness and low morale.

2.37 Birth

When a child is born there are usually a variety of reactions. On the part of the mother there is joy which may be followed by disillusionment as a result of the chores, the restricted social life and lonely days which may follow. The father is likely to be proud, but may become jealous later at the amount of the mother's time which is taken up with the child. These and other factors affect the mother/child and the wife/husband relationships. A considerable degree of maturity, that is, the ability to consider the other person's needs before one's own, is needed on the part of the parents if they are to provide the best environment for the child to develop. All the psychological needs are important but security and affection are paramount at this stage.

2.38 The first decade

According to John Locke the child is born into this world with a *tabula rasa* or clean table, that is, without any knowledge whatever and though this view has been challenged it is still held by many. Learning begins as soon as the nervous system responds to the changes in the environment. In the first three months vision is not acute and there is a lack of co-ordination. At about three months the child receives a co-ordinated image from both eyes. Recognition of objects is possible now. The sense of touch is present early on and the sucking reflex is said to be based on this. The newborn child is apparently less sensitive to pain than ten months later. The appreciation of pain thus involves education and is largely influenced by the parents' reaction. At birth the child is deaf, but high pitch sounds are heard soon afterwards. Mother's voice is recognized at three months and there is easy discrimination of sounds at one year. Taste and smell are absent at birth and begin to develop slowly from the two week stage onwards.

At about four months a child can turn its head on hearing a noise, focus its eyes on mother and sit up with support. On the emotional side it can show delight or distress. At five or six months it can grasp objects by the palm of the hand, find hidden objects and show fear or rage. Articulate sounds appear at about seven months and at this stage the child can sit up alone. At eight months it can stand up with help and can stand by holding on to furniture. At the nine month stage the child can remember things for one second. At ten months creeping is possible and it is also possible to grasp objects between the fingers and thumb. Imitation of syllables is also possible. The child may walk when led at this stage although it may be fourteen or fifteen months before the child walks alone.

At a year a child can show fear, disgust, rage, elation and affection and can say words such as 'Dada' and 'Mama'. Things can be remembered for about three to four seconds. It is possible for the child to speak several words at fifteen months and by eighteen months this is increased to over twenty, and at this stage things can be remembered for ten seconds or more. By twenty-four months the child is capable of considerable activity, has a good vocabulary and possibly has bladder and bowel control. It has been suggested that bladder and bowel control should be allowed to develop naturally and that undue fussing or excessive demands in this respect are undesirable.

Children are often very trying to their parents at the two year stage, so much so that they are referred to as the 'terrible twos'. Sometimes the child is stubborn and unfriendly and at other times anxious to please. At about this stage the child begins to ask questions and is anxious to tell about the world as he sees it.

The 'terrible twos' become the 'trusting threes'. Imagination begins to develop and this is very strong at the four year stage, but there may be some difficulty in distinguishing between the dream world and the world of reality.

There are a number of problems associated with the early years of life. These are to be expected and need not be taken too seriously unless they are obviously getting out of hand. Some of the problems encountered are:

a. *Crying fits*. Bright lights, loud noises, sudden movements, fears and loneliness all contribute to crying fits in younger babies. In older babies it may be boredom or mismanagement. Prolonged crying has a bad effect on the baby and the rest of the family. The cause should be sought in all cases and the baby should be picked up, but care must be taken over the picking up in case the baby over uses the system.

b. *Toilet training*. A child can sit on a pot at ten months, but this is probably too early to start toilet training. Normally a child has bowel control at two or two and a half years. Patience is required at this stage and the demanding mother is a bad trainer. At ten months a child has dry periods of up to an hour and by fifteen months this is increased to two hours. At about two and a half years, eighty per cent of children have full bladder control, that is, dry periods of up to five hours. In some cases bladder control comes later and up to twelve per cent of normal children have wet beds at four years.

Problems ensuing from faulty habit training are incontinence and enuresis. When these are present there may be an inherited factor, but most often it is due to faulty training. There may be sibling jealousy but this should only be temporary. Parental frictions and school anxieties also contribute. Various approaches have been tried in the treatment of incontinence and enuresis including rewards for dry nights and a bell system to ensure regular waking, but probably the most important is to see that the child's essential psychological needs are fulfilled.

c. *Temper tantrums*. Temper tantrums occur normally at about the three year old stage and may be due to bad management, over-tiredness, illness, boredom or fear. They are also an indication of inconsistent discipline on the part of the parents. A consistent approach and the fulfilment of the essential psychological needs helps.

d. *Fears*. Children are usually avid for information and often they take in more than they can comprehend. They thus need adult help and support and if this is not forthcoming the child is likely to become frightened and bewildered. Other causes of fears are loss of affection, ill-treatment, suggestion of the dark, mice or spiders and frightening stories. Fear is the best safeguard against danger and thus fears can serve a vital protective function. Excessive fear causes unhappines and interferes with normal development. A secure background helps the child to overcome fears.

e. *Stubbornness*. A young child resents intrusion and they often have little privacy. There is also the fear of change. A little tact and patience can help to overcome stubbornness.

f. *Nail biting*. Nail biting is a universal habit which is often associated with states of tension, but the habit may remain after the tension has disappeared. As far as possible tension states should be avoided and the essential psychological needs should be fulfilled.

g. *Head banging*. Head banging occurs in some children and this is often associated with the sleep and waking pattern. It is often better to leave such children alone.

h. *Jealousy*. Jealousy occurs at the arrival of a new member of the family. Children should thus be prepared for the new arrival and explanations given appropriate to age. Jealousy may also be aroused because of favouritism, physical or mental disability. It is important to avoid favouritism and to stress any virtues present.

Development during the early part of the first decade is eventful, sometimes stormy and sometimes disturbed. The behaviour settles and during the second half of the decade and up to puberty it is much more placid. Children are better able to deal with the world at this stage. They are able to count and read at seven years or before. By seven or eight they can tell the time and by ten they should be able to do simple arithmetic.

At the ten year old stage most children belong to a gang. This has a value in that it means that the child is away from parental over-protection and is an important stage in social development. There is also an anti-social aspect to children's gangs and it is a good idea if the activities are supervised as in the Scouts.

The main problem that arises at this stage and later is delinquency.

It is estimated that no more than four or five per cent of the child population, including those who are not caught, are delinquent. Delinquency is higher in urban than in rural areas. In a rural setting a child can let off steam, climb objects and throw missiles without causing much damage and without the likelihood of being caught. Similar behaviour in an urban setting quickly results in damage to property and trouble with the police. Overcrowding, poverty and poor parental control and the general social climate of the area all contribute to delinquency. Adequate play facilities and provision of clubs help with this problem.

Some children are unable to benefit from a normal education and are called *educationally subnormal*. Such children, whose intelligence quotient is usually less than 70 require special education. Others presenting problems are called *maladjusted*. A maladjusted child is one who is developing ways which have a bad effect on himself and his fellows and cannot without help be remedied by his parents and teachers in ordinary contact with him. Maladjusted is a comprehensive term which includes the juvenile delinquent, the autistic and the educationally subnormal child. It has been estimated that ten per cent of the child population are in this group.

A maladjusted child is less alert, more moody and more subject to behaviour problems and a variety of minor physical illnesses than the ordinary child. Parental relationships are likely to be poor and parental responsibility may not be taken too seriously or conversely there may be over-possessiveness on the part of the mother. The maladjusted child is said to live on an island separated from the mainland and the bridge has broken down. The main task in helping maladjusted children is to help to repair or replace that bridge. The help of the child guidance clinic may be necessary with some of the bridge building task. These clinics, which are staffed by child psychiatrists and social workers, are for the treatment of behaviour problems in nervous, unstable, and difficult children.

2.39 The second decade—adolescence

Following the relatively placid years before puberty comes the often stormy period of adolescence. Profound physiological changes take place at puberty. When these changes occur they are accompanied by rapid physical growth and the young person reacts to these changes. Menstruation commences in girls and there is development of the secondary sex characteristics. In boys a consequence of endocrine changes are facial blemishes (acne) and a 'breaking of the voice'. There is sometimes a degree of self-consciousness about these changes. There is often the associated difficulty of poor co-ordination due to temporary lack of integration on the part of the nervous system. This results in clumsiness such as dropping things, the breaking of dishes during washing up and standing on the feet of a partner whilst dancing.Such awkwardness causes tensions and embarassments.

Adolescents are often very idealistic and see the world in terms of black and white without intermediate shades. Compromise does not come easily. Such an attitude can cause difficulties. Other problems associated with adolescence are moodiness. This may be due to boredom, frustration, failure of romantic contacts and a feeling of inadequacy. Sex education is also important and sometimes there is a reticence on the part of parents to discuss this subject and it is left to the schools. A knowledge of the physiology of sex should be accompanied by an awareness of personal responsibility as a citizen and ethical maturity.

A good home, which is characterized by the giving of a large measure of independence to the children, mutual affection, participation in the family trials and tribulations and by welcoming the children's friends, contributes greatly to solving many of the adolescent problems.

During adolescence some children go to university and this involves leaving home and adjusting to being a 'new boy'. Others start work at this stage and likewise are 'new boys'. Arguments are likely to arise about the choice of work. Parents naturally tend to encourage a form of employment which involves training and usually little money at the beginning, but with prospects of security and a pension. On the part of the child there is sometimes the tendency to go for the big money straight away. Conflicts and scenes can result if parents try to impose their will in an arbitrary fashion. Gentle persuasive techniques are likely to be more effective and are certainly more pleasant.

2.40 The third decade—early adulthood

The second decade has been thought of as a time when young people make temporary relationships with members of the opposite sex, with more permanent relationships coming later. The third decade heralded the onset of adulthood and this for many meant courtship and marriage, but with the age of majority lowered to eighteen, it is likely that ideas may have to be revised about this. Just the same it is likely that events will follow the traditional pattern at least for a while. A degree of maturity on the part of both partners is essential for a successful marriage, hence the risk of marrying too early. A similarity of cultural interests is desirable. Home experiences are also important.

A considerable amount of adjustment is required in the early days of marriage. The sexual appetites of the partners may be different and adjustments must be made if one partner is not to feel that excessive demands are being made or conversely that desires are not fulfilled. There is usually a shortage of money and so much is needed. The husband finds that he cannot go out with the boys so frequently and the wife finds that she has less to spend on clothes and cosmetics.

The arrival of a child brings joy and pride but it also brings endless chores, anxieties and invariably social isolation. The baby may be ill or unwell and cry at night and keep its parents awake.

The third decade is the time when there are many problems and also many challenges which will require all the youthful energy available. In the field of work there should be promotion and in the academic world graduates are likely to be working for higher degrees. Promotion may be slow in coming and there may be impatience and frustration.

Marriage of course is not everybody's goal and a number of people of both sexes do not marry. Again adjustment is necessary and possible for such people. The energy available, which would be used in homemaking and family rearing, can be redirected for the benefit of mankind in fields such as religion, social and political activities.

2.41 The fourth decade—later adulthood

The fourth decade is often the decade of achievement. The person is generally approaching the top of his profession and is a person of authority and prestige. The finances should not be as strained as in the early days of marriage and the children are increasingly independent. Marital problems such as unfaithfulness, separation and divorce can occur at this stage.

2.42 The fifth and sixth decades—middle age

It is during this period that the first signs of ill-health appear. Hearing is less acute, spectacles may be needed for the first time, heart disease is common and there is a tendency towards obesity.

The family have left home by now and sometimes a gap is left behind.

In women the climateric is reached during this stage. The monthly periods cease and there are associated physiological and psychological changes. When ovarian activity decreases the pituitary activity must be directed elsewhere in order to maintain the balance of nervous and muscular energy. There is usually a period of imbalance and this is associated with fatigue, hot flushes and heart disturbances. The psychological manifestations are vague fears, groundless jealousies, anxiety feelings, compulsive acts and visceral complaints. In some cases the condition of involutional melancholia or agitated depression can result.

In men there is no well defined climateric as in women, but subtle changes resulting in imbalance and giving rise to similar consequences do occur, often at a later age.

This period of life can be enjoyable provided the couple have shared interests. It may be possible to take up hobbies and activities which could not be done when the children were at home. Preparation for retirement should take place at this time.

2.43 The seventh decade—retirement

It is a sad fact, that unless there has been adequate preparation, the long awaited retirement and pension is not enjoyed. This is particularly the case in a person whose work has been his whole life.

Retirement is an anti-climax, the person feels unwanted, the days are long and empty. Often the person grows careless about his appearance, withdraws from the world and sinks into a state of apathy resulting in physical and psychological deterioration. Adequate preparation for retirement can help to overcome these problems.

2.44 The eighth decade and onwards—old age

The improved health and welfare services have not really increased man's life span, but what has happened is that a greater number of people are living to the eighth decade and beyond. It has been estimated that there are over 2,000,000 people over 70 years in the community and the number is increasing.

In old age there is a general slowing down. The joints become stiff and arthritic conditions are common. The heart often becomes inefficient and failure ensues. There is an increased tendency to

3

respiratory infections, urinary infections and very often there is trouble with the bowels, mainly constipation. It has been observed that nearly fifty per cent of all old persons live alone and this gives rise to one of the greatest problems of all, loneliness.

On the mental side memory fails for recent events and there is a tendency to converse about the past. Ideas become set and there is reluctance or inability to change. Loneliness causes the person to look inwards and after a time this may lead to confusion.

Bereavement and widowhood can occur at any time, but obviously it is more likely to occur at this time. Although death is inevitable it still comes as a shock to most and causes great emotional upheaval. As well as remorse there is often an unjustified feeling of guilt. These factors and the fact that older people cannot, on the whole, adjust to changes so well means that the death of a partner is more upsetting than for younger people.

2.45 Summary
Mental processes are dependent on two things. First a healthy and an effectively functioning nervous system. The nervous system is subject to genetic and environmental influences during development and later on. Second, they are dependent on a healthy and effectively functioning mind. The mind is a term given to certain functions of the brain and has no physical structure, though we sometimes refer to the 'structure' of the mind in the same way as we refer to the 'structure' of a story, a play or a piece of music. There are a number of psychological needs which are required for the healthy development of the mind and a number of problems arise at the various stages. These range from crying fits, temper tantrums and nail biting in the early days to delinquency and adolescent moodiness later on. There are problems associated with marital adjustment, child rearing and establishing a career. Later on the problems are centred around failing health, retirement, bereavement, widowhood, a general slowing down, loneliness and concern with death. The provision of the psychological needs are important at all stages from the cradle to the grave. Many of the problems which arise are solved by the individual with the help of friends and family. Others cannot be solved within the family either because the problems presented are too great, or the family is not very helpful or, of course, the family may be non-existent. Professional help is sought or advised when the person can no longer cope and this is the basis of psychiatric treatment.

3

Mental health, mental mechanisms and mental reactions to illness

3.0 Introduction

We have seen from the last chapter that the brain and the mind are complex structures with many components. The general principle that the more parts there are in a machine the more there is to go wrong applies here. We have seen that each individual is subject to genetic and environment influences and we have seen that a whole variety of mostly minor upsets occur during development, ranging from crying fits, temper tantrums, enuresis, moodiness, delinquency and marital disharmony, to exceptional concern about oneself which occurs in later years. The majority of these upsets are self-contained and help is not sought and not required. In other words these people are mentally healthy. It would seem worthwhile to concentrate on mental health and to see what it means.

MENTAL HEALTH

3.1 Definition of mental health

If one looks through literature there are whole hosts of definitions of mental health. When there are many definitions it means of course that there is no general agreement and that the subject is difficult to define. It may be difficult to define but it seems essential to do so because if it is well done it should provide a base from which to consider mental illness. The World Health Organisation, Expert Committee on Mental Health (1951) defined mental health as follows: 'Mental health as the committee understands it, is influenced by both biological and social factors. It is not a static condition but subject to variations and fluctuations of degree; the Committee's conception implies the capacity in an individual to form harmonious relations with others, and to participate in, or contribute constructively to, changes in his social and physical environment. It implies his ability to achieve a harmonious and balanced satisfaction of his own potentially conflicting drives—harmonious in that it reaches an integrated synthesis rather than the denial of satisfaction to certain drives as a means of avoiding the thwarting of others. It implies in addition an individual whose personality has developed in a way which enables his potentially conflicting drives to find harmonious expression in full realization of his potentialities'. From this definition it seems that harmony is the keynote to mental health.

G. K. Chesterton (1874–1936) puts it much more briefly when he said: 'Of a sane man there is only one safe definition. He is a man who can have tragedy in his heart and comedy in his head.' There is no doubt that if the problems of the day are allowed to bear down too heavily on any individual, ruminations, gloom and fretfulness will follow. We have said earlier that dreams act as safety valves by providing a means of dispersing pent-up energy forces. Laughter and a sense of humour act in a similar way. They permit light relief from the problems and help to keep things in perspective.

3.2 Contributory factors

It is assumed that the infant is born mentally healthy, but it may of course inherit unhealthy tendencies. Mental health must be nurtured and cultivated if it is to be developed and maintained. A baby is at the mercy of its mother and is vulnerable to any afflictions that she may have. A baby in actual contact with an emotionally sick mother seldom escapes being affected. Babies respond best to calm, secure warm persons and are irritable and tense if the person is tense, excitable, nervous and insecure. In other words a mother or mother substitute who is secure within herself, is much more likely to be able to supply the psychological security which the child needs than one who is not. The relationship with the mother is very important because during the earliest phase of infantile experience the child is incapable of distinguishing the mother from himself.

A good mother gives the child a sense of confidence which permits him to exploit to the fullest his capacity and potential for growth. The premature introduction of bowel training or discipline generally confronts the child with obstacles that tend to warp his final adult form.

Events in early childhood are of vital importance to the development of the child because it is during this period that foundations for mental health are laid. As the individual develops there are a number of factors which contribute to mental health. There is the hereditary tendency which if present, can show itself at any time and is more likely to show itself if there are environmental stresses. These can include unhappy home conditions such as parental quarrelling, apathy or separation, poor housing, ov·.rcrowded conditions and a generally poor neighbourhood.

Learning takes place through precept and example and much

depends on the example set by the parents especially the mother. If she is the sort who fusses and flaps at every upset, has a high level of anxiety and is always anticipating doom and disaster, this is likely to be transferred to the child. A permanent state of tension, over-protection and excessive panic responses during childhood is likely to lay the basis of an adult neurosis.

Problems may arise at school such as bullying or victimization, or at work such as lack of satisfaction, bordeom and frustration due to slow or non-existent advancement. Later on there are family responsibilities which involve finding and making a home, keeping it in order, paying the bills and above all making decisions. A variety of things can go wrong and depending on whether the person has a vulnerable personality or not, rests the possibility of a breakdown. Most people can cope but many cannot. Those who fail to cope with such everyday stresses respond by succumbing to mental illness. Physical illness which is a threat to the person's security and independence, the abuse of drugs or alcohol, which happens too often, all contribute to mental illness and thus affect men tal health.

3.3 Characteristics of mental health

A mentally healthy person has a number of characteristics. He is well adjusted both in himself and to the outside world and his emotional and intellectual balance is not upset by internal complexes, conflicts or external stresses and is ready, willing and able to fulfil his role in society. He respects and has confidence in himself, and accepts, works with and to a large extent enjoys other people. He works, plays, has a family and social life and has an enthusiasm for living with a minimum of fear and hostility. He is reasonably even tempered, intelligently alert and has a happy disposition and is fairly efficient. The ability to love someone other than oneself is also important, as is to live within the bodily capabilities and productively without being a nuisance or a burden to society. There is a blend of emotions and character traits resulting in self control and conformity of habits. The mentally healthy person is able to adapt to change without setting up conflicts or causing other people to suffer pain or feel discomfort.

3.4 Maintenance of mental health

The maintenance of mental health depends on the presence or absence of hereditary factors which are likely to contribute to mental ill-health. It depends a great deal on the incidence and nature of the environmental stresses which are present and the individual's threshold for these. A low threshold means there is a likelihood that mental illness will occur and conversely a high threshold means that mental illness is unlikely to occur. The psychological needs are important at all stages of development and contribute greatly towards mental health. This does not mean, of course, that if the psychological needs are always met to the full, mental illness will not occur. Physical illness for example will still occur, much of it cannot be avoided, and may upset the mental balance. Drug and alcohol abuse, which affect mental health, is gaining momentum, particularly drug abuse. It might be said that if such people had their psychological needs met they would not be resorting to drug abuse. Such a statement would take some proving and until this is done we must accept the fact that whilst the psychological needs are important we must recognize that there are other factors.

There are a number of other factors which contribute to mental health and these are:

a. *Philosophy.* In the introduction we mentioned that philosophy tends to make the person more thoughtful and reflective and this is so. One is constantly amazed at the amount of bad fortune some people can withstand. Round-the-world sailors who are subject to great isolation and great loneliness will maintain that it is a personal philosophy which keeps them sane.

b. *Religion.* A religious faith and a religious belief are powerful allies in the face of adversity. From faith springs hope and where there is hope a current dilemma is more tolerable.

c. *Education.* Not everyone professes a religious belief, but everyone is educated. Education, therefore, has a wide and powerful influence on mental health. The overall aims of education are to prepare the person to be a citizen of the world and to help him to develop his intellectual resources to the fullest. It is this development of intellectual resources which is so important to mental health. Through education individual interests such as literature, music, art or natural history are developed and thus provide outlets for leisure time. Hobbies and recreation are vital for mental health. They are important during the work life, for the person with a hobby returns to work refreshed and with a clear mind to tackle the problems of the new day. It is even more important that the retired person should have an interest outside work for without such an outlet the days feel long and empty, boredom results and apathy follows. A long-earned retirement is not enjoyed. There are courses which prepare elderly workers for retirement and these serve a vital function.

3.5 Summary

The factors associated with mental health are happiness, vigour, full use of capabilities, integration of personality with a sense of freedom from conflict within oneself and harmonious adjustment to the environment. A personal philosophy, religion and education all contribute to the maintenance of mental health.

MENTAL MECHANISMS

3.6 Mental mechanisms

It is appropriate to introduce mental mechanisms at this stage, following a consideration of mental health and before mental illness is considered, because they also contribute towards mental health.

Mental mechanisms are likened to mental anaesthetics. This implies a reduction of sensibility and this occurs as far as painful experiences are concerned. It would be uncomfortable to have harsh reality constantly staring one in the face. In fact if this were to happen, mental health would most likely be seriously affected. The mental mechanisms which come to the rescue by supplying techniques for hiding away such realities, can be grouped as follows:

3.7 Techniques for substituting an attainable goal for an unattainable one

a. *Compensation.* When the mechanism of compensation is used, the individual covers up a weakness or defect by exaggerating the presence of a relatively less defective, or a more desirable characteristic. For example, dull boys who are poor at academic work may be good at games and will obviously be more inclined to discuss their ability at games than their lack of ability in the other direction. If the fact that they were a failure was permanently before their minds life would be uncomfortable if not unbearable.

b. *Sublimation (L. Sublimare,* to elevate). Sublimation is a commonly used mental mechanism. What happens is that an energy force is redirected to a more acceptable goal due to social pressure. For example the parental drive is redirected to teaching or nursing.

c. *Perversion (L. Pervertere,* to turn about). Perversion is the redirection of an energy force to an unacceptable goal and this occurs in sex habits.

d. *Day dreaming.* Day dreaming is employed when the individual cannot achieve a particular goal or dislikes exposure to competition and possible failure. A new goal is sought that is internal and therefore can be achieved, at least in a day dreaming fashion.

3.8 Techniques for improving the chances of reaching a natural goal

a. *Identification.* Identification involves putting oneself in the place of another. It occurs when there is an emotional tie which leads to the unconscious moulding of the personality after a model, for example, teachers or nurses. Identification is the basis of hero-worship.

b. *Regression* (turning back). When regression occurs there is a turning back to previous patterns of behaviour which were successful. For example when a new child arrives, an older one may resort to bed-wetting and perhaps crying more than usual. The child knows, though the mechanism is unconscious, that this form of behaviour was successful in the past in attracting parental attention and is now using it to ensure that the rival does not get more than his fair share. Regression also occurs in illness as we shall see when we consider mental reactions to illness.

3.9 Techniques for converting psychological stress into physical symptoms

Such techniques are an unconscious call for help and include:

a. *Compulsions.* When compulsions are present the person is forced to do repeated, absurd and pointless actions. Compulsions are biologically important because the stored stressful energy is allowed an outlet. A simple example of compulsive behaviour is fidgeting in the dentist's waiting room.

b. *Psychosomatic illness.* We have already mentioned psychosomatic illness in relation to the autonomic nervous system. Illnesses such as peptic ulceration, asthma and ulcerative colitis are all thought to have a psychological component which contributes to the disease process. The psychological stress is reflected in the affected organ and the organ is said to mirror the state of mind.

c. *Conversion hysteria.* When conversion hysteria occurs an emotional state is transformed to physical action which may result in blindness or paralysis. The classic explanation of this mechanism is the soldier going into battle. If he goes forward to battle he risks being injured or killed. On the other hand if he does not do his duty he risks being labelled a coward by his colleagues or worse still he may be shot for desertion. If the psychological stress, mainly fear, can be converted into physical action such as blindness or paralysis, this removes the soldier from danger and eases the stress.

d. *Accident proneness.* It has been estimated that 90 per cent of accidents in industry happen to 5–10 per cent of the workers. This is said to be due to the fact that such workers are hostile to themselves and to the environment. Repetitive work results in monotony and boredom. Accidents are a means of expressing a psychological plight and are really a call for help. We mentioned the economic aspects of industrial accidents in the introductory chapter.

e. *Suicide (L. Sui,* of oneself, *Caedere,* to kill). Suicide is an example of extreme hostility towards oneself and is a desperate call for help.

3.10 Techniques for ignoring the existence of a conflict
Stresses and conflicts can be substituted or converted, but they can also be ignored and there are a number of mechanisms available for doing this:

a. *Repression (L. reprimere,* to press back). Repression is the rejection of unacceptable drives and their associated ideas so that they are driven from the conscious to the unconscious mind. Such a mechanism allows an experience to be forgotten. An example of this is a person who has cancer and is aware of it, and then carries on normally ignoring its existence.

Suppression (*L. Supprimere,* to press down) has, as can be seen, a very similar meaning to repression. In psychological terms repression is an unconscious process and is therefore a mental mechanism. On the other hand suppression is said to be a conscious process and is therefore not a mental mechanism.

b. *Reaction formation.* Reaction formation depends on the fact that past experience colours present behaviour. If there is a strong conflict between wishes which have been repressed because they are unacceptable, the conscious mind may develop a strong bias to the exact opposite of the repressed wish. Thus a person with guilty feelings about sex may develop into a prude and condemn all sexual matters.

c. *Indirect expression of the experience.* This occurs in matters of sex. If the individual is incapable of establishing a normal relationship or is in some way frustrated and unfulfilled then an indirect means of expression is sought. This is the basis of the Peeping Tom and the 'what-the-butler-saw' mentality, as well as the basis for pornography generally.

d. *Rationalization.* Rationalization involves the discarding of what we actually are and putting a reasonable excuse in its place. For example, blaming the teacher for failing an examination.

3.11 Techniques for separating two antagonistic aspects of a conflict

a. *Dissociation.* Dissociation is the 'splitting off' of a part of the personality to avoid conflict. The undesirable facet of the conflict is forgotten. Dissociation techniques involve loss of memory, fugues, sleep-walking and functional paralysis. Perhaps the term fugue as used in this context needs a word of explanation. It has nothing to do with music but involves a period of complete loss of memory, when the individual disappears from his usual haunts. The period may last for several days or more and when the person comes to, he may find that he is many miles from home and, though he made contacts and generally lived during the time of the fugue, his mind is completely blank and he cannot remember the events during the episode.

b. *Multiple personality.* Conflicts can be avoided by taking on a personality to suit the situation. Take the case of the suburban housewife who, though having a happy family life, longs for a bit of excitement. She leaves home and has an affair with an artist type and they live a somewhat bohemian existence in contrast to her usual mode of life. When she returns home, as she does, she assumes her suburban personality again and never the twain shall meet. An example of a case of multiple personality is depicted in 'The Three Faces of Eve' by Eve Beauchamp.

c. *Projection.* Projection is a commonly used mental mechanism and involves blaming someone or something for personal deficiencies and lack of achievement. A simple example is the case of the bad workman who blames his tools.

3.12 Techniques for retreating from a conflict

a. *Shyness.* A degree of shyness and the associated modesty is a desirable attribute. But a degree of shyness which results in avoiding, evading or withdrawing from a problem, whilst it offers a solution of a sort, can be a handicap.

b. *Hyperactivity.* Hyperactivity allows a means for pent-up energy to be used up. It can be observed that some people are idly busy or 'fussing' under stress.

c. *Drug addiction.* Drugs and alcohol allow a temporary withdrawal from reality. In fact the pressures of modern day living, with the fierce competitiveness associated with the so-called rat race, are often put forward as a reason for the increasing abuse of drugs and the increased incidence of alcoholism. The withdrawal from reality given by drugs is only temporary and when the person returns the original problem exists and there is an additional one, which is, the after effects of the drug or the alcohol.

3.13 Summary
Mental mechanisms in normal persons are useful as mental anaesthetics and contribute to mental health. Intense stresses and conflicts interfere with the enjoyment of life and impair efficiency by removing the person from reality. If the removal is great the person will be unable to cope and the inability to cope, as we mentioned in the summary to the previous chapter, is the basis of psychiatric treatment.

MENTAL REACTIONS TO ILLNESS

3.14 Mental reactions to illness
Illness affects the physical, the mental and the social side of life. In fact the whole person is involved. We shall now consider how people react to illness generally before considering specific mental illnesses.

Disorganisation of the pattern of life is the first effect of illness, apart from any pain or discomfort which may be associated with the particular disease. If the person is admitted to hospital there is separation from the *family.* For most people the family is the focal point of security. There is separation from *work* which provides financial security. Being away from work may bring financial worries or it may affect the person's future with regard to promotion prospects. Illness also causes separation from the *community.* For some people social interests are very important and a loss of these can be upsetting.

3.15 Hospital life

The sick person is at a disadvantage, for in addition to the problems just mentioned he has to cope with hospital life and all its peculiarities at a time when he is least able or least inclined to do so. Before admission to hospital the person was fully responsible for himself and perhaps for many others. Now he is expected to enter a new type of relationship and he has, to some extent, to depend on other people. Then there are the rules and regulations. These may be necessary for the overall efficiency but they may be irksome to the individual.

3.16 Relationships

A number of factors affect relationships in hospital. First there is the image of the hospital. Image seems to be an overworked word these days, nevertheless it embodies an important concept. The public view of hospitals generally is influenced by the Press and the mass media. Organ transplants and the dramatic transfer of such organs from one hospital to another naturally creates a favourable image. On the other hand allegations of neglect or even cruelty which are sometimes made, counter this.

Next there is the image of the particular hospital. This may have been gained by previous first-hand experience or second-hand from ex-patients or visitors.

Another factor is the type of person. Some people have a happy, optimistic and well-adjusted outlook to life. It is easy to get on with such people. With others it is not so easy.

Nurses and doctors form the hub of hospital life therefore the nurse-patient and the doctor-patient relationships are all important as are the relationships between the patient and the other personnel. Of all the personnel involved the nurse is the central figure; because of her closeness to and longer contact with the person, she is more exposed to his anxieties. It is unfortunate that some nurses are disliked from the start; this may be due, for example, to the 'halo effect'. Juniors who are adjusting to hospital life may be under stress themselves and this can easily be felt by the sick person. It is therefore essential that nurses should be as emotionally detached and thus as objective as possible.

Last but not least there are the other people in the ward. They can have a positive or a negative influence, usually positive. The influence of suggestion is considerable and the patients themselves deal with their fellows who 'play up'.

3.17 Communications

This is an extremely communication conscious era and of course communications are very important in hospital. In recent times much attention has rightly been given to this aspect of hospital life.

Illness and admission to hospital usually give rise to anxiety and questions such as: 'What's the matter with me?', 'Will I recover?' 'Will I be crippled?' 'Will I be able to earn my living?' These are all important questions for the sick person and answers should be forthcoming. If you are new to caring for the sick and therefore inexperienced several of these questions will be outside your ability, others will be beyond your professional mandate and you must not attempt to answer them. You should assure the patient that you will ask the person whose job it is to answer, to talk to them. Dealing with questions is a skilled job because it is of the utmost importance to the sick person. Tact and understanding are needed and the following points should be kept in mind: the cultural background, the intelligence, the temperament and personality of the person, as well as the nature of the illness. The hospital policy should also be observed.

3.18 Individual responses to illness

Many people accept illness in their stride and do not over react to it. As we would expect the mental mechanisms come to the aid of many more. Others react in a variety of ways depending on their make-up.

a. *Denial*. Denial is not an uncommon reaction. Here the person says there is 'nothing wrong with me' because it would be too frightening to accept the fact. It is also found that people deny mental illness and say 'it's all physical' because a physical illness is thought to be more acceptable than a mental one.

b. *Suppression*. When we considered the mental mechanisms we said that suppression is not one because it is a conscious process. Suppression is found as a reaction to illness. This is a conscious attempt to remove from the conscious mind, thoughts or feelings which cause anxiety and guilt. This process is accompanied by a considerable amount of tension and the skilled observer will recognise that all is not well.

c. *Rationalization*. When employed in relation to illness the person usually comes up with the explanation that his illness is due to overwork, the weather or any such socially acceptable reason rather than admit to insecurity, feelings of inefficiency or guilt. The mechanism does not alter the disease process in any way, but it does provide an excuse and an escape route.

d. *Regression.* When we considered mental mechanisms, we mentioned the reaction of a child at the arrival of another and saw that behaviour often regresses, as a means of getting attention. This successful reaction is used in relation to illness. Personal responsibility is rejected and there may be associated impatient and demanding behaviour. The nurse's attention is frequently sought and there may be sulking and tears and the person may demand to be washed, fed and so on.

e. *Overdependency.* Overdependency is really another example of regression. The person does not attempt to solve his problems, he expects other people to do so for him. His attitude is that by putting himself in the hands of doctors and nurses he has transferred his problems to them and they should now solve them. Long term illnesses tend to produce overdependency and this should be avoided if at all possible because it makes rehabilitation difficult.

f. *Phantasy* (*G. phantasia*, appearance). Fantasy and phantasy are synonymous. Fantasies and day-dreams provide a means of substituting an attainable goal for an unattainable one. The substituted goal is an internal one. Some people react to illness by retreating into a fantasy world. The fantasies revolve around art, religion or literature and in his fantasy world the person is very important. His everyday feelings of inferiority and inadequacy are more than adequately compensated.

g. *Aggression.* Illness sometimes provokes an aggressive reaction. Many people keep aggressive tendencies under control and thus they remain latent for a long time. Although it is the nurses and those in close contact with the person who feel the brunt of the aggression, the cause lies elsewhere. Taking it out on other people is termed displaced aggression.

h. *Apathy.* Apathy is not an uncommon reaction to illness. This may be caused by extreme frustration which leads the person to feel abandoned and unwanted. Apathy causes the person to be socially isolated and is to be particularly guarded against in long term illness, though people with short term illnesses can also be affected.

i. *Depression.* There are many emotions felt in relation to illness and sadness is certainly one. If the person feels so much sadness that he feels ill then he is depressed. The reaction may be no more than a 'touch of the blues' or it may be more serious. There may be guilt feelings, feelings of unworthiness and of having 'let everybody down'. The depression which is a not unusual reaction to illness is unlikely to lead to suicide, but this possibility should never be forgotten.

j. *Negativism.* Negativism means a lack of co-operation which is often very subtle. The person may outwardly agree and then annoys by doing nothing or even 'throwing spanners in the works'. It is said that negativism is a form of aggression which is indirectly expressed.

k. *Paranoid feelings.* Some people react to illness by becoming suspicious and hostile and these feelings are sometimes projected on to other people. Such people often employ the technique of *scapegoating*, that is, blaming someone else or something, often the hospital, as being the source of all their difficulties. In some people this reaction can progress to a state where the person believes that the hospital staff are conspiring to harm him. Such a reaction is a delusion and, as we shall see later, is a common symptom in mental illness.

3.19 Long term reactions

The variety of reactions considered so far apply in the main to people with short or medium length illnesses, though they can continue should the illness be a long one. There is another reaction which is solely found in people with long term illnesses. Such people become overdependent on the hospital and virtually cease to make decisions. Initiative disappears and complete conformity replaces it, resulting in apathy and dejection. Such a reaction which is found in other institutions as well as hospitals dealing with long term illnesses is called *institutional neurosis*. This is a serious reaction and efforts are being made to prevent it occurring. The Mental Health Act 1959 which is framed to provide better community care and facilities was an important step in this direction.

3.20 Summary

Illness causes serious disruption to the individual's life. It gives rise to specific symptoms which may be distressing and it leaves the person physically weak, psychologically dependent and socially isolated. It is not surprising that something with such all embracing effects produces reactions. These reactions vary with the individual and the circumstances and a number have been mentioned. In order to bring effective help to the sick person, nurses and others concerned should have an understanding of these reactions. If the processes are understood it is easier to accept them and understanding also provides a base from which these reactions can be modified.

4

Bodily reactions to mental stress

4.0 Introduction

If we accept the fact that any illness affects the whole person, and most people do, then there must be bodily reactions to mental stresses, just as there are mental reactions to physical illness. The term *psychosomatic* is used for such reactions and means *mind* and *body*. The concept is not new, though the term is, and has received varying support since the practice of medicine began. That great English physician Thomas Sydenham (1642–89) expressed the basis of the reaction well when he said—'Tears unlet will make other organs weep'. Sydenham, sometimes known as the English Hippocrates, recognized that emotions could be indirectly expressed through the various organs of the body.

4.1 The mechanism of the reaction

In order to appreciate the mechanism of the reaction it is necessary to look again at the factors which contribute to human behaviour. It will be recalled that these include sensory stimuli which produce responses, drives, emotion and past experiences. The total of the person's responses is his behaviour.

There are a variety of expected responses to any stimulus depending on the hereditary make-up and the personality of the person. In the case of psychosomatic reactions the person often 'swallows his feelings' and then uses his body as a means of expressing emotion or emotional conflict that is 'blocked'. This expression of states of emotional turmoil which is unconscious, is referred to as psychosomatic. Organ language is a term applied to the various phenomena which appear.

4.2 Organ language

Examples of 'organ language' which are found in everyday use are 'muddle headed' in relation to mental confusion, 'broken-hearted' and 'warm-hearted' in relation to the heart. 'You make me sick', 'I'm sick of you', 'sick with fear', 'weak stomached' or 'strong stomached' are used about the stomach. 'Paralysed with fear', 'blind with rage', 'shaking with emotion' and 'blowing your top' are further examples of commonly used 'organ language' terms.

4.3 Experimental evidence

Loose 'organ language', graphic though it may be, would in itself
be insufficient to support the psychosomatic theory. There is experimental evidence available to give it support. This is found in the work
of two American doctors, Wolff and Wolff (1947). They made a
series of observations on a man called Tom, who as a result of a
childhood operation had a gastric fistula. As a result of the fistulla
part of Tom's stomach was outside the abdominal wall and was
thus readily observable. The doctors observed and reported the responses of Tom's stomach to emotional states. They reported that in
conditions of fatigue and depression, the mucous lining of the
stomach looked blanched, and both the gastric secretions and the
movements of the organ were reduced. From these observations
the effects of emotion on gastric digestion can be readily deduced.
When other emotions were present, such as anger, the stomach lining
became red and engorged with blood, the movements and the secretions were increased. This last reaction forms the basis of the psychosomatic explanation for peptic ulceration.

4.4 Organs affected

When we considered the autonomic nervous system, we mentioned
that any organ supplied by the autonomic nervous system could be
affected by a psychosomatic condition and this means practically
every organ in the body. In individual cases only one organ is usually
affected. Such an organ is referred to as the *constitutional target
organ*. As the term constitutional is synonymous with heredity, it
implies that there is a hereditary factor involved and this is so. This
explains why some people respond to mental stresses by succumbing
to raised blood pressure, others to peptic ulceration and others to
ulcerative colitis. It is accepted that responses are peculiar to the
individual but in general personality types are associated with each
response. Migraine sufferers are usually exacting and meticulous in
their work. Those who respond with peptic ulceration are usually
worriers. Sufferers of ulcerative colitis are usually extremely conscientious, exceptionally sensitive to criticism and tending to be
over orderly and over tidy.

4.5 Types of reaction

There are two types of reaction and these depend on the effect on
the 'target organ'. If the reaction causes little physiological disturb-

ances and no permanent tissue damage in the target organ, the reaction is said to be *transient*. If on the other hand the physiological disturbances are considerable and pathological changes take place in the target organ, then the reaction is said to be *deep seated*.

4.6 Transient reactions

Fear, which is accompanied by tachycardia, increased respiration rate, vasoconstriction of the skin, sweating, the cold sweat type, pilo-erection, dilation of the pupils, dry mouth and muscular tremors, is an example of a transient reaction. Grief is accompanied by tears, excess nasal secretion, skin pallor, reduced muscular tone and movements and is another example of a transient reaction. So is constipation of psychogenic origin, dyspepsia, sweating and migraine. Other examples are palpitations without evidence of heart disease and simple blushing. There is no clear cut division between the transient and the deep seated reactions and some transient ones may become deep seated. This depends on the length of time a reaction lasts.

4.7 Deep seated reactions

The deep seated reactions can be considered systematically. In the following conditions it is thought that there is a major psychosomatic component contributing to the disease process, though of course those who do not subscribe to the psychosomatic concept would disagree.

A. The Skin. *a*. Neurodermatitis.

        b. Eczema.

B. Respiratory system. *a*. Asthma.

C. Cardiovascular system. *a*. Essential hypertension.

        b. Coronary thrombosis and angina.

        c. Fainting attacks, though there may be other reasons.

D. Gastro-intestinal tract. *a*. Peptic ulceration.

        b. Ulcerative colitis.

        c. Anorexia nervosa.

        d. Obesity.

The last two reactions are examples of completely opposite reactions. Anorexia nervosa occurs in young girls who are concerned about their weight. There is a complete loss of appetite and such girls will actually starve themselves to death unless medical help intervenes.

At the other end of the scale people respond to stress by over-eating and as a result become obese, with all its associated problems.

E. Endocrine system. *a.* Thyrotoxicosis.
              b. Diabetes mellitus.

F. Reproductive system. *a.* Excessive, irregular or painful menstruation without any organic cause.
              b. Sterility for which no cause is found.
              c. Impotence in men.

G. Muculo-skeletal system. *a.* Rheumatoid arthritis.
              b. Backaches without any other cause.

4.8 Principles of treatment

The principles embodied in any form of treatment were well stated by E. L. Trudeau (1848–1915), the American physician in his quotation: 'To cure sometimes, to relieve often, to comfort always'.

In the case of psychosomatic illnesses, as in the case of most illnesses, these can be taken in reverse order.

4.9 Comfort

There are two sources of comfort. First there is the comfort brought about by the treatment of the physical symptoms which are foremost in the person's mind and the principal reason why help is sought. Antihistamine preparations bring immediate comfort in eczema, antacids help with the hyperacidity of peptic ulceration and hypotensive drugs bring comfort from the unpleasant effects of raised blood pressure.

Secondly there is the psychological comfort brought about by explanation and reassurance. For this to be effective *rapport* must be established between the person and his doctor, nurses and other staff. Rapport means that the person has confidence in those around him and is willing to co-operate in treatment.

4.10 Relief

Physical rest, which does not necessarily mean rest in bed, as prolonged bed rest saps the person's energy and brings a long list of complications in its trail, and psychological rest usually achieved by the aid of sedatives or tranquillizers bring about a relief of symptoms. Sometimes of course more specific therapeutic measures have to be used. These may include surgical intervention such as partial gastrectomy for peptic ulceration or removal of the colon for ulcerative colitis.

4.11 Cure

A cure can only be accomplished if the cause of the illness is sought out and eradicated. This, in theory, may be done by *psychoanalysis* but in practice this form of treatment is extremely time consuming and the results are not always proportional to the time spent. Psychotherapy, which when carried out on an individual basis takes the form of a therapeutic interview and when conducted on a group basis takes the form of a therapeutic discussion, is commonly used. In these techniques mental probing takes place which causes the 'bottled up' or 'swallowed emotions' to be released. Such an emotional release which is likely to be accompanied by tears is called *catharisis*. This emotional release can be brought about more quickly using drugs and the process is called *abreaction*. The technique will be mentioned later when we consider methods of psychiatric treatment. It helps the person to come to terms with his problem for the first time for, as we mentioned, the psychosomatic process is unconscious. If the person is to be cured completely all the pent-up emotions must be released and this is sometimes difficult.

4.12 Auto-immunity

It has been said that the psychosomatic theory has never received universal support. It has had ardent supporters and equally ardent detractors and it is again threatened. A new theory has been put forward to explain the cause of the conditions we have just described as psychosomatic and this the theory of auto-immunity. The basis of this theory is that people suffering from these illnesses develop antibodies against their own tissues. These antibodies destroy some of the body tissues in specific target organs. The pathological changes which take place in the stomach or duodenum in the case of peptic ulceration or the colon in the case of ulcerative colitis are said to be due to these antibodies. Such diseases are sometimes called the 'I hate me diseases' as there is an element of self destruction in the process.

4.13 Summary

The basis of psychosomatic reactions is that the expression of emotion or emotional conflict is blocked and is indirectly expressed through the various organs of the body. The indirect expression of emotion through the body is called 'organ language'. A variety of reactions are possible, but the individual reaction depends on the site of the constitutional target organ. Treatment is aimed first at relieving symptoms and then seeking out the cause. The psychosomatic explanation put forward for these reactions has been substituted by some by the auto-immune explanation. No doubt research will ultimately provide the answer, but in the meantime it is an exciting prospect, and one worth a little personal speculation, to see which theory stands up to scrutiny and thus survives.

5

Observation, examination and investigation

OBSERVATION

5.0 Introduction

Observation is one of the nurse's or indeed any other helper's most vital functions. Observations which must be accurate and reported either verbally or in written form, are essential to the doctor to help him in his diagnosis of new cases and as a guide to progress, or otherwise, in persons already diagnosed. The method of observation should be systematic and comprehensive and the following outline is put forward as one way of achieving these double objectives. It involves going from the general to the particular.

5.1 General activity

The person's general activity should be observed and it should be noted whether it is retarded or accelerated, furtive, restless or obsessional.

5.2 Appearance

The general appearance, posture, dress, mannerisms of a person tell a lot about him and are considered from two points of view:

a. *Facial*. It can be observed whether the person is calm or frightened, suspicious, grimacing, vacant, is mask-like, shows signs of pain, misery or is dreamy, shocked, deluded or hallucinated.

b. *Dress*. The choice of clothes and the mode of dress tells much about the person. Points to watch are neatness or untidiness. Are the clothes smart in fashion and decorative, or are they old fashioned and dirty? We shall consider which of these observations are particularly appropriate when individual conditions are considered later.

5.3 Conversation

It is sometimes said that when we open our mouth we put our foot in it. Certainly our mode of conversation reveals a lot about us. Points to watch for are whether the conversation is unusually slow or fast, spontaneous or hesitant, childish and self-centred, or guarded. It may also be incoherent, sarcastic or abusive or may reflect delusions or hallucinations.

5.4 Mood

The prevalent mood is a good guide to the person's state of mind. It can be readily observed whether the person is happy or sad, anxious, afraid and changeable or aggressive. The person may be apathetic and indifferent or suspicious and incongruous.

5.5 Attitude

Attitudes are extremely important and may be affected by many things including illness. These may range from a co-operative, tolerant and helpful to a negative, demanding, impulsive and resentful attitude. Other attitudes are submissiveness, over dependence and apologetic, or the person may be withdrawn, reserved and suspicious, plausible and scheming or grandiose. It is obvious that only a few of these attitudes will be found at any one time. For example in depression the prevalent attitude is that the person is withdrawn and apologetic, whilst conversely in mania, the attitude is likely to be a demanding and an impulsive one.

5.6 Intellect

There are many means available for measuring intellectual function and we shall consider these later, but from ordinary observation it is possible to get a general impression of the person's intellect. It is possible to tell whether the person appears bright or dull, though this is somewhat subjective and such an assessment is open to error. For example a person who is depressed or who is suffering from myxoedema may appear dull, but the illness may be masking an excellent intellect. Observation should reveal whether the person has insight or not, and it should reveal something of the quality of his judgement, memory, reasoning and orientation.

5.7 Eating habits

We have frequently said that states of mind have bodily consequences and observation of the appetite patterns in the various conditions confirms this. In depression there is a loss of appetite whilst young people with schizophrenia may have insatiable appetites —bulimia. People with paranoid conditions may refuse food suspecting it to be poisoned and people whose intelligence is affected either by subnormality or age may have dirty eating habits. Observation of the fluid intake is even more important because a very inadequate water intake results in dehydration and serious illness.

5.8 Sleeping habits

Observation of the sleeping habits is of the utmost importance and the sleep patterns in depression are essential for diagnosis because different varieties of depression produce different patterns as we shall see later. The total hours of sleep, the time of getting to sleep and the waking time should be observed. It should also be observed whether it is continuous or, intermittent, heavy or restless and noisy, whether it was disturbed by dreams or whether there was sleep-walking. It should also be noted whether sedation was used or not.

5.9 Physical state

Observation of the physical state must be done concurrently with observations on the mental state if a comprehensive picture is to be obtained. Pain is a symptom of a number of physical conditions and the nature, character and frequency of the pain should be noted. Likewise many physical conditions produce changes of temperature and this should be taken and recorded. The remainder of the observations should be carried out systematically:

a. *Nervous system.* The main observations here are the responses to sensation which indicate whether the sensory part of the system is working and the power and co-ordination of the muscles which indicate the functioning of the motor part of the nervous system. If the person is able to walk the gait is very important because the various sensory and motor lesions produce characteristic gaits. Involuntary movements, tremors and twitchings should be noted.

b. *The Cardiovascular system.* The pulse and the blood pressure tell a great deal about the functioning of the cardiovascular system and should always be recorded and reported. Breathlessness, palpitations and colour changes at the extremities should be noted.

c. *The Respiratory system.* The presence or absence of a cough should always be noted and so should the nature, volume and characteristics of any sputum produced.

d. *The Gastro-intestinal system.* In addition to the appetitite already mentioned it should be observed whether there is nausea, vomiting, diarrhoea or constipation. The weight should also be recorded and any losses or gains reported. The condition of the teeth is important and so is abdominal distension. It should be observed if there is incontinence.

e. *The Urinary system.* The volume, the nature and characteristics of the urine should be observed. Urgent action should be taken if the volume is small, less than 1,000 ml. in 24 hours, or if blood is present. It should be observed whether there is enuresis or urinary incontinence.

f. *The Endocrine system.* There are no particular observations which can be made on this system but a normal hair distribution is an indication that the system is working well. A combination of observations may lead to a diagnosis involving part of this system. If it is found that a person has a frightened look, is emotionally labile and has an increased pulse rate, further investigation may reveal that the person has over activity of the thyroid gland—thyrotoxicosis.

g. *The reproductive system.* The menstrual history is important and observations should include whethei the periods are regular or irregular and whether the losses are above or below average.

h. *The skin and appendages.* The skin is said to mirror what is happening within the body therefore observations of this organ are important. It should be observed whether it is intact or broken, clean or dirty, infected or inflamed or whether it is coarse or fine. The skin for example is very coarse in people of subnormal intelligence and in people suffering from endocrine conditions such as myxoedema. The hair and the nails are also affected in these conditions. The hair is scanty, exceptionally coarse and dry, and the nails crack.

5.10 Group activities

It is important to note whether the person participates in the activities within the hospital. Does he take part in occupational activities and group discussions? People who suffer from schizophrenia for example may avoid such activities or may assume a passive role if they participate at all.

5.11 Response to treatment

The response to treatment should be observed. It is important to know if the treatment is having the desired effect and that it is not accompanied by any unwanted or unpleasant side effects. This is particularly important in the case of drug treatment and we shall consider the effects which should be watched for later. The response to other treatment should also be noted. In the case of electroconvulsive therapy there is some loss of memory for events around the time of treatment, but prolonged amnesia would be considered an unwanted effect and might result in that form of treatment being discontinued. The responses to habit training, psychotherapy or social activities are equally important and should be observed and reported.

5.12 Summary of observation

Accurate, objective, meticulous and comprehensive observations are of vital importance and should be considered as one of the nurse's and other helpers', most important function. Observations which should be unobtrusive and discreet, the person should not be seen or feel to be observed, should always be reported either orally or in writing. Written observations are preferable because they are more permanent and if one nurse is called away other members of the team can easily take up where she left off. There should be a hand-over report of course. It is unrealistic to commit facts to memory as the memory often plays tricks.

EXAMINATION

5.13 Examination of the nervous system

Examination of the nervous system begins by the taking of a complete history which should reveal personality changes and disorders of function, if present. The examination of the nervous system is the doctor's job, though the nurse usually prepares what is required and also assists. Very often the doctor is only too pleased to demonstrate and explain what he is doing and this is certainly the best way to learn. The account given here gives the scope of the examination and it should help to understand it. There are many approaches but the one considered here begins by examining the higher functions and works downwards to the reflexes and includes tests for:

A. Cerebral function.
B. Cranial nerves.
C. Cerebellar function.
D. Motor system function.
E. Sensory system function.
F. Reflex function.

5.14 Cerebral function

a. General behaviour. The examiner first looks for defects in learned cultural aspects of behaviour such as peculiar gestures or speech, facial expressions or mannerisms and the appropriateness of activity. The degree of rapport with the examiner is assessed.

b. Level of consciousness. The examiner looks to see if the person is alert, is quick or slow to respond to verbal, visual and other stimuli. A note is made whether the patient is drowsy, is in a stupor or a coma.

c. Intellectual performance. Memory is assessed during history-taking and the store of information is estimated. The amount of schooling the person has had is an index of his premorbid performance. Orientation for time, place, person and so on is ascertained. The retention of numbers and the subtraction of 7s from 100 acts as a memory and concentration test. The ability to reason is tested by asking the meanings of well known proverbs such as a 'stitch in time saves nine'.

d. Emotional reactions. The emotional reactions are observed and it is noted whether the person is tense, hostile, or depressed and whether the reactions are appropriate or bizarre. It is also noted if the person is subject to emotional outbursts.

e. Thought content. The examiner checks to see if there is undue preoccupation or excessively recurring thoughts and whether replies to questions are appropriate and relevant. He also looks to see if answers are repeated, if there are any fixed ideas, delusions or hallucinations.

f. Sensory interpretation. It is ascertained whether the person can recognize what he hears, sees and touches. Failure of this function is called *agnosia*.

g. Motor integration. Motor integration is essential for the performance of skilled acts such as opening and closing a safety pin, speaking or writing. Failure of this function is called *apraxia*.

h. Language function. The ability to understand spoken language is tested by observing the response to simple instructions such as 'touch your nose'. The ability to understand the written word is assessed by asking the person to read a passage from a newspaper or book. Failure of this function is called *aphasia*. Combined tests involve sound recognition (whistling, snapping of fingers) speech comprehension, recognition of body parts, drawing a shape, identification of objects (coins, keys), comprehension of writing (news-paper) and listening to a sample of a person's speech.

5.15 The cranial nerves

When we considered the nervous system we did not mention the cranial nerves in any detail. We shall now consider them in an applied fashion. There are twelve pairs of these nerves which arise from various parts of the brain stem (Fig. 5.0). These nerves are known by numbers and by names as follows:

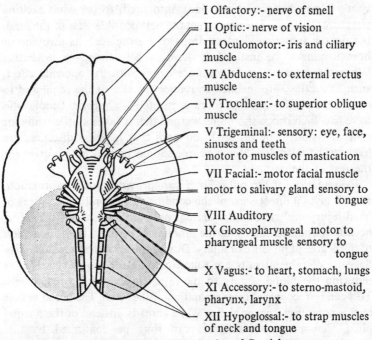

I Olfactory:- nerve of smell

II Optic:- nerve of vision

III Oculomotor:- iris and ciliary muscle

VI Abducens:- to external rectus muscle

IV Trochlear:- to superior oblique muscle

V Trigeminal:- sensory: eye, face, sinuses and teeth motor to muscles of mastication

VII Facial:- motor facial muscle motor to salivary gland sensory to tongue

VIII Auditory

IX Glossopharyngeal motor to pharyngeal muscle sensory to tongue

X Vagus:- to heart, stomach, lungs

XI Accessory:- to sterno-mastoid, pharynx, larynx

XII Hypoglossal:- to strap muscles of neck and tongue

Fig.5.0. Diagram to show origin and distribution of Cranial nerves.

I THE OLFACTORY NERVE. The olfactory nerve is the nerve concerned with the sense of smell. It is tested by observing the person's ability to discriminate between two contrasting smells such as tobacco and coffee.

II THE OPTIC NERVE. The optic nerve is concerned with vision. There are several aspects of vision which are examined separately:

a. The Fundi. (*L. Fundus*, bottom). When the doctor examines the fundi of the eyes he is simply examining the bottoms of the eyes and an instrument called an ophthalmoscope is necessary to do this.

When an ophthalmoscope is used to examine the fundi, a pink glistening membrane containing blood vessels can be seen. More detailed examination reveals the presence of a yellow spot (macula lutea). Within the yellow spot is an area called the fovea centralis and this is the point of acute vision. Near the yellow spot is a disc-like structure called the optic disc. This is the point where the optic nerve enters, also the retinal artery, and in contrast to the yellow spot no vision is possible at this point and is known as the 'blind spot'. If possible you should look into fundi to see what exciting structures they are. In order to get the best possible view of the fundi the doctor sometimes orders drops of a drug such as atropine or homatropine to be instilled in the eyes beforehand—a *mydriatic*. When the examination is complete drops with the opposite effect, such as eserine, are instilled to reduce the size of the pupil and to enable the person to focus more accurately—a *myotic*. People who have had such drops should be warned that it takes a little while for normal vision to be restored and until that happens distances are likely to be misjudged. Such people should be told not to drive for the rest of the day.

Examination of the optic fundi can provide much information. First it gives a direct view of the condition of the retina. In cases of head injury and raised intra-cranial pressure, oedema of the retina occurs—papilloedema—and the amount of oedema is an indication of the degree of pressure or injury. During the ageing process excessive deposits of mineral salts are found coating the blood vessels thus reducing the blood supply to the organ by narrowing the vessels. This can be recognized by examination of the fundi. The blood vessels in this condition appear as fine white threads, instead of the normal pink. Cerebral anteriosclerosis can thus be confirmed by this examination. Venous congestion, exudates and haemorrhages may also be recognized.

b. Visual acuity. Visual acuity is usually assessed by a *Snellen* chart. This chart, which was designed by the Dutch physician H. Snellen (1834–1908), contains several rows of letters at varying sizes, starting with very big ones at the top and scaling down to very small ones at the bottom. From examination of a number of subjects with normal vision it was found that they could read the sixth row of letters at a distance of six metres and the visual acuity is expressed as 6/6. The distance, represented by the bottom figure, remains constant and the figure on the top row represents the number of the row which the subject was able to read. A visual acuity of 3/6 means that the person's eyesight is only fifty per cent efficient. Each eye is tested separately and the subject is given a piece of cardboard or something similar to cover the other eye. There is also a book of small print for assessing near vision.

c. Colour vision. About 1 in 20 of the population, mainly men are colour blind and the degree varies. Some can recognize most colours except those colours such as green, yellow and orange which are mixtures of colours and are similar. In 1917 a Japanese Ophthalmologist called Shinobu Isihara designed a series of coloured patterns to detect colour blindness. They consist of abstract designs of various colours and superimposed on these designs are numbers outlined in colours which colour blind people have difficulty with or cannot appreciate. The subject is asked to say or write the number he sees and when none is seen it is possible not only to pick out difficulties, but the exact colours involved.

d. The visual field. It is sometimes found that in one position the person may be able to see quite well and in other positions vision is defective. The entire area taken by vision is the visual field and defects of this field can be detected by asking the person to follow finger movements with his eyes. This method reveals gross defects and a more accurate method such as the use of a perimeter gives more precise information.

III THE OCULOMOTOR NERVE. The oculomotor nerve is concerned with the movement of the eye. It is the motor nerve to all the eye muscles except the lateral rectus and the superior oblique. It also supplies the para-sympathetic fibres to the sphincter of the pupil and the ciliary muscle.

IV THE TROCHLEAR NERVE. The trochlear is the motor nerve to the superior oblique muscle which rotates the eyeball outwards.

V THE TRIGEMINAL NERVE. The trigeminal nerve has four branches:

   a. The ophthalmic is a sensory nerve to the cornea, ciliary body, lacrimal glands, nasal mucous membranes, the eyelids, the forehead and the nose.

b. *The maxillary* which is sensory to the cheek, side of nose, upper jaw and teeth, mucous membranes of the mouth and the maxillary sinus.

c. *The mandibular* branch is sensory to the mandible, the lower teeth and the skin in front of the ear.

d. *The motor* branch innervates the muscles of mastication and the temporal muscles.

Sensory function of the fifth nerve is tested by using wisps of wool, dull and sharp pin pricks and by applying hot and cold objects to the skin with the subject's eyes closed. The corneal reflex may be tested with wisps of wool.

The motor branch of this nerve is tested by palpation of the temporal and masseter muscles, observing for jaw deviation and by testing the subject's ability to close his mouth against resistance.

VI THE ABDUCENS NERVE. The abducens is the motor nerve to the external rectus muscle which rotates the eyeball outwards.

The cranial nerves III, IV and VI are examined as a unit by inspection of the eyelids, observing the eye movements and the movements of the pupils. Nystagmus, a condition in which involuntary rolling of the eyes occur, involves this group of muscles. Finally, the reaction of the pupils to light is tested. An ordinary torch may be used for this purpose and the pupils should come to a pinpoint when exposed to a bright light. When the light is removed the pupils should return to their normal size. In conditions such as head injury or poisoning the pupils are dilated.

VII THE FACIAL NERVE. The facial nerve has two divisions:

a. *The motor division* which innervates the facial muscles, the scalp, the auricle of the ear, the buccinator and the stylohyoid muscles.

b. *The sensory division* innervates the anterior two thirds of the tongue, the soft palate and the salivary glands.

This nerve is tested by asking the subject to look up, to wrinkle the forehead and any asymmetry is noted. The subject is asked to keep his eyes closed against resistance, to show his teeth, to blow out his cheeks and to whistle.

VIII THE VESTIBULO-COCHLEAR (AUDITORY). The vestibulo-cochlear nerve has two divisions and is the nerve of hearing.

a. The cochlear division is concerned with hearing. This part of the nerve may be tested by whispering or by the use of a watch to test auditory acuity. Weber's test and Rinnie's test are used as a test of sound conduction. Both tests involve the use of a tuning fork. In Rinnie's test a vibrating tuning fork is placed over the mastoid process and kept there until the vibrations cease. If the tuning fork is then placed in front of the ear vibrations should again be felt. This means that the air conduction of sound is better than bone conduction and this is the normal reaction. In Weber's test a vibrating tuning fork is placed centrally on the head and between the ears. If the bone conduction is normal the vibrations should be felt equally well in both ears.

b. The vestibular division supplies the semi-circular canals and is responsible for the maintenance of balance. This is achieved by means of tiny chalk-like balls (otoliths) which balance on hair-like structures (cilia) within the semi-circular canals. As long as the otoliths remain in contact we maintain our balance. If a person turns several times in one direction, for example, in dancing, then otoliths become dislodged and dizziness follows. In order to prevent this happening ballet dancers and similar performers can be observed to deliberately and regularly turn their heads in the opposite direction of the movement—counterpoise.

The vestibular division is not normally tested in an ordinary examination, but it may be tested using the *caloric* test. For this test the subject must be seated and water of different temperatures is introduced to the ear. The normal subject will feel dizzy if any temperature is too high or too low, hence the need for the subject to be seated. When water is removed the subject soon loses the feeling of dizziness.

The outer part of the ear and the tympanic membrane are examined by the use of an auriscope.

IX THE GLOSSOPHARYNGEAL NERVE. The glossopharyngeal nerve supplies sensory innervation to the posterior part of the tongue, the tonsils and the pharynx. It also provides motor innervation to the pharyngeal muscles. The motor part is tested by eliciting the 'gag' reflex which is obtained by stroking each side of the pharyngeal wall.

Cranial nerves VII and IX are concerned with the sense of taste. The following items are necessary to test this sense:

a. A 5 per cent solution of cane sugar—sweet.

b. A saturated solution of quinine sulphate—bitter.

c. A solution of citric acid—sour.

d. A 1 per cent solution of sodium chloride—salt.

The tongue should first be dried and then small pieces of blotting paper dipped in the various solutions are painted on the tongue. If the areas where the various tastes are appreciated are mapped out it is found that:

a. At the tip, sweet and salt are appreciated.

b. At the sides, sourness is appreciated.

c. At the back, bitterness is appreciated.

d. At the centre of the tongue no taste sensation is appreciated.

X THE VAGUS NERVE. The vagus nerve has already been mentioned in relation to the automonic nervous system. The vagus is a wandering nerve and supplies sensory innervation to the back of the ear, the pharynx, the larynx, the thoracic and abdominal viscera. It is tested by testing the ability to swallow, for example, by giving the subject a drink of water. The movements of the vocal chords, the palate and the uvulva are tested by asking the subject to say 'AH'.

XI THE SPINAL ACCESSORY NERVE. The spinal accessory nerve supplies motor innervation to the sternomastoid and trapezius muscles. It is tested by palpation of the muscle and by pressing down on the shoulder to test the strength of the trapezius muscle. The strength of the sternomastoid muscle is tested by asking the subject to turn his head to one side whilst at the same time opposing the motion.

XII THE HYPOGLOSSAL NERVE. The twelfth and final cranial nerve is the hypoglossal. This is a motor nerve to the strap muscles of the neck and tongue. It is tested by asking the subject to put out his tongue and observing for deviation, atrophy and tremors and its strength.

5.16 Cerebellar function

The cerebellum is concerned with balance and co-ordination and these functions may be tested as follows:

a. The subject is asked to touch his nose and it is noted whether the movements are smooth and without tremor or ataxia. The speed, rhythm, power and co-ordination is observed.

b. The subject's ability to gauge distances is assessed by asking him to touch the examiner's finger which is placed in several different positions.

c. Co-ordination is tested by asking the subject to run his heel up and down his shins and also by asking him to make a figure of 8 in the air with his toes.

d. The subject should be aware of his position in space with his eyes closed. This is the basis of Romberg's sign which is used to test cerebellar function.

e. Finally as a test of co-ordination, the subject is asked to walk heel to toe and then normally. This sequence is repeated a few times and normal subjects can cope with this test perfectly well, but it will not be possible for subjects with disordered cerebellar function.

5.17 The motor system function

There are 31 pairs of spinal nerves with origins in the spinal cord (Fig. 5.1). It is not proposed to give details of these nerves in the same way as the cranial nerves. Instead the motor function and the sensory function of areas of the body are considered.

a. The body muscles are examined for size and signs of atrophy. The symmetry of posture and the muscle contours and outlines are observed. The muscles of the limbs are compared for size using a tape measure.

b. The muscles are examined for tone and the examiner checks to see whether they are soft and flabby or firm and tense. Movements are observed and note is made of whether they are spastic, rigid or cogwheel.

c. Involuntary and abnormal movements are sought by observing the outstretched limbs for choreiform movements and dystonic twitchings.

d. Muscular strength is assessed by flexion and extension of the joints and lifting the arms over the head. The strength on both sides is compared and the subject is asked to raise his head and limbs against resistance. The subject is asked to rise from a knee-bent position and to walk on his toes and then on his heels.

5.18 The sensory system function

Sensory function is assessed by examining the superficial and the deep sensation. Superficial sensation may be assessed using wisps

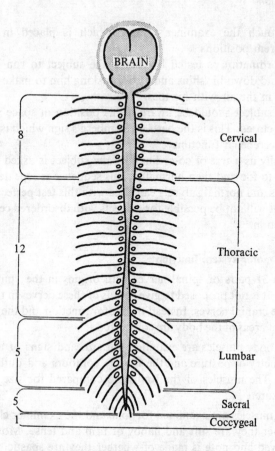

Fig.5.1. Diagram of spinal cord and peripheral nerves.

of wool or Von Frey hairs if available. Deep sensation may be assessed by the application of pressure. A note is made if there are any areas where no sensation is felt—anaesthesia, or areas where there are disorders of sensation such as tingling or 'pins and needles'—paraesthesia. The ability to appreciate temperature variation is assessed by applying test tubes of hot and cold water of known temperature to the skin. The vibration sensation is tested by placing a vibrating tuning fork over bony prominences such as the ankle. Steroagnostic function is tested using common objects such as coins, keys and so on. Bradaesthesia, the recognition of numbers written on the hands is tested by using a pencil.

5.19 Reflex function

A patella hammer is used to elicit the majority of the reflexes except the eye reflexes. There are superficial and deep reflexes as follows:

A. SUPERFICIAL

Reflex	How elicited	Response	Spinal segment involved
a. Plantar	Stroking sole of foot	Plantar flexion of toes in babies and in diseases of the pyramidal tract The toes are extensor	S.1 & 2
b. Cremasteric	Stroking of thigh	Drawing up of testicle	L.1 & 2
c. Upper abdomen	Stroking near costal margin	Retraction of same side of epigastrium	T.8 & 9
d. Lower abdomen	Stroking below umbilicus	Retraction of same side of abdominal wall	T.9 & 10
e. Conjunctival	Touching cornea (wisp of wool)	Winking	5 & 7 Cranial
f. Pupillary	Flash light	Contraction of pupil	3 Cranial

B. DEEP—UPPER LIMBS

Reflex	How elicited	Response	Spinal segment involved
a. Biceps	Tapping of Biceps tendon	Flexion of forearm	C.5 & 6
b. Triceps	Tapping of Triceps tendon	Extension of forearm	C.6, 7 & 8
c. Wrist (supinator)	Tapping extensor tendons just above the wrist	Jerking up of the hand	C.6

DEEP—LOWER LIMBS

Reflex	How elicited	Response	Spinal segment involved
a. Knee	Tapping of patella tendon	Kicking forward of leg	L.2, 3 & 4
b. Ankle	Tapping of Achilles tendon	Plantar flexion of foot	S.1 & 2

Abbreviations

C = Cervical segment of spinal cord
L = Lumbar   „   „   „   „
S = Sacral   „   „   „   „
T = Thoracic   „   „   „   „

Some reflexes involve up to three nerves; others such as the wrist involves only one. In the case of the cranial nerves abbreviations are not used and the word 'cranial' is written in full.

5.20 Summary and list of equipment

A neurological examination provides a great deal of information and the findings should help the doctor to formulate his diagnosis. Some of the reactions are of particular interest to the nurse for if she is caring for an unconscious person she will be expected to test for some of these reactions, such as the response to commands, skin sensation and the reaction of pupils to light, as part of her standard observations. It is therefore important to become proficient in these skills, as a person's life may depend on the early recognition of changes in function.

A list of equipment and the function of each piece will now be given as an aid to the nurse when assembling the equipment for this examination. Allowances must be made for local practices and if there is a procedure book available it should be consulted.

Equipment	*Function tested*
Safety pin	Motor integration
Pencil and paper	
Newspaper or book	Language function
Tobacco and coffee	Smell
Homatropine and eserine drops	Optic fundi
Ophthalmoscope	
Snellen chart	Visual acuity
Isihara pattern book	Colour vision
Perimeter	Visual fields
Torch	Pupil reaction
Wisps of wool or Von Frey hairs	Sensations
Sharp and dull pins	
Test tubes of hot and cold water	Temperature reaction
Auriscope	Ear
Tuning fork	Sound conduction and vibration
Spatula and torch	Mouth and throat
Different tasting liquids:	Taste
Sugar solution—sweet	
Acid „ —sour	
Quinine „ —bitter	
Salt „ —salt	
Glass of water	Swallowing
Coins and keys	Steroagnostic function
Pencil	Bradaesthesia
Patella hammer	Reflexes
Tape measure	Compare muscle size

INVESTIGATION

5.21 Investigation

By the time the doctor has taken a full history and examined the person, he has made his diagnosis or at least a provisional diagnosis. Sometimes a number of investigations are necessary in order to clinch the diagnosis and to exclude other possibilities. The nervous system can be investigated from two points of view, the physical and the psychological. Physical investigation involves radiological, chemical, microbiological, serological and the electrical aspects of the system, whilst psychological investigation is aimed at assessing the intelligence and the personality type of the individual.

5.22 Physical investigations

A. RADIOLOGICAL (X-RAYS). There are a number of these investigations which may be done:

a. Straight X-ray. Whenever there is a head injury or an accident involving the loss of consciousness an X-ray photograph of the skull is taken. This enables fractures to be seen which may not be detectable on ordinary examination. In cases of a space occupying lesions of the brain, say a tumour, this form of X-ray is often useful. No special preparation is necessary before this investigation other than to ensure that the person is at the X-ray department at the appointed time.

b. Air Contrast photographs (encephalography). This procedure involves the introduction of air, by means of a lumbar puncture needle, into the subarachnoid space of the spinal cord. The air rises and enters the ventricles if there is no obstruction. The procedure is carried out with the person sitting up and may be followed by a headache due to a reactionary increase of the intra-cranial pressure. Explanation and reassurance are the best preparations for this procedure. Afterwards the person should rest in bed for twenty-four to forty-eight hours depending on local custom.

c. Air contrast photographs (ventriculography). This is a more elaborate procedure which is carried out in the operating theatre under local anaesthesia. A small burr hole is made in the skull on either side of the midline and a needle is introduced into the ventricles. Cerebrospinal fluid is withdrawn, the intra-ventricular pressure is measured and air is then injected. X-ray photographs are taken in various positions and the ventricles are outlined as translucent areas. This investigation is carried out in people with suspected brain tumours and who are likely to have already raised intracranial pressure. The procedure thus carries the danger of collapse or convulsions and coma may follow as a complication of this procedure. The preparation is that for an operation. Consent must be obtained. The scalp has to be shaved beforehand and consent must be obtained before this is done. Pre-operative medication is given and all the notes, records and previous X-rays should accompany the person to the theatre. The person should be nursed flat after the procedure for twenty-four to forty-eight hours.

d. *Opaque contrast media* (myelography). Sometimes an opaque contrast substance is injected into the spinal theca in order to outline the space around the spinal cord and to pinpoint protrusions of the intervertebral discs or spinal tumours. The preparation and after care is similar to that of a lumbar puncture which will be mentioned later.

e. *Angiography.* The blood vessels of the brain can be outlined by the injection of an opaque material such as diodone into the carotid or vertebral artery. The injection is carried out under a local anaesthetic by direct puncture of the blood vessel. Sometimes it is done through a small incision in the neck over the site of the carotid artery. Following injection of the dye a series of X-ray photographs are taken. This has to be done very quickly because the dye soon disappears into the circulation. This investigation reveals the presence of aneurysms or thrombosis in the cerebral blood vessels. The preparation is similar to that for a ventriculography and the complications are also similar.

f. *Isotope tracers.* Sometimes isotopes such as P^{32}, an isotope of phosphorus, are used to define the outlines of a cerebral tumour. An isotope which will be taken up by the suspected tumour must be used. The isotope solution may be taken orally or it may be injected into the bloodstream. A geiger counter is then used to map out the area emitting radioactivity; this is the area of the tumour.

B. CHEMICAL. Samples of blood and cerebrospinal fluid are necessary for chemical examination. The blood may be examined for any substance which is in the body or enters the body. The principal investigations are:

Chemical	Normal range
Alkali reserve (as bicarbonate)	24–32 m Eq/L
Chloride	97–107 m Eq/L
Glucose (fasting)	70–110 mg/100 ml
pH (hydrogen ion concentration)	7·3–7·45
Potassium	3·8–5·1 m Eq/L
Protein	6·0–8·0 g/100 ml
Sodium	137–149 m Eq/L

Hormone, enzyme and vitamin concentrations can be estimated and some of these are of particular interest in relation to the nervous system. For example the vitamin B group of vitamins are called the anti-neuritic vitamins. Deficiency of these vitamins seriously affects the functioning of the nervous system. The presence of poisons, drugs, or alcohol—the breathalyser and associated blood test—can be determined and measured.

As the chemicals of the body are found in solution in the plasma, in the majority of cases, it does not matter if the blood clots as the cells are not required; the majority of specimens for chemical investigation may be collected in plain bottles. Samples of cerebrospinal fluid are also collected in plain bottles. A guide to the collection of specimens will be given later, but the nurse's main duties are to see that the specimens are properly labelled. Numbers should be used as well as names, for it is possible to have two people with the same names and initials. Specimens should be delivered promptly to the laboratory, for the best results are obtained from fresh specimens.

There is a great deal of chemical research in progress at the moment to try to find a chemical basis for some mental disorders.

C. MICROBIOLOGICAL. Micro-organisms such as viruses, bacteria and spirochaetes can affect the nervous system and give rise to infection—meningitis—or abscess formation. The spirochaete of syphilis causes an infection which may involve the brain or the spinal cord. Specimens of cerebrospinal fluid are necessary if the infecting organism is to be isolated and identified.

D. SEROLOGICAL. If there is an acute infection the pathologist looks for the organism responsible. In the case of latent infections he examines the serum for the presence of antibodies and there are a number of such serological investigations used in connection with diseases of the nervous system:

a. *The Wassermann reaction.* The reaction depends on the ability of complement, a protein substance normally present in serum, to 'fix' an introduced antigen. (An antigen is something which stimulates the production of antibodies). The reaction may be represented as follows:

Antigen + Suspected Syphilitic + complement→   Breaking up of
Serum containing   (Free)   red Corpuscles
red blood corpuscles   (Haemolysis).
from an ox or sheep.

Complement not fixed so haemolysis took place. This is a negative reaction and means that the person is not suffering from syphilis.

Antigen + Suspected Syphilitic + complement→   No haemolysis.
Serum containing red   (Fixed)
blood corpuscles from
an ox or sheep.

The complement was fixed so no haemolysis took place. This is a positive reaction indicating that person has a syphilitic infection.

The Wassermann test not only gives a positive or a negative result but also gives an idea of the quantity of antibodies present as a number of different concentrations are used. A positive reaction in a low concentration indicates a high level of antibodies.

b. The Venereal Disease Reference Laboratory Test (The V.D.R.L.). The V.D.R.L. test depends on the fact that antigen/antibody reactions produce cloudiness—flocculation. Because it is simpler and therefore quicker to carry out, the V.D.R.L. test is often used now instead of the Wassermann test. The result may be positive or negative and when a positive result is obtained it is expressed as + if weak and + + + + if strong.

c. The Kahn test. The Kahn test works on the same principle as the V.D.R.L. test and provides a result which is graded in a similar way.

E. LUMBAR PUNCTURE. We have just seen that a lumbar puncture is necessary for the introduction of air and dyes in order to examine the nervous system, and it is also necessary in order to obtain samples of cerebrospinal fluid for chemical, microbiological and serological examination. It is now time to consider this procedure.

a. Reasons for lumbar puncture

1. *Diagnostic.* It may be used to obtain diagnostic information in cases of tumours, head or spinal injuries, infections or suspected congenital lesions.

2. *Relief of pressure.* It is sometimes used to relieve pressure as for example in meningitis or uraemia, but this is not done very often because removal of fluid may result in the brain stem being drawn into the foramen magnum and being injured as a result—'coning'.

3. *To introduce drugs and other substances.* Streptomycin may be introduced in the treatment of tuberculous meningitis, because streptomycin injected in the usual way does not cross the 'blood brain barrier' and thus does not reach the infected meninges. As we mentioned, air or dyes may be introduced for diagnostic purposes. Spinal anaesthesics may also be introduced, but these are rarely if ever used nowadays.

b. Equipment. Local practice varies considerably and if there is a procedure book available it should be consulted. If there is a C.S.S.D. (A Central Sterile Supply Department) it is likely that a complete sterile set will be supplied. If not the following equipment should be provided.

A dressing pack with towels for draping the area, gauze and woollen swabs and lotion containers. A basic set of two dressing forceps, two dissecting forceps and scissors should be supplied. The lumbar puncture needle and the manometer for measuring the pressure should be available—the pre-sterilized disposable variety are most commonly used. A cleansing lotion depending on the doctor's choice and local custom, should be provided. Some doctors like a dye-containing antiseptic such as iodine to mark the site of the puncture. A needle and syringe together with a local anaesthetic such as 1 per cent novocaine will be required. A pathological investigation request form and two plain specimen collection bottles should be available. Two are required because the first sample may be contaminated by blood due to injury caused by the needle. Bed blocks will be needed if the foot of the bed is to be raised after the procedure and if this cannot be done by mechanical means.

c. Method. As always the procedure should be explained to the person beforehand and his questions answered. There are two positions which can be used. First sitting back to front on a chair or lying in the left lateral position in the bed. If the bed position is used the person's neck should be flexed and the legs drawn up to give better access to the lumbar area of the back.

d. Site. When the area has been cleansed and anaesthetized, the needle is introduced at a point between the third and fourth or the fourth and fifth lumbar vertebrae. These points are located by draw-

ing a line from the iliac crests to the midline. The point of inter-
section is the spine of the fourth lumbar vertebra, a dye-containing
substance can be used to mark this point.

The dura mater ends at the lower border of the second sacral
vertebra and the spinal cord ends at the lower border of the first
lumbar vertebra. The subarachnoid space also continues to the
same level as the dura mater. For this reason a needle can be introduced without damaging the spinal cord.

e. Nursing care after a lumbar puncture. Following the procedure
the person should be made comfortable and nursed in a flat position
or with the foot of the bed elevated. Headache is the immediate
complication which arises and should be relieved as prescribed by the
doctor. Infection may occur as a late complication, but should not
arise if a good aseptic technique is practised.

The equipment used should be cleaned and made ready for future
use or returned to the C.S.S.D.

f. Normal cerebrospinal fluid. Normal cerebrospinal fluid is a
watery and slightly alkaline fluid and contains:

Chlorides as sodium chloride	710–750 mg/100 ml.
Glucose	50–80 mg/100 ml.
Protein	15–40 mg/100 ml.
Cells	0–5 lymphocytes/C.M.M.
Urea ⎫ Creatine ⎭	Small amounts

The specific gravity is 1·005 to 1·008, the volume is 120–150 ml.
in an adult (approximately 10 ml. are removed at lumbar puncture)
and it exerts a pressure of between 80 and 120 mm. of cerebrospinal
fluid.

g. Alteration of cerebrospinal fluid in disease.

1. *Cerebrospinal fluid appears cloudy* in infections except in infections due to viruses. The pressure is also raised in infections. A tumour
along the circulating channels may obstruct its flow and this can be
checked by the Queckenstedt test. This is done during the procedure
of lumbar puncture by compressing the jugular veins for ten seconds.
Normally the pressure rises quickly by 100 mm. of cerebrospinal
fluid or more and then falls quickly to normal. In cases of spinal
block due to obstruction such as a tumour, no such rise in pressure
occurs.

2. *Tuberculous meningitis.* In tuberculous meningitis the white cell

count may range from 100 to 300 per cubic millimetre, the glucose and the chloride levels are lower than normal. In this type of meningitis it is not always possible to isolate the causative organism.

3. *Meningococcal meningitis.* The cerebrospinal fluid in meningococcal meningitis is usually very cloudy, the white cell count may be as high as 1,000 per cubic millimetre, and as in the tuberculosis, the glucose and chloride levels are below normal. The organisms may be isolated. The picture is somewhat similar for pneumococcal, streptococcal, staphylococcal and influenzal meningitis.

In virus infections no organisms are seen and the cerebrospinal fluid is often described as 'sterile'. In poliomyelitis the white blood cells are increased and the protein content is raised. The position is somewhat similar in encephalitis lethargica, though here the protein tends to be normal.

In early syphilis the white cells are increased and the Wassermann reaction or the V.D.R.L. is positive. In late syphilis the white cells may not be affected but the Wassermann reaction remains positive. In syphilis which causes General Paralysis of the Insane (G.P.I.), the protein content is increased and, of course, the Wassermann reaction remains positive.

F. ELECTRICAL (ELECTROENCEPHALOGRAPHY, E.E.G.)

a. The electroencephalogram (E.E.G.). The E.E.G. works on the principle that excitable cells such as nerve cells have what is called an action potential. When there is a potential, or a potential difference, as it is called, between two points, an electric current will pass from the high to the low potential. For normal electrical activity the cells must be healthy. It follows, therefore, that abnormal or diseased cells will give a pattern different from normal. This form of investigation was perfected by the German doctor Johannes ('Hans') Berger (1873–1941) who published the results of his researches in 1929.

The electrical potential between the cells of the brain are very small and have to be considerably amplified by the machine. The electrical energy thus amplified is converted to mechanical energy which makes a tracing on specially prepared graph paper. The following are the principal wave frequencies used:

Delta: 0·5–3·5 cycles a second. Tumours give rise to these low frequency waves.

Theta: 4–7 cycles a second. These are found in the parietal area of the brain.

Alpha: 8–13 cycles a second and are found in the occipital area
          of the brain.
Beta: 14–30 cycles a second and are found in the frontal area
          of the brain.

b. Diagnostic use. The E.E.G. is used extensively as an aid in the
diagnosis of epilepsy, the localization of brain tumours and the
assessment of brain damage following injury. Recently the E.E.G.
has been used as a means of confirming death in cases of potential
donors of organs, such as the heart, to be transplanted into other
people. This is a highly emotive and controversial subject and not
everyone agrees that the E.E.G. is the best method of confirming
death for this purpose. When there is no life there is no electrical
activity and the recording appears as straight lines on the paper.

c. Preparation. The big machine and the mass of electrodes may
frighten many people and sometimes it is confused with electroconvulsive therapy. Other people think of the machine as a lie detec-
tor, an intelligence test or a mind-reader. The person should be
reassured on these points because it is essential to have his co-operation. Some people are concerned about where the electricity is coming
from. It can be explained or demonstrated that everyone has electricity
in their bodies. For example the cracking heard when hair is combed
is due to electricity.

The person should wash his hair beforehand as dirt and grease
may affect the reading. Normal meals may be taken unless there is an
instruction to the contrary.

d. Factors affecting the E.E.G.

1. *Age.* A new born child produces a very slow pattern of 0·5
cycles per second. At one year this is increased to 5–8 cycles a second.
The adult pattern is found at 8–10 years of age.

2. *Muscular activity.* Simple muscular activity such as opening
and closing of the eyes upsets the pattern.

3. *Sleep.* The wave patterns are slower during sleep and sometimes
in specialized investigations, recordings are taken continuously
throughout the night.

4. *Blood sugar level.* The brain cells require a continuous supply
of energy in order to function. A low blood sugar (hypoglycaemia)
level may precipitate a convulsion, hence the reason for seeing that
the person has his usual meals beforehand.

5. *Endocrine function.* There is a relationship between the occur-

rence of seizures and the endocrine controlled salt retention which tends to occur in the premenstrual period.

6. *Drugs.* Antihistamine drugs may be responsible for producing an abnormal recording. Barbiturates give rise to fast waves and may mask slow abnormal activity. Ideally the subject for E.E.G. should not be receiving any drugs; if this is not possible the doctor responsible should be given full details of the medication taken in the period before the recording.

7. *Electroconvulsive therapy (E.C.T.).* One or two treatments with electroconvulsive therapy (E.C.T.) do not usually affect the E.E.G. If the person has had several treatments, slow waves may follow but these disappear a few weeks after the treatment is discontinued. As with drug treatment it is important for the E.E.G. specialist to have the person's E.C.T. history, if any.

5.23 Psychological investigations

A. INTELLIGENCE. Intelligence has been variously defined and those definitions include overall mental efficiency. This definition incorporates or implies many of the other definitions such as the capacity to meet new situations, or to learn to do so, the ability to perform tests or tasks involving the grasping or relationships and the ability to grasp and understand abstract concepts. The degree of intelligence is proportional to the complexity of the relationships grasped or the abstractness of the concepts understood. Intelligence is therefore not a single entity but has a number of facets which are called abilities. The term ability implies proficiency at the particular task. Abilities include mechanical ability, i.e. ability to mend bicycles, cars, electrical appliances and to make models. Mathematics, language and music are all activities requiring special ability.

Intelligent acts are said to involve three things:

a. The perception of the important aspects of the environment.
b. The ability to hold this information received and then to reorganize it.
c. The solving of the problem by reaching the best possible solution having weighed up all the pros and cons.

Observation of the requirements for intelligent acts led the English psychologist C. E. Spearman (1863–1945) to formulate his two factor theory of intelligence and these are:

a. The general factor—G factor.
b. The specific factor—S factor.

The general factor is the summation of several special factors. The person who is able to solve a variety of problems involving mechanical aptitude, language and mathematical function, has a high level of general intelligence. Such a person may have a particular aptitude for mathematics and thus can be said to have a well developed S factor for this subject. But it is possible the same person may not be very proficient in music and has a poorly developed S factor for music.

B. DISTRIBUTION OF INTELLIGENCE. Examination of intelligence distribution curves in the population (Fig. 5.2) shows that the majority

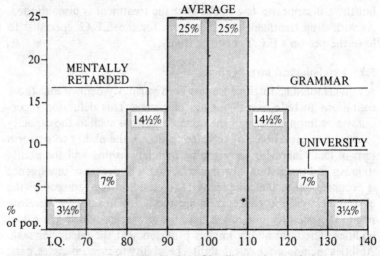

Fig.5.2. Histogram to show distribution of intelligence in population.

of the population are of average intelligence and their intelligence quotients (I.Q.s) lie within the 80 to 120 range. Children with I.Q.s below 70 are not considered to be likely to benefit from an ordinary education and said to be subnormal and these are a comparatively small group. At the other end of the scale there is only a small number of people with an I.Q. of 140 or more and these people are in the genius class. People in the average group do unskilled, semi-skilled and skilled jobs depending on which end of the scale their I.Q. lies. In order to go to Grammar school the pupil needs an I.Q. of more than 110. After school such people join the professions such as teaching, accountancy, banking, nursing and engineering. To benefit from a university education the student should have an

I.Q. over 120. Such people take up law, medicine, science, religion, top administrative posts in the Civil Service and so on.

This does not necessarily mean that a person's I.Q. can be assessed by the nature of his work. It is unlikely that a person with low intelligence will get to university, or if he does, remain there to graduate. On the other hand it is possible to find extremely intelligent people doing so-called lowly jobs. Achievement is not based on intelligence alone, there are factors such as perseverence, emotional stability and lack of opportunity due to economic deprivation. The British system of education, providing, as it does, free education according to the person's ability and irrespective of background, has done much to rule out the economic factor as a brake to achievement.

C. MEASUREMENT OF INTELLIGENCE

a. What is measured? The measurement of mental function or psychometry as it is sometimes called, is an ordinary biological measurement which can be compared with the chemical serological or electrical measurements which we considered in the section on physical investigation. Like the physical measurements, the mental measurements provide data for comparison with the person's own previous performance or with that of other people.

Intelligence tests measure two things:

1. The information which the subject has retained from past experiences.
2. The ability of the subject to cope with the experiences and the problems of life.

The first of these is influenced by education (the environment), whilst the second is not.

We have mentioned earlier the debate that exists about the hereditary/environmental contribution to intelligence and it will be remembered that some of the participants in the debate placed the hereditary contribution as high as 90 per cent whilst others rated it at 38 per cent. It is accepted that both aspects contribute, though the size of the contribution of each is in dispute. Intelligence tests must be designed to cover both. In practice this is so and we shall mention which aspect is to be measured when the individual tests are considered.

b. How is it measured? Intelligence is measured by the use of a number of tests, often referred to as a battery of tests. There are junior and adult versions of these tests. The results provide the mental age of the individual in relation to the performance of other people in that age group and the intelligence is calculated as follows:

$$\frac{\text{Mental age (M.A.)} \times 100}{\text{Chronological age (C.A.)}}$$

Thus a child with:

$$\frac{\text{Mental age} = 12 \times 100}{\text{Chronological age} = 10}$$
$$\text{I.Q.} = 120$$

The $\frac{\text{M.A.}}{\text{C.A.}}$ is multiplied by 100 to avoid the clumsiness which the use of decimals or fractions would give. As the chronological age (the actual age) and the mental age are different entities, the result obtained when they are divided by each other has no units and is therefore called a 'Quotient'.

Whenever a test or group of tests is chosen, there are two criteria which must be met:

1. It must be a valid test. A valid test measures what it is required to test.
2. It must be a reliable test. A reliable test gives the same result when set by two or more testers to large and different groups of subjects.

To ensure fairness to the subjects, all tests are subjected to the closest scrutiny and a period of three years is allowed to lapse before a new test is accepted for general use. Other considerations are the ease of application and the ease of marking the test. For instance, it may be easier to use a test which is suitable for groups of subjects as well as individuals.

The following are examples of intelligence tests found in use:

1. *The Wechsler intelligence test*. There are two separate versions of this test; the children's version which is abbreviated to W.I.S.C. (Wechsler Intelligence Scale for Children) and the adult version abbreviated to W.A.I.S. (Wechsler Adult Intelligence Scale). This is a comprehensive battery of tests and includes assessment of the information store, comprehension ability, arithmetical reasoning and the range of the vocabulary. These factors depend on whether the person was educated or not—environment. For those without

education but with good inborn intelligence there are tests such as picture completion, block design and the assembly of objects.

2. *The Stanford-Binet test.* This was first a French test but has been revised by L. M. Terman and J. G. Merrith, both Americans. There is also a children's and an adult version of this test.

3. *Raven's Matrices* (Fig. 5.3). This test has been designed to test the subject's native intelligence as it is not affected by the educational

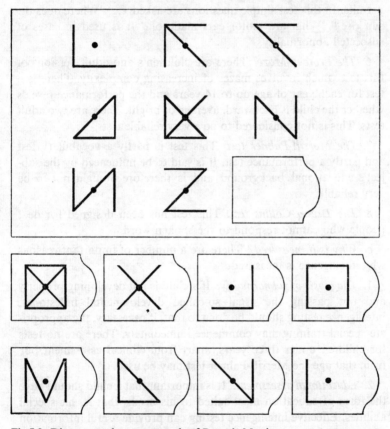

Fig.5.3. Diagram to show an example of Raven's Matrices.

status or the social training of the subject. A book of patterns is used and the patterns increase in complexity as the test goes on. The patterns on each page are incomplete and at the bottom of the page there are a number of alternative choices, of which only one is correct, for the subject to choose from.

4. *The Mill Hill Vocabulary.* In contrast to the Raven's Matrices, the Mill Hill Vocabulary test is purely a test of vocabulary and as such it is dependent on the subject's educational background. It is sometimes used in conjunction with Raven's Matrices and it may also be used in cases where language function is a particular asset for a job.

5. *The Kent Oral test.* This is a very simple and a very quick oral test and should be backed up with one of the other tests when time permits. In this test simple questions are asked e.g. 'Where does the sun rise?' 'What are motor cars made of?' It is used in cases of suspected abnormality.

6. *The Proteus Maze.* There are children's and adult versions of this test which involves mazes of increasing complexity. There is a test for each year of age up to 14 years and the performance reveals whether the child is backward, average or bright. There are two adult tests. This is not considered to be a very reliable test.

7. *The Merrill-Palmer test.* This test is partly a vocabulary test and partly a performance test. It is said to be influenced by the subject's educational background and is therefore thought not to be very reliable.

8. *The Drever-Collins test.* This test has been designed for deaf people who cannot respond to the spoken word.

c. Why is it measured? There are a number of important reasons why intelligence is measured:

1. *Diagnosis of subnormality.* If a child is not developing properly and not passing the usual so-called developmental milestones, intelligence testing should be done so that, if necessary, the appropriate special training may commence immediately. There are no tests for children under three years, apart from clinical assessment, but from that age the Merrill-Palmer test may be used.

2. *Educational assessment.* It is important that a child should have the form of education most suited to his needs, that is, his special abilities. Effective intelligence testing can provide useful information when a decision about a child's educational future is being made.

3. *Vocational/Employment Selection.* Just as it is important to select the right form of education, it is equally important to select the right form of vocation or employment. This is important for the employer and the employee and many employers have an Industrial Psychologist on their staff to help with personal selection. The Indus-

trial Psychologist sets specially designed aptitude tests for the particular job under consideration and prospective employees take these tests. Intelligence tests only form part of an aptitude test.

4. *Assessment of the effects of injury.* Head injuries affect intelligence and in the case where injuries are considerable, road traffic accidents for example, it is important to have an accurate assessment so that retraining and rehabilitation may be planned to the best advantage.

5. *Assessment of disease processes.* Physical diseases such as tumours of the brain affect intelligence and the degree can be assessed by intelligence testing. Diseases such as Huntington's chorea, Picks and Altzheimers disease all produce presenile dementia and thus affect the intelligence. In old age there is some falling off of intelligence, but this is by no means always the case. In old age accompanied by cerebral arteriosclerosis there is a considerable falling off of intelligence with resulting dementia. The future management of such people is aided if the functioning level of intelligence is known.

Intelligence and other psychological tests are done by the psychologist and the nurse's main contribution is to see that the person is at the department at the appointed time. A number of tests have been mentioned, but the list is by no means exhaustive. You should try and see what is in use in your hospital and if you have the opportunity you should practise some of them, such as the performance tests. This piece of advice is based on the old Chinese proverb: 'If I hear I forget, If I see I remember and if I do I understand'. It is worth making friends with the psychology department.

B. PERSONALITY

a. Personality types. Earlier when we considered the factors which contribute to the individual's personality, we saw that there were many. Starting with Aristotle who described the temperaments, many workers have described personality types and among these is Jung who gave us the introvert and extrovert types. The introverted type was shy and withdrawn, whilst the extroverted type was forthcoming of the hail-fellow-well-met approach and enjoyed social contact. Sheldon sought a relation between body build and personality types and gave us what he called somatypes. The somatypes fell into three groups:

1. *Ectomorphs.* Such types had a preponderance of ectodermal

tissue which gives rise to the skin and the nervous tissue. The ecto-morph was mentally active and was a thinker rather than a doer.

2. *Mesomorphs*. This type had a preponderance of mesodermal tissue which gives rise to muscular tissue. The mesomorph was there-fore full-blooded, energetic and tended to take up athletics.

3. *Endomorphs*. The endomorph had a preponderance of endo-dermal tissue which gives rise to the internal organs such as the intestines. Such types were large gutted and fat with a love of com-fort. They also tended to be jolly people and correspond closely to Jung's extroverts.

Shakespeare also observed personality types and body builds and seems to have deduced a relationship, when in Julius Caesar he said: 'Let me have men about me that are fat; Sleek-bodied men and such as sleep o' nights; Yon Cassius has a lean and hungry look, He thinks too much; such men are dangerous'.

Kretschmer worked on personality types in relation to body build and described three types as follows:

1. *Schizothymes*. People of this personality type were found to be tall, thin, tending to think a lot and be rather secretive. Such people were said to have a schizothymic personality and should they develop a mental illness it would be likely to be schizophrenia. This type corresponded with Jung's introverts and Sheldon's ecto-morphs.

2. *Cyclothymes*. Such people were short, fat, easy going and sub-ject to mood swings ranging from happiness to sadness. People with this personality type were said to be cyclothymic and were likely to develop either a manic or a depressive type of illness. The cyclothymic personality sometimes called the pyknic personality corresponds with Jung's extroverted type and with Sheldon's endomorphic type.

3. *Dysplastic*. Kretschmer called those who did not fit into his other two types as dysplastic and this type of personality was often a mixture of the other two types.

Professor H. J. Eysenk of the Institute of Psychiatry, worked out a body build index as follows:

$$\frac{\text{Height} \times 100}{\text{Chest diameter} \times 6} = \text{body build index.}$$

The body build index theory never received a great deal of support and does not seem to be used or referred to very often now.

Cannon, who coined the term homoestasis which means the constancy of the internal environment of the body, made observations of the effect of endocrine function of personality. In the section on observation we made reference to this in relation to thyrotoxicosis.

b. Assessment of personality.

1. *Reports.* School reports are taken into account when a person wants to go on for further education or to take up employment. In the case of nurses, the ward reports provide a form of personality assessment. References nearly always ask for information about the person's character, reliability, trustworthiness and so on and are also an attempt to assess personality. Objective reports and references are useful and provide much valuable information. Unfortunately some are too subjective to be of any use.

2. *Interviewing.* Interviews, like reports and references, are often used to assess personality and again because of their lack of objectivity they tend to be unreliable. From an interview it is possible to tell if the person has any physical defects and his speech and mode of dress can be observed, but assessments may be affected in many ways. Very few men are immune to the presence of a very pretty girl and older women often take an instant dislike to such girls. The interviewee may have a characteristic such as race, religion or colour that is disliked by the interviewer. A private interview is desirable in many cases because a panel of interviewers tend to have a frightening effect on some people. On the other hand a panel can have the effect of increasing objectivity by the dilution of any subjective attitudes which may exist.

3. *Questionnaires.* The use of questionnaires is the most commonly used method of assessing personality. Questionnaires are quick and easy to apply and supply a great deal of information. They can be given to large groups of people and they are easy to mark. Many of the questions are of the 'yes' or 'no' variety. Examples of questions which may be asked are:

'Do you worry too long after an embarrassing experience?'
'Do you feel diffident when you meet strangers?'
'Do you often feel tired for no good reason?'
'Do you adapt easily to new situations?'

It is possible to determine the predominant personality traits of the person from these tests provided, of course, that the test used is considered both valid and reliable. Introverted or extroverted traits can be recognized and so can neurotic tendencies. The traits forming the cyclothymic or the pyknic personality types are readily observed. There are a number of personality tests available and they include:

    a. The Minnesota Multiphasic Personality Inventory (M.M.P.I.). The M.M.P.I. is a card-sorting questionnaire and includes over 500 items. The conclusion is based on the way in which the subject sorts these cards.

    b. The Maudsley Personality Inventory (M.P.I.). The M.P.I. consists of the 'yes' and 'no' type of questions such as the examples given above.

4. *Projective Tests.* The basis of these tests are people's tendencies and willingness to make up stories about what they see. In other words people project their attitudes on to the environment. When shown the same ink blot some people will see images of skeletons, wizened old ladies or monster-like giants, whilst others may see images of pleasant sights such as the dancing girls and so on. What the person sees is influenced by his personality and it is his personality or facets of it which is under consideration. The tests are easy to set, but they are difficult to work as there are no right or wrong answers. There thus must be a subjective element creeping into such an assessment. Some projective tests found in use are:

    a. The Thematic Apperception Test (T.A.T.) In the T.A.T. the person is offered a number of cards containing a variety of pictures including two or three of human figures. The person is asked to tell a story about the picture on a card. The stories are assessed and the examiner looks for personal meanings which may be related to the person's illness. It will be seen again that assessment cannot rule out the subjectivity of the examiner. Despite this it is said that such a test is useful for discovering dominant emotions, unsatisfied drives and emotional conflicts.

    b. The Rorschach Ink Blot Test. In the Rorschach test, the subject is shown a series of ink blots printed on separate cards and he is asked to describe what he sees. He is allowed to turn each card any way he wishes. Notes are made of the length of time taken to make a response, whether he is concerned with parts of the picture or the whole, and whether he concentrates on any particular colour.

A person with a mother-in-law problem may interpret every image as being a grotesque, evil and witch-like old lady. Someone who is depressed sees everything in dull, dark grey colours. People suffering from the condition known as schizophrenia may see very bizarre images which are usually incomprehensible to the average person. Again there are no right or wrong answers; the examiner looks for recurring themes as well as for unique responses.

   c. The Lowenfold World Technique. This is a simple form of a projection test which is used for the assessment of mentally subnormal children. The subject is provided with a sand-tray, paints and toy equipment and is asked to make whatever he likes with these materials. Personality traits can be discovered from the objects made and the choice of colours used.

   Personality is assessed for much the same reasons as intelligence is measured. There are many facets to the personality and this precise assessment difficult. But the information obtained can be of use in the overall assessment of the person. Personality is very important in nursing and some hospitals use formal methods of assessment, mainly the use of questionnaires, to supplement the usual methods of reports and interview. As the efficiency of personality tests increases it may be possible to select those who are most suited to nursing and thus reduce wastage.

5.24 Summary of examination and investigation

In this chapter we have seen something of the scope offered to those caring for the mentally ill. There is a wide range of human observations which can be made. During examination there are opportunities to observe normal function (physiology) and disordered function (pathology). In addition to observations and examinations all the resources of science and technology are available in order that a correct diagnosis may be made. The job is demanding, exacting and calls for great attention to detail, but it is also immensely interesting and exciting.

6

Principles of treatment

6.0 Introduction

We have now set the scene by considering the normal arrangement of the brain and the mind, the mental and physical reactions to stresses and the methods of observations, examination and investigation. Before considering the different illnesses, we shall consider the principles of psychiatric treatment so that the reader will have an understanding of what is involved when treatment is mentioned in relation to a particular illness.

6.1 Factors contributing to mental illness

The factors contributing to mental illness are many. Often there are a variety of factors which contribute to mental illness, though one or two are likely to predominate in any particular case.

6.2 Methods of treatment

The treatment of any illness depends on the cause. If the cause is known a specific treatment, if available, can be given. In the case of many mental illnesses, as we shall see later, the causes are not known and therefore the treatment is aimed at relieving symptoms. There are a number of such treatments which produce a dramatic effect in the person's condition, even though their precise mode of action is not always clear:

A. General.
B. Psychological methods.
C. Chemical methods.
D. Electrical methods.
E. Occupational methods.

F. Surgical methods.
G. The therapeutic community.
H. Other methods.
I. The eclectic approach.

6.3 A. General methods

If environmental stresses, either in the home or at work, are a major contributory factor in the causation of a particular illness, then admission to hospital may allow an escape from these stresses and thus provide rest. Admission to hospital is, of course, a stressful event in itself and everyone concerned must be aware of this and every effort must be made to reduce stress. Loneliness may be a contributory factor and the friendship and companionship of other people may be therapeutic in itself.

Mental illness often results in a neglect of personal habits. Ordinary hygiene may be neglected; this aspect is put right by admission to hospital. Diet is also important. People who live alone often cannot be bothered to cook proper meals, people who are depressed before admission usually have lost all interest in food and people with paranoid ideas may reject food on the grounds that it is poisoned. Economic factors are also involved. Old people living on a small fixed income often have little money to spend on food. The result is malnutrition and specific nutrient deficiencies, particularly of vitamins. A good balanced diet is essential for all, but it can be therapeutic in some instances as well.

As well as correcting the effects of these socio-economic factors, efforts must be made to remedy them as part of the person's rehabilitation. This is in the province of the Psychiatric Social Workers and the Mental Welfare Officers. They can mobilize the social services on the person's behalf. Help may be needed with housing. The person may be entitled to supplementary benefits and so ease the financial strain. There are also a variety of local authority services such as meals on wheels and the home help service which are invaluable when required. The social worker can also put the person in touch with the appropriate local voluntary organization. These measures help to reduce environmental stresses and thus contribute to the prevention of further illness of the same nature.

6.4 B. Psychological methods

There are four interpretations of human behaviour as follows:

a. Hormic (*G. horme*, an urge). This interpretation is based on the theory that behaviour is determined by inborn drives, tendencies and dispositions. This theory was put forward by William McDougall (1871–1938). He made observations and concluded that behaviour was based on instincts (drives) and he put forward a number of these such as food seeking, self preservation, aggressiveness, sex and the gregarious instinct. These instincts are no longer fashionable and are now called drives. This interpretation has no particular application in the treatment of mental illness though of course this aspect is included in other approaches.

b. Psychoanalytic. The psychoanalytic theory was put forward by Sigmund Freud (1856–1939). Freud was first a neurologist of some repute before he concentrated on mental diseases. This came about when he observed that a large number of people sent to him as a neurologist had no definable neurological illness, but could be relieved of their symptoms by hypnosis which involved the recall of painful memories. Freud later abandoned hypnosis and used the technique of 'free association' allowing the person to ramble on with his thoughts when in a state of relaxed consciousness and interpreting the data. He published his first account of his work *Studies in Hysteria* in 1895 and is said to be the founder of psychoanalysis.

We owe to him the idea of the unconscious mind and he gave us terms such as the id, the ego and the super ego. Over and above the ego he put the super ego or what we call conscience. The super ego develops out of the ego and determines what is morally acceptable to the ego. Some experiences are repressed. It will be recalled that repression is a mental mechanism. The repressed experiences disappear from the conscious mind, but live on in the id (the unconscious mind). These repressed experiences together with the inborn drives contribute to behaviour. Sometimes the repressed material is such that it produces symptoms. It is the job of the psychoanalyst to uncover the nature of this material and to help the person to come to terms with it. The psychoanalytic approach is concerned with the individual's difficulties of adjustment to life and uses the idea of repressed wishes and motives.

c. Behaviourist. I. P. Pavlov (1849–1936), the Russian physiologist who experimented with dogs, and the American physiologist J. B. Watson (1878–1958) were among the leading behaviourists. This approach explains behaviour in terms of stimulus and response. We perceive stimuli through our senses and we make the appropriate responses. Some of these responses become automatic and these are what Pavlov described as conditioned reflexes. Pavlov's dogs were shown food and there was an anticipatory increase in the flow of saliva. A bell was rung at the same time. Later is was possible to initiate the salivary response without the presence of food but simply by ringing the bell.

The behaviourist approach does not recognize the unconscious mind, though it does take into account that attitudes and expectations affect behaviour; it aims at bringing psychology more closely in line with the basic sciences of biology, chemistry and physics. The person's self observation of his feelings and experiences are important.

Application of this approach is made in a variety of conditions such as sexual abnormalities, drug abuse and compulsive gambling.

   d. Social. The social interpretation of behaviour is a 20th century creation. This theory has for its basis that man is a social animal. The approach is concerned with the interactions of groups rather than individuals and uses the techniques of mass observation; it studies the nature, similarities, differences and relationships of groups.

   The anthropologists made a leading contribution in this field and this is not surprising since the study of anthropology includes the human being in his bodily form (physical), his racial characteristics (folk), and his social development (social). Contributors to this field were B. Malinowski (1884–1942), a Pole who settled in England and made a number of expeditions to New Guinea, Margaret Mead, a well known American anthropologist and O. A. Oeser who studied unemployment problems in Dundee.

   There is considerable application of this approach. It is the basis of the therapeutic community put forward by Maxwell Jones (1952) and the basis of administrative therapy put forward by D. H. Clark (1958). We shall give these approaches to psychiatry further consideration later.

6.5 Psychoanalysis

Psychoanalysis is based on Freud's psychoanalytic theory and is practised by a psychoanalyst, who may be a psychiatrist with a special training in the subject, or a non-medically trained psychologist also with special training. We mentioned earlier that material unacceptable to the ego is repressed, but this material lives on in the id (the unconscious mind) and it may later influence the person's behaviour to the extent of producing symptoms. The mechanism is an unconscious one and the person has no idea as to what is at the root of his symptoms. It is the function of the psychoanalyst to trace the origins of these conflicts. This exercise does not, of course, make the symptoms vanish overnight, but it does help to give the person a self-understanding and this is sometimes called *insight*. With the acquisition of insight into the problem, the person can usually more readily accept his symptoms and put them in perspective.

   Very often an intense relationship is established between the psychoanalyst and the subject which is either a love or a hate relationship. Powerful emotions which have been pent up in the unconscious mind may be released and may be transferred on to the therapist. This process, which also occurs in other situations, is simply called *transference*.

Psychoanalysis as a form of treatment is very expensive in terms of time and money. It involves a series of long interviews to uncover the hidden material. For these reasons it is not a commonly practised form of treatment. The shorter and equally effective method of psychotherapy, to be mentioned later, is the common form of psychological treatment. Psychoanalysts in training undergo a training analysis so as to prepare them for the problems they are likely to meet in practice.

6.6 Psychotherapy

Like psychoanalysis, psychotherapy is based on the Freudian or psychoanalytic interpretation of human behaviour. It is not as time consuming as psychoanalysis and it is a commonly used form of treatment and it depends on the relationship between the therapist and the person. The methods range from listening, reassuring, and counselling to suggestion, persuasion and support. *Ventilation*, that is, the release of bottled up emotions takes place. These emotions are transferred to the therapist and this is an important element of psychotherapy. Special techniques such as the use of hypnosis and the use of drugs—narcoanalysis—are also used.

Psychotherapy has two aims. On a superficial plane it aims at giving support as well as being re-educative and reconstructive. Here listening, reassuring, and counselling feature largely. Suggestion and persuasion, although used, are not used as frequently as popularly thought, because as we have said earlier ready-made solutions are unlikely to have any long term value. The person must, therefore, be helped to find his own solutions. On a deeper plane the aim is self understanding and maturation of the personality. This is a lengthy process and it may take years to achieve. There are two types of psychotherapy:

A. Individual psychotherapy.
B. Group psychotherapy.

6.7 Individual psychotherapy

Individual psychotherapy involves a face to face relationship between the therapist and the person. It consists of a series of private interviews and the aim may be superficial or deep, according to the person's problems and needs. The indications for this form of treatment are anxiety states of any type, hysteria, obsessional neurosis and alcoholism. The results are variable. Sometimes a person obtains complete relief from a short course of psychotherapy. In others, results are more difficult to achieve.

6.8 Group psychotherapy

Group psychotherapy evolved from the need to treat large numbers of Military personnel with war neurosis during the second World War. It was introduced partly because of the time saving involved and partly because it can be considered as a form of treatment in its own right. Group psychotherapy can take many forms. For example ward meetings, which are a common feature in the everyday life of a psychiatric hospital, groups involved in art therapy, psychodrama, musical appreciation, work parties of various sorts and outings all come within the gambit of group psychotherapy. They are all exercises in human relationships and individual interactions.

Group psychotherapy, the effects of interpersonal interactions, aims at developing the social skills, discipline, self-expression and self-reliance of the individual and thus contribute to the person's recovery in this way. There are also special forms of group psychotherapy known as 'sensitivity' groups. These techniques are used by business men. The participants criticize each other strongly with no holds barred. The object is to improve the social effectiveness of the individual and generally broaden his shoulders. Similar techniques are used for psychotherapists in training. There are also special interest groups such as Neurotics Anonymous, Gamblers Anonymous and Alcoholics Anonymous.

Group psychotherapy sessions are different from any other form of meeting. The group, consisting of six or eight people and certainly not more than ten, form a circle with the object of giving equality to all the members. The meetings are very informal and there is no agenda, no chairman, no minutes and no procedure rules. The therapist may act as a catalyst to 'spark off' discussion or he may remain absolutely quiet. If he adopts the latter approach there may be long silences when it is possible to hear a pin drop. During such silences great tension is built up and the atmosphere is described as 'electric'. The person under the greatest pressure is the one who breaks the silence. This may be done by an emotional outburst with the person leaving the room or by a verbal tirade involving something or somebody. Some of the ensuing discussion can be of the near-the-quick type and is sometimes distressing. On the other hand states of distress are uncovered, emotional tension is relieved and often the person feels much better as a result.

The indications for psychotherapy are all the psychological illnesses with a neurotic basis. It is also used for those with particular problems such as sexual difficulties, alcoholism, delinquency, marital problems and conditions such as asthma. Psychotherapy is not considered appropriate for people with so-called psychotic illnesses and those with personality disorders (psychopaths), though attempts have been made to use it for this latter group. When groups are selected there should be an element of compatibility from the point of view of age, intelligence and social background. This form of treatment is generally unsuitable for the elderly.

6.9 The nurse and psychotherapy

The role of the nurse in relation to psychotherapy varies from hospital to hospital. In some, nurses participate in meetings, whilst in others they do not. Sometimes the nurse is given the status of an observer and at other times a charge nurse may be the only professional contributor as may happen in an alcoholic unit. The Committee that produced the report 'Psychiatric Nursing Today and Tomorrow', were aware of the variations in practice and have recommended that there should be research into the personal and psychotherapeutic role of the nurse.

Nurses, particularly nurses in training, have to assume the role assigned to them by the policy makers of their employing authority. If the role is to be an active one the nurse should be well prepared for this. The nurse should be fairly experienced before participating so that her own anxieties about the 'newness' of hospital life have disappeared. A theoretical knowledge of groups is desirable beforehand and this should include an understanding of the philosophy behind the treatment, its aims, its methods, its indications and its associated problems. It must be recognized that any group is made up of individuals and these may attract or repel each other. Generally opposites attract and likes repel. It must also be considered that there will be a variety of motivations and ambitions. Some will want to dominate and lead, and others may be passive but subtly attempt to manipulate. It will be seen that there are a variety of forces involved which can affect the behaviour of the members of the group. This is what is meant by *Group dynamics.*

For the nurse who is adequately prepared, aware of the dynamics involved and alive to the pitfalls such as manipulation, an active role in group psychotherapy should not present any problems, but it should provide an interesting and fascinating opportunity to observe human behaviour in action.

6.10 Hypnosis

The technique of hypnosis has been available for nearly two hundred years. It was first practised by Anton Mesmer (1734–1815) an Austrian physician, who started using it about 1772. He described a power which he called 'animal magnetism'.

Hypnosis is based on suggestion and depends to a large extent on the confidence the subject has in the therapist and also on the motivation of the subject. For hypnosis the person may lie on a bed or couch, or sit on a chair. Relaxation is important. The subject is asked to gaze fixedly at a 'fixation object' such as a pencil, a coin or a spot on the ceiling whilst the therapist makes suggestions of relaxation and sleep. He is told that he is feeling drowsier and drowsier and gradually his eyes close. The subject is not asleep in the ordinary sense because he can hear what is being said, answer questions and obey instructions.

Hypnosis is helpful in a variety of conditions such as hysteria, amnesia, alcoholism, psychosomatic disorders such as asthma and eczema and stammering. It has been used, but not extensively, instead of anaesthesia for dental extractions. It has also been used during pregnancy and labour to alleviate apprehension and as an anaesthetic in the final stages. It is also of value in relieving pain which occurs in terminal cancer.

Nurses new to psychiatric nursing often wonder why this method of treatment is not more commonly used, for it is possible to undergo a three year training without ever seeing hypnosis used. There are a number of reasons for this. First it takes time, secondly alternative methods are likely to be as effective and thirdly it depends on the therapist's training in the subject, his attitudes towards it and his experiences with it in the past.

6.11 Narcoanalysis

Narcoanalysis is a form of psychotherapy in which drugs are used as a form of short-cut in order to obtain emotional relief—*catharasis.*

It is readily observable that people under the influence of alcohol or recovering from a general anaesthetic tend to talk more readily. Many are also more suggestible. This is the basis of narcoanalysis. Drugs such as Sodium Amytal, Sodium Pentothal, Sodium Brietal or methedrine are used. The drug of choice is given intravenously in sufficient quantities to produce a drowsy dreamy state, sometimes called the twilight state, but not sufficient to promote sleep. Such drugs are popularly known as 'truth drugs'.

When the subject is relaxed the therapist, who has already taken a full history of the subject's illness, goes over various aspects of the person's life. Some sessions may be calm and unproductive but others may be stormy with violent emotional reactions. Such an emotional reaction is called an *abreaction*. Take for example cases of military personnel who, in wartime, have seen their friends and colleagues killed and mutilated in horrific conditions. Such material is too unpleasant to keep in mind for too long and so mental mechanisms come to the rescue and the material is repressed. Such material may give rise to symptoms later and when the emotions are released by abreaction there is likely to be a violent response. The therapist makes a note of the subject's answers and attitudes and these are discussed with him later with the object of giving him self-understanding. The technique is also used in conditions of amnesia in order to help the person to discover who he is.

As in psychotherapy generally, the role of the nurse in this form of treatment varies. Some therapists prefer to be alone with the subject during these sessions so that he will be able to talk more freely. On the other hand some reactions may be violent so that it is necessary to have one or more nurses present. It is usually the custom to let the person 'act-out' the episode, rather than restrain him, as this often brings relief. You must of course follow the hospital policy in this matter, but if you get the opportunity to witness narcoanalysis you should not miss it.

The nurse will be required to prepare the necessary equipment and this includes the drug or drugs chosen by the doctor, a syringe and needle, rubber tubing for a tourniquet, swabs and a cleaning lotion. The response to drugs is often unpredictable, therefore, it is wise to have drugs and oxygen available for emergency resuscitation.

Lysergic acid diethylamide (L.S.D.) was used for narcoanalysis at one time, but since it is suspected of causing brain damage, its use has been discontinued except for research purposes.

6.12 Behaviour Therapy

This method of treatment is based on the behaviourist interpretation of human behaviour and employs established learning theories. Unlike the psychoanalytical approach which seeks reasons for the illness, the behaviourist approach is to relieve symptoms, irrespective of the cause. There are a number of different types of behaviour therapy.

A. DESENSITIZATION (DECONDITIONING). Desensitization is particularly useful where phobias are a problem. The subject is slowly accustomed to the phobic situation while he is relaxed. The therapist draws up a list of the most frightening and the least frightening situations. He is then asked to imagine the least frightening of these and proceeds to the more frightening as treatment progresses. For example, a person who has a phobia about travelling in buses may first be asked to think about the experience. Later he may be shown photographs of buses. He might then be taken to a stationary bus and later be taken for a short ride accompanied by the therapist. Gradually the distances are extended and eventually the person ventures out on his own knowing that he may contact the therapist by telephone should he panic.

There are many indications for this form of treatment, as one American observer listed over 100 phobias. The best results are obtained where the phobias are not complicated by presence of other symptoms.

B. AVERSION (NEGATIVE CONDITIONING). Desensitization helps the person to cope with a situation which previously frightened him. Aversion treatment tries to do the opposite, that is, to prevent the particular form of behaviour by associating that behaviour with unpleasant stimuli. A variety of techniques are used. Alcoholics may be given the drug apomorphine which causes the subject to vomit, in conjunction with quantities of his favourite alcoholic drink. The subject vomits and if vomiting continues to be associated with the intake of alcohol, then it is hoped that the subject will develop an aversion for alcohol. Electricity may also be used. A transvestite, this is a man who likes dressing up in women's clothing, is given a controlled electrical shock which is safe but somewhat unpleasant, when so dressed. Again if the wearing of such clothes becomes associated with unpleasant stimuli, then it is hoped that the practice will be stopped. Similar methods have been used for homosexuals, compulsive gamblers, drug addicts, alcoholism and smoking.

C. OPERANT CONDITIONING. This is a relatively new form of behaviour therapy and works on the reward or punishment basis. Any form of behaviour is reinforced. Correct behaviour is rewarded by giving praise, points, money or some other reinforcement. Incorrect behaviour is punished. This does not mean physical punishment, but it means that praise is withdrawn and is replaced by disapproval, points may be lost or a fine may be imposed if there is money involved.

This method has been useful in the training of subnormal and autistic children. It is also useful in the retraining of people with schizophrenia who have become institutionalized. A few years ago such a person who had spent 30 years in a mental hospital and had a course of operant conditioning made front page news. There were headlines such as 'Man Mute for 30 years Speaks'. Operant conditioning can produce such results but it is expensive in terms of time and thus of money.

The role of the nurse varies in this form of treatment. Very often there are only two people involved in a treatment session, the subject and the therapist. The subject must have complete confidence in the therapist. In the case of sexual deviation many people are extremely sensitive about their problem and may be reticent to discuss the subject. There is a case for limiting the number of people involved. A nurse is not often involved and her role is a supporting one. The clinical details of those in the nurse's care must always be treated as confidential. Because of the nature of the conditions requiring behaviour therapy, the need for confidence is increased.

6.13 Chemical methods

William Osler (1849–1919) said, 'the desire to take medicine is one of the features which distinguish man the animal from his fellow creatures. It is really one of the most serious difficulties with which we have to contend'. If this was true in his time it is certainly true of today. The Sainsbury Committee, which examined the pharmaceutical industry in 1967, found that there are over 3,000 different therapeutic substances available. In addition to legitimate therapeutic use, there is also considerable abuse of certain of these substances as we shall see later.

The use of chemicals in the form of drugs is considerable in the field of psychiatry. We shall now consider some of the drugs which act on the nervous system generally and then those with a specific psychiatric function.

6.14 Pain relievers (analgesics)

Painful impulses are transmitted by the sensory part of the nervous system to the cerebral cortex. Some people squeal when exposed to minor degrees of pain whilst others can withstand, what would be considered by some, as exceptional pain without complaint. This variation in response is explained by the introduction of the pain threshold concept. The first group of people above are said to have a low pain threshold whilst the latter have a high one. The use of analgesics is aimed at raising this pain threshold. Aspirin, which is available in many forms, and paracetamol, a drug of similar effect but with less side effects, are the most commonly used analgesics. These drugs are suitable for relieving pain arising in the skin, muscles and joints.

Severe pain arising in the viscera of the body such as that associated with coronary thrombosis, renal colic, post-operation and malignant disease, require more powerful drugs such as morphia or pethidine to bring relief. These more powerful drugs, often called *narcotics*, have a double action. First, like aspirin and similar substances they raise the pain threshold and secondly they alter the mental reaction so that pain is no longer an unpleasant sensation. These drugs have powerful actions but they also have powerful side-effects. They depress the functions of the vital centres such as respiration so much that it presents a threat to life. Dependence, which as we will see later is a serious problem, also results.

Anaesthesia, which involves the use of a variety of chemical agents in liquid or gaseous forms, is an extension of analgesia. The substance, or the combination of substances used, causes a loss of consciousness and thus a loss of sensibility to pain and permits potentially painful procedures to be carried out without the person being aware of it.

6.15 Anxiety relievers (sedatives)

Anxiety is a common feature of everyday life and a degree of anxiety seems to be necessary as a protective mechanism in order to prevent us from doing foolish things, in particular taking unnecessary risks. On the other hand anxiety has been said to be the poison of human life and certainly prolonged anxiety states detract from the enjoyment of life. A sedative relieves anxiety without producing sleep. A drug commonly used for this prupose is phenobarbitone. This is also used as an anticonvulsant. Amylbarbitone is another drug which may be used as a sedative. In fact small doses of any of the hypnotics in the next section will produce a sedative effect. Whether a drug is a sedative or an hypnotic depends on two things. First the length of time it takes the drug to act, phenobarbitone and amylo-barbitone are both long acting barbiturates. Secondly the size of the dose; larger doses are required to produce sleep.

6.16 Sleep inducers (hypnotics)

Sleeplessness or *insomnia* is fairly common in everyday life and many people have to have chemical help in order to sleep. It is a common feature of a number of mental illnesses and is a particular problem in depression. Macbeth described sleep as 'chief nourisher in life's feast'. If sleep does not occur naturally it is important to give the person every assistance possible, including drugs so that it may be achieved.

There is a wide range of drugs available for the treatment of insomnia which fall into two groups:

1. Non-barbiturates.
2. Barbiturates.

1. NON-BARBITURATES

a. Chloral. This is a form of chlorinated alcohol and was first used in 1869 as an alternative to opium and alcohol. Chloral produces sleep within half an hour and there is no hangover. When taken in solution it has a horrible taste so that a little fruit juice should always be added. Chloral is also available in tablet form as dichloral-phenazone (Welldorm) and produces similar effects.

b. Paraldehyde. Paraldehyde is an aliphatic aldehyde which is an irritant as well as having an offensive smell and was first used for medicinal purposes in about 1882. It may be given orally or by injection. If a large dose has to be given by injection, two separate injections should be given, for if a large volume is injected into a site there is a risk of chemical abscess formation. Whichever route is used to give the drug, a proportion of it is excreted in the breath, so that after taking it a person may smell for up to 24 hours. There is usually little in the way of a hangover, but some people do become dependent on the drug.

c. Glutethimide (Doriden). This drug is chemically related to the barbiturates. It leaves no hangover and its effect lasts for about six hours.

d. Nitrazepam (Mogadon). Nitrazepam is a quick acting non-barbiturate hypnotic. It may be used for insomnia associated with anxiety states.

2. BARBITURATES. This group of drugs was first introduced to the medical world in 1903 and is now the most commonly used group to produce sleep. The drugs used as hypnotics are pentobarbitone sodium (Nembutal), quinalbarbitone sodium (Seconal), butobarbitone sodium (Soneryl), amylobarbitone (Amytal). Barbiturates are also used at the beginning of a general anaesthetic because they cause immediate loss of consciousness by producing immediate sleep. Drugs used for this purpose are thiopentone sodium (Pentothal) and methexitone (Brietal). When a short light anaesthetic is required one of these drugs is used in conjunction with a muscle relaxant such as suxamethonium (Scoline). This is the form of the anaesthetic used for electroconvulsive therapy. A list giving the doses, the length of action and some of the side-effects of these drugs will be found in Appendix 3.

People become dependent (addicted) to barbiturates and there is widespread abuse of this group of drugs. We shall consider this later in the chapter on alcohol and drug abuse.

6.17 Anti-epileptic drugs (anticonvulsants)

Epilepsy in itself is not a mental disorder but the fact that 1 in 200 of the population are epileptics and that some epileptics suffer concurrently from psychological illness as well, means that there will be a number in any mental or mental subnormality hospital.

Phenobarbitone was the first anticonvulsant drug and is still commonly used. Other examples are primidone (Mysoline) phenytoin sodium (Epanutin) and ethosuximide (Zarontin).

When an epileptic fit occurs there is a massive release of nervous impulses which bombard the skeletal muscles of the body. These muscles are so stimulated that they respond with numerous powerful contractions. This is a fit or a convulsion. Anticonvulsants such as phenobarbitone have a sedative effect on the nervous system. They are used to prevent such releases of energy and if this is not possible, they modify the effect and the result is a less forceful fit. This is the basis on which anticonvulsants work.

A list of these drugs, their indications, dosage and side effects will be found in Appendix 2.

6.18 Anti-Parkinson drugs

Parkinson's disease was first described in 1817 by James Parkinson (1755–1824) in a small book entitled 'An Essay on the Shaking Palsy'. We have already mentioned this condition in relation to the function of the basal ganglia in an earlier chapter. The main features of this disease are uncontrolled and unco-ordinated movements which produces a peculiar gait and a 'pill rolling' tremor of the hands.

Like epilepsy this is a disorder of the nervous system rather than the mind, though there may be an associated depression. There are likely to be a number of people in any mental hospital with this condition as a naturally occurring disease. It is likely that there will also be a number with drug induced Parkinsonism. This occurs as a side effect of the tranquillizers in use such as chlorpromazine. Everyone is aware of this side effect and efforts are made to prevent it happening by giving an anti-Parkinson drug prophylactically. Even so and because of individual responses to drugs, the complication sometimes arises.

Some of the common drugs used for the treatment of Parkinsonism are ethopropazine (Lysivane), benzhexol trihexyphenidyl (Artane), orphenadrine (Disipal), procyclidine (Kemadrin) and benztropine (Cogentin). The site of action of these drugs is thought to be the reticular formation which was mentioned in an earlier chapter. Their action is anti-cholinergic, for in Parkinson's disease there is too much acetycholine, in particular in the reticular formation, and this causes the excessive salivation which occurs. Another drug L. Dopa has been introduced recently. Further experience will be needed before this drug can be fully assessed.

6.19 Tranquillity inducers (tranquillizers)

In theory a sedative should relieve anxiety without producing sleep. In practice it does not always work like that. Moreover drugs which in the past were used as sedatives were mostly barbiturates and these produce dependency. Researchers have for some time been looking for a drug which would produce a tranquil mind without producing sleep or causing the person to become dependent. During this search it was observed that the drug promethazine (Phenergan) which was used as an anti-histamine preparation had some of these properties. Further research led to the discovery, in 1951, of the drug chlorpromazine. This was the first tranquillizer and though many others have been discovered since then, it is still in common use twenty years later. Chlorpromazine and similar tranquillizers are particularly useful in the control of hyperactive behaviour which is associated with some mental illnesses. Tranquillizers also produce drowsiness and sleep in some subjects but in many cases it is possible to work out the minimum therapeutic dose which will control symptoms and which will not cause sleep, and thus allow the person to carry on with his everyday activities.

Chlorpromazine (Largactil) is an effective tranquillizer which is tolerated by most people. It has a number of side-effects which may be troublesome. It causes peripheral vasodilation of the blood vessels which results in a lowering of the blood pressure. The increased blood flow to the skin means excessive heat losses resulting in a lowering of the body temperature. It potentiates the effects of other drugs. This can sometimes be used to advantage by giving chlorpromazine with an analgesic such as morphia. The pain relief obtained from the combination is much greater than that which would be obtained from morphia alone. Like all other drugs it is detoxicated by the liver and in a small number of subjects it causes jaundice. It may give rise to drug-induced Parkinsonism. Some subjects when taking chlorpromazine become exceptionally sensitive to sunlight, photosensitivity, and may develop skin rashes.

Chemically, chlorpromazine belongs to the phenothiazine group and there are a number of other tranquillizers which are derived from this group and these are:

a. Promazine (Sparine)
b. Acepromazine (Notensil)
c. Flupromazine (Vespral)
d. Fluphenazine (Moditen)
e. Fluphenazine enanthate (Modecate)
f. Prochlorperazine (Stemetil)
g. Trifluoperazine (Stelazine)
h. Thiopropazate (Dartalan)
i. Thioridazine (Melleril)

This list is by no means exhaustive. You will readily observe this for yourself before long. Only well tried drugs are included because not all of those introduced stand the test of time.

In addition to drugs of the phenothiazine group, there is another group called the butyrophenomes, which are proving effective in the control of hyperactive behaviour. These are:

a. Haloperidol (Serenace)
b. Trifluperidol (Triperidol)

Both of these are effective in the control of acute mania and are sometimes used in the treatment of severe schizophrenic reactions.

There are a number of other drugs which have a place in the treatment of mental illness. They are all powerful drugs but relatively speaking they are less powerful than the phenothiazine group and are sometimes called minor tranquillizers. Drugs so designated include:

a. Chlorodiazepoxide (Librium). This is said to be useful when phobias are a problem
b. Diazepam (Valium)
c. Hydroxyzine (Atarax)
d. Meprobamate (Equanil)

6.20 Mood elevators (antidepressants or thymoleptics)

Specific drugs for the relief of depression did not appear until 1957. Before that people who were depressed were treated with one of the amphetamine group of drugs. Imipramine (Tofranil) is chemically related to the phenothiazine tranquillizers and was discovered in the course of a search for new tranquillizers. It is an effective drug in the treatment of depression. It has a number of side-effects including a dry-mouth, gastro-intestinal upsets and sometimes rashes. There are a number of other drugs which have a similar action to imipramine and these are:

a. Amitriptyline (Tryptizol)
b. Nortriptyline (Aventyl)
c. Desipramine (Petrofran)

In addition to the antidepressants already mentioned there is another group called the monoamine oxidase inhibitors (M.A.O.I.). In an earlier chapter we mentioned that the chemical transmitter at the post-ganglionic nerve endings of the sympathetic part of the autonomic nervous system, is noradrenaline. This noradrenaline is produced in response to the impulse travelling along the nerve and the noradrenaline so produced is destroyed by an enzyme called monoamine oxidase. There are other substances such as serotonin which is broken down by this enzyme. It has been found that if the breakdown of these naturally occurring substances is greatly slowed down by the introduction of another substance, the person's mood is uplifted. This is the principle of the action of the monoamine oxidase inhibitors.

There are a number of side-effects associated with this group of drugs. They include irritability, insomnia, restlessness, sweating, hyperprexia. Great care must be taken if these drugs are to be given in combination with any others. This applies especially to alcohol. They also react unfavourably with any foods containing pressor amines such as tyramine. Foods which contain these amines are cheese, yogurt, broad beans, yeast extracts (Marmite), meat extracts (Bovril) and alcoholic drinks.

Examples of this group of drugs are:

a. Phenelzine (Nardil)
b. Isocarboxazid (Marplan)
c. Mebanazine (Actomol)
d. Tranylcypromine (Parnate)
e. Paraglyine (Eutonyl)

6.21 Vitamins

Vitamins are substances which are normally present in sufficient quantities in a balanced diet, and are essential for normal metabolism. The nervous system has a special need for vitamins of the B group. If B_1 (aneurine) is deficient beri-beri occurs, if nicotinic acid is deficient, pellagra occurs and if B_{12} (cyanocobalamin) is deficient pernicious anaemia occurs. An excessive intake of alcohol upsets the vitamin B supplies in the body. Alcoholics become particularly depleted by B_1 (aneurine, also called thiamine) and this is replaced by injection. There is a drug called chlormethiazole (Heminevrin) which is almost identical chemically to aneurine, but has not vitamin activity. In the last few years this drug has been introduced for the treatment of alcoholism.

Sometimes, though not often, gross deficiency of aneurine leads to a form of beri-beri with demyelination of the nervous system which is accompanied by psychological symptoms. This is called *Wernicke's encephalopathy.*

6.22 Insulin

Insulin is a hormone produced by the β cells of the islets of Langerhans in the pancreas and plays an important part in the metabolism of glucose in the body. Glucose contains energy, but in order that the energy may be used by the body, the glucose must enter the cells of the body. Insulin is necessary for this important step to take place. If insulin is not present or if it is prevented from carrying out its function by 'anti' substances such as glucagon, the concentration of glucose in the blood increases—hyperglycaemia, and the concentration of glucose excreted in the urine is increased—glycosuria. Glucagon, like insulin, is produced by the pancreas.

In a mental hospital you may have in your care people with diabetes and a concurrent psychiatric problem, and insulin may be prescribed as a treatment for the diabetes. It is found that in normal people small doses of insulin (10–20 units) given half an hour before meals has the effect of stimulating the appetite. This is called *modified insulin treatment*. It may be used in the treatment of anorexia nervosa, weight loss associated with alcoholism and in some cases of malnutrition.

In the past large doses of insulin were given to people suffering from schizophrenia. It was thought that the hypoglycaemia which resulted had a beneficial effect; it was sometimes called *insulin shock treatment*. This form of treatment has been abandoned for about a decade because of its questionable efficacy.

In this section we have been principally concerned with the principles of chemical forms of treatment. We shall return to the practical aspects later. In Appendix 1 we shall set out the indications, dosage and side effects of some of the principal drugs used in treating mental disorder.

6.23 D. Electrical methods (electroconvulsive therapy, E.C.T.)

Electricity was not always used for 'shock' treatment, as it is sometimes called, for chemicals were used at first. The originator of 'shock' therapy was Dr. L. J. Meduna of Budapest. In 1934 he put forward the hypothesis that as epilepsy rarely occurred in a person suffering from schizophrenia there might exist an antagonism between the two conditions. On this basis he began to produce convulsions in such people using drugs such as camphor in oil or cardiazol, with the object of relieving symptoms. Drugs proved an unsuitable means of producing convulsions and people began to look for alternatives.

Two Italian psychiatrists, U. Cerletti (1877–1963) and L. Bini (1911–1964), investigated the use of electricity for this purpose and administered the first E.C.T. in April, 1938. Electricity was found to be far more satisfactory for the production of convulsions and has been in constant use, subject to some modifications, since then.

a. Indications for E.C.T. E.C.T. was developed for the treatment of schizophrenia, and though it is still used for this purpose, it is more commonly used for the treatment of depression. It may also be used in the treatment of mania. It is less commonly used in neurotic illnesses except where there is an accompanying depression. Apart from coronary thrombosis, cerebral arteriosclerosis and heart failure there are few contra-indications, though care must be taken with pulmonary tuberculosis. Old age is not an obstacle to treatment, indeed excellent results are obtained in old people. It is a safe form of treatment. In a study involving a quarter of a million cases, there were only nine deaths and six of these had fairly severe physical illnesses. For fit people the risk is amost nil.

b. Method of treatment. The preparation, which includes explanation and reassurance, is similar to that for any operation. A four hour fasting period is essential before treatment in order that the stomach is emptied of food. If this is done there will be no danger of food particles being inhaled into the lungs should vomiting occur. Premedication is given an hour before, usually atropine which has the effect of making the mouth and air passages dry. The person should be told about this so that he is not surprised by it when it happens. Dentures, if any, and valuables are put safely by. Written consent for the procedure must be obtained beforehand. A bed or a couch may be used for the treatment.

A general anaesthetic in the form of Pentothal or Brietal is given intravenously and this is followed by a muscle relaxant such as Scoline or Brevidil. When the muscles are relaxed a gag is put in the mouth to avoid the person biting his tongue. The headbands containing the electrodes at the ends are dipped in an electrolyte solution, such as sodium bicarbonate, to facilitate the passage of electricity, before being placed over the temporal areas of the head. A current of 200 to 400 milliamps is passed through the body for one second from a voltage of 150 volts. If the right dose of the muscle relaxant for that person has been given, then only mild twitchings of the muscles are seen instead of a strong convulsion, but the treatment value is the same.

Analeptics such as adrenaline, coramine and aramine should be ready in case of need. So should oxygen and a suction apparatus. Oxygen is given for a short period following the muscle relaxant because these drugs also relax the respiratory muscles. The convulsion also temporarily interferes with breathing, it is therefore wise to enrich the oxygen content of the blood at this stage.

Recovery is rapid and frequently takes less than 10 minutes. The person is able to get up and have breakfast in about 20 minutes. Many people with depression have poor appetites but in the period following E.C.T. it is usually possible to persuade the person to eat a good meal. Following breakfast the person is usually ready to participate in the day's activities. These activities often have to be modified if the person is very depressed. A course of treatment usually consists of 6–12 treatments.

c. Complications. As far as is known the brain suffers no damage as the result of E.C.T. Most people have some degree of amnesia following treatment. They cannot remember what happened immediately before as well as during and for a short period afterwards. This is usual, but in addition there might be forgetfulness for names and dates, particularly in elderly subjects. This memory disturbance, which is sometimes distressing, clears up in a few weeks when the course of treatment has finished. Dislocations and fractures, especially fractures of the vertebrae, occurred in the early days but are virtually never seen now. Cardiac failure could occur if too strong a current were passed but as most machines are incapable of passing a sufficiently large current, this is unlikely. Respiratory complications can occur through blockage of the airway.

d. How does it work? It is not fully understood how E.C.T. works, but it is thought to act on the thalamus and the hypothalamus. It is postulated that the reaction which occurs in depression, or mania, depends on the pattern reaction or 'set' of the autonomic nervous system and the endocrine system which are both controlled at the level of the thalamus and hypothalamus. The electric current produces autonomic changes which occur during the coma with the effect of adjusting the 'set' to normal. This goes some way to explain the apparent paradox of how it is possible to use the same treatment for contrasting illnesses such as depression and mania.

The effect of the treatment on depression is often dramatic. A tormented, agitated, weeping, suicidal person is transformed into a

calm, vigorous, active and happy person. Insomnia disappears, the
appetite improves and the weight increases.

  e. The machine. There are battery and mains models available.
An A.C. Mains Model is most commonly used. This acts as a step-
down transformer. It steps down the voltage from 240 volts, as
supplied by the mains to 100 to 150 volts. There is usually a red
light on top which shows that the instrument is switched on and a
white light which lights when the treatment is actually being administered. Some models have an ammeter to measure the amount
of current used. Others have a switch to increase the voltage, but
this cannot be increased beyond a certain limit, usually 150 volts.

6.24 E. Occupational methods

'Employment is nature's best physician and is essential to human
happiness', the great Galen is reputed to have said in about A.D. 170.
We have mentioned before the great personal satisfaction which can
be derived from useful employment, apart from the monetary reward.
There is great misery and unhappiness associated with unemployment, apart from the profound economic effects which result. All one
has to do is to read about the unemployment problems of the 1930s,
or better still to speak to people who have lived through it to confirm
this.

  Adequate employment facilities in a mental hospital are important
for a number of reasons.

  a. The majority of people with mental illnesses are physically fit,
except in the acute stage of the illness when there may be loss of
energy and anorexia, as occurs in depression. It is important to provide meaningful employment for those who are capable, so as to
provide an interest and to prevent boredom. If a number of physically
fit people live closely together friction is likely to occur and aggression may follow. If the energy is used in useful work activities this is
less likely to happen.

  b. Many people with mental illness steadily withdraw from the
environment into a world of fantasy, as happens in schizophrenia
for example. Such people become increasingly preoccupied with
morbid ideas, morbid thoughts, delusions and halucinations. The
long-term aim of treatment will be to remove these symptoms, as far
as possible, or to help the person to come to terms with them.
In the meantime an occupation which provides an interest also
provides a diversion for mental energy and thus produces a respite
from the symptoms.

c. If a person is out of work for even a little while and the work habit is lost, it is often difficult to start again. Many mental illnesses tend to last longer than physical illnesses. It is therefore important to have a means of restoring the work habit before the person is discharged and returns to work in the community.

d. Some people with mental illness are difficult to rehabilitate and spend a long time in hospital. In the past, because of lack of facilities and the absence of a stimulating programme, such people lost initiative and volition; they became apathetic and dependent on the hospital and as a consequence, rehabilitation was made even more difficult. Such people were said to be *institutionalized* or suffered from *institutional neurosis.* This can, to a large extent, be prevented by a purposeful, imaginative, varied and dynamic work programme.

OCCUPATIONAL THERAPY. Occupational therapy has a number of aims:

a. Diagnostic. It is possible to observe the person in a variety of situations and over a relatively long period in the occupational setting. These observations can be of value when the doctor is formulating his diagnosis.

b. Assessment. By setting projects of various types such things as concentration, persistence and initiative can be assessed. Such information is valuable, if not vital, in placing in a job or when discharge home is being considered. It is also important when further training in a Government Training Centre, Industrial Rehabilitation Unit or Sheltered Workshop is to be recommended.

c. Re-education. Re-education, or the revival of lost skills can be undertaken as part of occupational therapy. For example a typist whose speed, accuracy and touch has been affected by disuse can be given an opportunity to regain her previous standards of efficiency. This can be done in the department initially and later the person may be given a job in one of the offices as a preparation for resuming gainful employment outside hospital.

A housewife may have lost some of the skills involved in household management and many occupational therapy centres are equipped with modern flats where the elements of home-making can be practised.

For a workman it is possible to arrange a realistic workday. This usually takes place in the Industrial Therapy Department. A member of the staff known as the 'Industrial Liaison Officer' or with some similar title, arranges contracts with industrial concerns to do work for them; this is frequently assembly work. In some hospitals those attending the Industrial Unit, clock-in as they would in ordinary employment, and are paid a wage which by law has to be under £2 a week. If the figure earned were more than this sum, National Insurance Contributions would have to be paid and thus add to the administration involved. It is not possible or necessary to provide occupations appropriate to each person, though this should be attempted if at all possible. The establishment of a consistent work-habit is the prime object of this form of rehabilitation.

In any form of treatment it is important to review methods, assess progress and in the light of this to plan for the future. In the occupational/industrial setting this is done by joint staff policy meetings. These are held weekly, or more frequently, and are attended by doctors, nurses, occupational therapists and others concerned with the rehabilitation programme. Sometimes the Disablement Resettlement Officer (D.R.O.) attends as well and provides a vital link with prospective employers. The D.R.O. is an Officer of the Department of Employment at the local Employment Exchange. He is aware of vacancies available locally and nationally and is thus in a unique position to contribute towards rehabilitation. The D.R.O. is trained in vocational guidance and he may recommend and arrange for a person to attend an Industrial Rehabilitation Unit (I.R.U.). Alternatively, if the person needs retraining, he may recommend a period at a Government Training Centre (G.T.C.).

6.25 The relationship between nurses and occupational therapists

Team-work is essential in any sphere of activity and it is absolutely essential in hospital life. Because occupation is such an important part of the person's treatment and rehabilitation, it is important that nurses and occupational therapists should work closely together. Each have separate contibutions to make, but they are such that they can complement each other. The nurse is in closer contact with the sick person than any other member of the therapeutic team and thus knows him better. The occupational therapist has made a special study of the best ways of providing work activities which will make the greatest contribution to the person's rehabilitation. A blending of both these contributions in a co-operative spirit, considerably enhances the quality of the service provided.

6.26 F. Surgical methods

Surgical operations of the brain and nervous system are common.

For example congenital lesions such as *spina bifida* or *hydrocephalus* may be corrected surgically. Infections resulting in abscess formation may need surgical intervention. Surgery is often needed to correct the results of injury. Severed peripheral nerves can be successfully rejoined. The brain may be the site of *benign* or *malignant neoplasms*. Primary malignant neoplasms of the brain are not common. Those which occur are of a secondary nature and come from other sites in the body, the lungs for example. Cerebral vascular accidents are common in the later years of life. The most common of these, 'stroke' is not amenable to surgery, but cerebral *aneurysms* usually are. In the subdural type of haemorrhage where blood is trapped and cannot escape, drainage helps. In Parkinson's disease, which is a degenerative condition of the nervous system, there are surgical procedures which bring much relief. There are several surgical approaches to the treatment of this disease, but each involves the selective destruction of areas of the basal ganglia; relief of symptoms follow dramatically.

So far the surgical approaches mentioned are concerned with the organic aspect of the nervous system, though of course they may have mental consequences. Mental disorders without any detectable organic basis are sometimes called *functional*. This covers the majority of mental illness and there is a surgical approach for such conditions.

In 1935, A. C. de Egas Moniz of Lisbon injected alcohol into the frontal lobes of the brain to release emotional tension. This was the forerunner of the *prefrontal leucotomy* operation. In 1949 Egas Moniz shared the Nobel Prize 'for his discovery of the value of prefrontal leucotomy in certain psychoses'. The operation of leucotomy was used for psychotic disorders, but this is no longer the case. The principal indication now is severe *obsessional compulsive neurosis* which does not respond to any of the other treatments available.

How does it work? It will be recalled from an earlier chapter that one of the many functions of the frontal lobe of the brain, is initiation of motor function. In the case of obsessional neurosis an excessive amount of motor impulses are initiated, so that the person is compelled to repeat certain acts so frequently that he has little time left to do anything else. These repetitive acts may range from handwashing to constantly checking that the gas is turned off, or to avoiding the cracks when walking on the pavements. At operation, a number of the nerve fibres coming from the frontal lobe are cut so that the number of offending impulses transmitted is greatly reduced and the symptoms are relieved as a consequence. To cut the right number of fibres is a matter of fine judgement. If too few are cut the operation will be ineffective and if too many are cut the person's psychomotor activity may be reduced to an unacceptably low level, resulting in retardation and withdrawal.

The operation of prefrontal leucotomy is performed very infrequently and when it is the person is usually transferred to the local neurosurgical centre. For these reasons an account of the preparation or the nursing care involved is not given.

6.27 G. The therapeutic community

The concept of the therapeutic community is based on the social interpretation of human behaviour which we mentioned earlier in this chapter. It involves the self-evident fact that experiences from the environment affect behaviour and that these experiences involve other people. The sharing of experience is thus the crux of the matter. It follows that every aspect of the hospital structure and function, and the behaviour and attitudes of the staff and others have a potentially therapeutic effect.

Until the advent of the therapeutic community, mental hospitals were run on a hierarchical basis. There was a physician superintendent in overall charge of the hospital and there was a distinct line of command. Policies were formulated at the highest level, with or without discussion, and instructions were passed downwards. These were expected to be obeyed even though they were not always fully explained 'They' decided, 'they' directed, 'they' said, was the fashion and the recipients were certainly given no say.

In the therapeutic community this state of affairs is altered. All members of the community, staff and patients alike, contribute towards the formulation of policy. In some communities all the members have equal voting rights and it may happen that the patients might out vote the staff on a policy issue. In other communities the formulation of policy may be limited to relatively minor things or alternatively senior staff may retain the power to vote decisions which are too much out of line with hospital policy. The main feature of the therapeutic community is that it is *administration by participation*, and it does not mean anarchy. In fact when the 'they' complex has been removed and everyone is involved in the decisions, the overall standard of behaviour improves. People who have previously directed their energies towards 'they' in an aggressive and destructive way, now use these energies in a constructive manner for the benefit of the community. In some hospitals the patients are so involved in the running of their affairs that the term 'patient government' has been used.

The success of a therapeutic community depends mainly on the freeness of its channels of communication. This communication must be two-way, upwards as well as downwards. There must be involvement when decisions are made, but this alone is not enough. It is important to know the effects of these decisions at the grass-roots; there must be 'feedback'.

The affairs of a therapeutic community are conducted in a series of meetings. We have already mentioned group dynamics in the section on group psychotherapy. Group dynamics will of course operate in meetings held in a therapeutic community, but the conduct of the meeting is somewhat different. These are business meetings and what the participants say is not examined in the way it would be if they were conducted on the psychoanalytic interpretation of human behaviour. Problems are discussed, grievances are aired and decisions are reached. There is a chairman, who may be a patient or a member of staff, a secretary and quite often, though not invariably, minutes are kept. The rules of the group are formulated and the standards of behaviour are prescribed; the time that people should be in by and the time of lights out are examples. Chores are allotted usually on a rota basis. Some people fear that if this state of affairs were allowed nothing would get done and that the standards of behaviour degenerate. This is not true. Every group sets its own standards and rules and these are higher than those of any individual. The therapeutic community by a combination of participation, good communications and feedback, and by the social pressures involved through the operation of group dynamics has the effect of raising individual standards of behaviour.

The improvement of individual behaviour is not the only advantage to flow from the therapeutic community method of conducting a hospital. Many people with mental illness, particularly those with neurotic illnesses, have difficulty in reaching decisions. Admission to hospital where all the person's needs are met and where decisions are made by the 'authorities' provide an excellent means of escaping from the harsh realities of life, but make no contribution to the person's rehabilitation. Being involved in a therapeutic community the person has to become involved in decision making and some find this difficult at first and may try to opt out. For this reason most therapeutic communities have one absolute rule and that is attendance at meetings is compulsory. Ultimately the majority can see the value of such involvement.

The other major advantage of the therapeutic community approach is that it keeps the person mentally alert and actively involved in his environment and thus contributes towards the prevention of institutional neurosis.

The role of the nurse in a therapeutic community is clear. Nurses like others are an integral part of the community and as such they must participate fully. Adequate preparation is necessary and a knowledge of group dynamics is essential in order to appreciate what is happening and to be prepared for the inevitable pitfalls associated with this approach. Some nurses find the therapeutic community concept difficult to accept at first but ultimately the majority readily see its advantages.

6.27 H. Other methods

We have said before that mental illness, or indeed any form of illness, cannot be considered in isolation. If a person is mentally deranged because of a fever, a thyroid crisis or has an infection associated with puerperium, then of course the underlying condition must be treated concurrently. Likewise a person presenting with General Paralysis of the Insane will need a course of an appropriate antibiotic such as penicillin.

The social side of life must also be considered. We have mentioned Psychiatric Social Workers, Mental Welfare Officers and voluntary workers, but the religious aspects must not be forgotten. In sickness, religion often takes on a new dimension and many people derive enormous help from the appropriate religious minister. The effect of a religious minister can be twofold. By his training and experience he is usually an expert at listening and counselling; in fact superficial psychotherapy. Secondly he can reinforce a religious faith and the effects of this are such that they cannot be overlooked in any illness.

Things such as patients' clubs, dances and similar activities generally have a beneficial effect. Holidays are important for those who have to spend a considerable time in hospital. These can be conventional seaside holidays and are usually arranged in the off-peak season for economic reasons. Alternatively, exchange holidays with other hospitals either in this country or abroad can be arranged. It might be thought that an exchange holiday is somewhat of a busman's holiday, but the change of environment, personalities and routines involved provide stimulation and interest and are usually enjoyed.

6.29 I. The eclectic approach

For descriptive purposes we have described each method of treatment separately, but you may have seen or you will see that several of the methods may be used for one person. The general methods apply to everyone. A person who is depressed may be prescribed E.C.T. in conjunction with the appropriate antidepressant drug. At the same time he is likely to be having psychotherapy and be engaged in occupational activities. He is thus having something from each of the methods available which are appropriate to his needs. This is what is known as the eclectic approach and it is the one most commonly used.

6.30 Summary

Although the volume of information available about mental diseases is considerable, there are still some fundamental facts, such as the cause of many of these illnesses, which are unknown. There are however a large number of methods at our dispcsal for the relief of symptoms. These range from general methods such as diet and rest to psychological methods which may include psychoanalysis, individual or group psychotherapy and behaviour therapy. There are a wide range of chemical substances in the form of drugs, which may be used and electricity is used for E.C.T. Occupational methods are important and surgical methods are sometimes, though rarely, indicated. The therapeutic community approach is being increasingly adopted and the social and religious aspects are important in many instances. Many hospitals use what is appropriate from each method and this is the eclectic approach.

7

Principles of nursing

7.0 Introduction

In the previous chapter we considered the methods of treatment which are available to the mentally ill and the nurse's role in those treatments. We shall now consider the nurse's own contribution, first in relation to other members of the therapeutic team and then in its own right.

7.1 The therapeutic team

A nurse is required to have many qualities and the ability to get on well with other people ranks high among these because many people contribute to a person's treatment and rehabilitation. The therapeutic team is big and all of its members will require access to the patient at some time. The majority work from 9 a.m.–5 p.m. so that some planning is required in order to coordinate these services. A new admission will see both the junior doctor, the registrar and the consultant. Pathology and psychology tests are likely to be ordered and so is an X-ray. The occupational therapist needs to plan a work programme and the social worker may have a social problem to work out. Dental treatment, physiotherapy or chiropody may also be indicated. A nurse will have to see that all these people have access to the person. At the same time she will have to ensure that, in the early days in particular, the day is not wholly taken up with appointments. Thus a nurse acts as a buffer between the helpers and the helped.

The skill of a therapeutic team depends mainly on the personalities of the nursing staff. If a nurse is friendly, helpful and approaches her work in a spirit of co-operation, she is most likely to be successful. Good personal relationships, which mean a great deal of give-and-take, are essential as a lubricant for the efficient working of the therapeutic team and are vital for the efficient management of a sick person's day.

7.2 Admission to hospital

For any person admission to hospital is a big step and it provokes a variety of reactions. Fear and anxiety often rank foremost among these. A nurse must be aware of this and do what she can to make the procedure as stressless as possible. First impressions are said to be important and people expect a nurse to be cool, calm and collected. She is expected to execute her duties in a quiet, unobtrusive and efficient manner. But quietness, unobtrusiveness and efficiency are not enough, there must also be warmth or emotional tone. The 'social climate' should give a sick person a feeling of security. This is conveyed as much by actions, and gestures as by words of greeting. A nurse must inspire confidence and if she can do this she will be making an important contribution to the person's peace of mind.

7.3 Types of admission

Since the introduction of the Mental Health Act 1959, the majority of people enter hospital informally. Like any person who is feeling unwell they see the family doctor. He arranges for an appointment to be made, often at the out-patients department of the local general hospital, with a psychiatrist. The person may be admitted immediately if his condition warrants it or he may be put on the waiting list until a vacancy becomes available. Alternatively if he cannot or will not attend for an out-patient appointment, arrangements may be made for a *domicilliary visit*. The psychiatrist decides whether admission to hospital is indicated or not. If it is, an offer of informal admission is always made first. Should this be refused, and of course it sometimes is, then a compulsory admission is recommended. A summary of the types of compulsory admissions is set out as follows:

MENTAL HEALTH ACT 1959 COMPULSORY ADMISSIONS

Types of Admission	Category	Sec.	Persons Authorized	Doctors	Forms	Duration
Police	All Classes	136	Constables	Nil	Nil	72 hours
Emergency	All Classes	29	Any relative or Mental Welfare Officer	1	Application and recommendation form	72 hours
Already in hospital	All Classes	30	Consultant in charge	1	1 Section 30 form	3 days (including day of order)

Types of Admission	Category	Sec.	Persons Authorised	Doctors	Forms	Duration
Observation	All Classes	25	Nearest relative or M.W.O. or person authorized under Sec. 52 or 53	2	ditto	28 days
Treatment	Psychopaths or sub-normal only if under 21. Mentally ill or severely sub-normal of any age	26	ditto	2	ditto	1 year
Hospital order	Patients convicted of criminal offences	60	Assize Court Quarter Session	2	Hospital order forms	As specified in order

The legal aspects will be considered in greater detail later, but it will be seen that people can be admitted following an emergency application (Section 29) and application for admission for observation (Section 25), and an Application for treatment (Section 26). Section 30 applies to a person who is already in hospital and though not well enough insists on being discharged. Application may be made to have the person detained under the terms of one of the other sections. Sometimes people with mental illness become involved with the law and if there are psychiatric grounds for doing it, the person may be ordered to be detained in a psychiatric hospital for treatment. Such a person would be admitted under the terms of Section 60 (court order). Should the court consider that there is a risk of the person repeating his crimes, if not restricted to hospital, then the terms of Section 65 may be applied. This means he cannot be granted leave of absence, be transferred or discharged, without reference to the Secretary of State. In the case of a person who is already serving a prison sentence, and who is then found to be suffering from mental illness of a degree which warrants detention in hospital for medical treatment, the Secretary of State can order his transfer to hospital under the terms of Section 72.

There are other ways of being admitted to a psychiatric hospital. A policeman may bring a person for admission whose behaviour is such that it gives ground to suspect mental disorder. Such a person would be admitted under the terms of Section 136. A person may avoid or by-pass all the other routes and simply walk into the hospital and ask to be admitted. A hospital is by no means bound to accept such people, in fact the hospital has the right to refuse any admission, but in practice each case is considered on its merits and some people are admitted in this way.

7.4 Reactions to Admission

There are many possible reactions to admission to hospital. There is fear, there may be justifiable fears of the known and unjustifiable fears of the unknown. On the other hand the nature of the illness may produce apathy. There is often a feeling of insecurity because of concern about what is going to happen in hospital and about the outcome of the illness. There may be a feeling of hopelessness at having let down the family and friends, this may occur in the bread-winner or the housewife. There may be resentment over the loss of independence associated with admission. Some people react to stressful situations by being aggressive, demanding and expecting instant results. Others react to the situation with equanimity and make the most of their plight. The reader is referred to Chapter 3 where the reactions to illness are considered in more detail.

7.5 The reception

Because admission to hospital is such an important step, everything should be done to make it as smooth as possible. Sometimes there is advance information available about future admissions and this should be studied. This will not of course be the case in emergency admissions.

Somebody should be allotted the job of receiving the admission. The person should be welcomed, like any guest would be, in a friendly and warm way so as to make him feel at home. It is a good idea to have a short chat before getting down to the formalities of admission. Such a chat is by no means a waste of time, it creates a good impression for the person being admitted and it gives the nurse an opportunity to begin observing the various facets of the person's behaviour. Needless to say, like all observation, this must be done unobtrusively. The new admission should be introduced to the ward staff and others present. He should be taken on a tour of the ward and

shown where things are kept and he should be introduced to his
fellow patients. The ward routine, meal times, times of rising and
lights out and visiting times should be explained. Many hospitals
have a booklet giving such information but even so there are still
likely to be many questions. Some of these questions will stem from
more deep-rooted anxieties and others will stem from the person's
need to talk. In reply to questions it would be easier and quicker
to tell the person to study the booklet and that he would find the
answers there. This is an undesirable approach because it implies
that the staff really have not time for such mundane matters. On the
contrary the situation provides such an excellent opportunity for
establishing rapport that it should not be missed.

7.6 Dealing with personal hygiene

Many mental illnesses result in a withdrawal from the environment
and in a deterioration in the standards of personal care. This means
that a number of admissions will be in need of a bath and it is also
likely that some will be harbouring fleas or lice. Careful examination
and a bath is therefore indicated. You should follow the rules of
your hospital with regard to bathing and these are usually to be
found in the form of a notice in the bathroom or possibly in the
procedure book. The general principles are that privacy should be
ensured, apart from the supervision of the nurse. This supervision
should be as unobtrusive as possible, but such supervision is necessary, for though the person may not wholly like it, it may save a life
by preventing accidents and suicide. If an ordinary bath or shower
is used, the cold water should be turned on first. The temperature
of the water should be in the range of 37 to 40 ° C (98 to 104 ° F) and
no further hot water should be added once the person has begun to
have a bath.

A nurse should carry out a systematic examination of the person.
The hair should be carefully examined for lice and the condition of
the skin should be noted. The nurse should look for cuts, bruises,
swellings, infections, rashes and discharges. Any findings should be
reported immediately to the ward sister or charge nurse. If an infesta-
tion (the presence of lice or fleas) is discovered, the person's clothes
may need to be treated or destroyed, but a nurse should not do this
on her own account; permission should be obtained from the
appropriate person in the hospital.

7.7 Assisting at medical examination

A full medical examination is carried out soon after admission to hospital and the nurse has a number of functions in relation to this procedure. It is her job to see that all the equipment is available and in working order. The batteries and bulbs of torches and instruments such as the ophthalmoscope and the auriscope should be tested beforehand. She works with the doctor during the examination, she sees that the person is in the right position, instils eye drops beforehand, if ordered, and assists a person who is unsteady on his feet to walk so that his gait may be observed. The nurse will be able to report to the doctor her own observations and so contribute information which may be helpful in the formulation of a diagnosis. It is usual for a nurse to chaperon a man doctor when he is examining a woman. The nurse can also learn much from the procedure and no opportunity should be lost to increase knowledge or to consolidate existing knowledge.

The majority of the equipment required is already mentioned in the section on neurological examination. In addition a sphygmomanometer is needed to measure the blood pressure, a proctoscope may be needed to examine the rectum and a vaginal speculum is needed when a vaginal examination is indicated. Gloves or finger stalls and a lubricant are required for a manual rectal examination.

7.8 Dealing with relatives

We have mentioned that patients react in a variety of ways to illness; so too do relatives. When we considered the factors contributing to a mental illness we saw that they included environmental stresses. These stresses may well be the person's near relatives. It has been said that it is not always the most sick member of the family who is admitted for treatment. However, this is the person's environment and the environment to which he must be rehabilitated. Some doctors are so conscious of this that they aim to treat the whole family rather than individual members of it.

With hindsight, some relatives see how they contributed to the illness and feel guilty and want to make amends. This sudden gush of guilt-motivated sympathy may be as upsetting to the person as their previous errant behaviour. Some relatives feel that they have let the person down and failed, but through the mental mechanisms this sense of failure is projected onto something or somebody else, usually the hospital. Other relatives are glad to have the patient out of the way, but they may make perfunctory visits. It should be mentioned that not all relatives present problems, many are perfectly reasonable and understanding and appreciative of the medical and nursing treatment. The nurse should, however, be aware that problems can and do arise.

The nurse should deal with relatives in a friendly, courteous and kind manner. She should try to answer questions which are within the scope of her knowledge and she should be careful not to get out of her depth. Questions which she cannot or should not answer should not be left; the relative should be passed on to the appropriate person, possibly the doctor, so that an answer may be obtained. This applies particularly to questions about prognosis.

7.9 Dealing with visitors

There are a great number of possible visitors. Apart from the person's friends and work colleagues who may make social visits, there are such people as lawyers who may be called in so that the person may make a will or to deal with some other legal matters. Business partners or associates may call to discuss business problems. The Personnel Officer from the person's place of work may call, so might his local religious minister. On the official side, the police might wish to interview him and occasionally patients are visited by the Lord Chancellor's Visitors.

The decision as to whether the person should receive visitors or not, rests with the doctor who is likely to seek the nurse's advice. Visitors, like relatives, should be received in a pleasant and friendly manner. As much privacy as possible should be given, but at the same time the nurse should keep a weather-eye on what is going on. Business discussions may be harassing and care must be taken that the person is not being pressurized, into making a will for example.

7.19 Dealing with complaints

Complaints seem to be inevitable. In an organization involving so many people some misunderstandings are bound to arise. Secondly there is the nature of some mental illness where the tendency to complain is an integral part of the process. Thirdly, there is the effect of a legal order. Only a small percentage of patients in a mental hospital, say 20 per cent or less, are detained by a legal order. But those who are often have a grievance and tend to complain. Legal orders, while still absolutely necessary in some cases, are a stumbling block in the nurse-patient relationship; she represents authority and 'they'. Because she is in the front line and therefore closest to the person she receives the brunt of his complaints,

Dealing with complaints is a very important duty. The nurse should try to understand the underlying mechanisms which are operating; if she does this she is less likely to become annoyed. Minor complaints such as the absence of toilet paper or that the tea is cold can obviously be dealt with locally and so can many similar complaints. Other complaints should be passed on either to the nursing officer responsible for the ward, the doctor or the general administration as appropriate. There must be, above all, free channels of communication so that no complaint is lost and therefore ignored.

7.11 Dealing with property

Considerable care is required when dealing with property because if mistakes are seen to occur in such mundane matters, then people cannot be blamed for suspecting incompetence in other areas. Many items of property have a sentimental value and much distress is caused if these are mislaid. Sometimes patient's memories are faulty and they may claim to have brought items to hospital which they have not. Others may make such claims in the hope of obtaining compensation and others still may do so just to make trouble. Therefore, for a variety of reasons a careful check should be made of the property and all the items should be recorded.

The type of property book varies considerably. The flimsy perforated type which allows a number of carbon copies to be made is often used. The property should be checked and signed by two people, then one copy may be given to the patient to keep. The policy concerning the amount and type of property to be retained also varies and depends in part on the person's condition. Valuables such as items of jewellery, bank books, cheque books and similar documents as well as money, are usually deposited for safe-keeping in the appropriate administration office and a receipt is obtained which should be kept safely. Some people will object to giving up such personal items. If this is the case the hospital rules about property, which usually state that the hospital accepts no responsibility for property other than that handed in for safe-keeping, should be brought to the person's notice.

The question of whether the person should wear his own clothes is a matter of hospital policy but the general tendency is that it is allowed. This has a beneficial psychological effect on the person and the practice should be encouraged. Losses of private clothing do occur and cause inconvenience and bad feeling, therefore, all items should be clearly marked. It is particularly important for clothes to be marked before being sent to the hospital laundry.

7.12 Observation

Observation is the prime function of the nurse. It should be unobtrusive, discreet, efficient, comprehensive and detailed. Accurate observations are invaluable to the doctor in the formulation of his diagnosis and are equally as invaluable to the nurse, because changes can be detected early enough for corrective action to be initiated and so provide much job satisfaction.

The method of observation has been outlined in a previous chapter and should be followed unless you have been taught an alternative method in your training school.

7.13 Reports

It is important that all observations made should be reported. The reports take two forms:

a. Oral
b. Written

You may be required to give an oral report to a number of people. You should always give a hand-over report to the nurse who takes over from you. Anything unusual about the person should be reported immediately to the ward sister or charge nurse. The doctor or the Nursing Officer may ask for a report of the nurse's observation.

A written report is made to cover each 24-hour period. In the case of new admissions considerable detail is required and less in the case of people who have been in hospital for some time. Reports should be as brief as possible and this is a facility which a nurse must develop. In order to do this the most important points must be selected. In the case of someone who is depressed it is important to know if suicidal ideas were expressed or what the appetite is like; in the case of someone with schizophrenia it is important to know how much the delusions or hallucinations, if present, are upsetting the person. In an older person who is being habit-trained as part of his rehabilitation, it is important to know if he has been incontinent, and if so, how many times. This is positive reporting, that is, reporting action on the happening side of the person's activity. Negative reporting, is reporting something which might have happened but did not. For example reporting that an epileptic did not have a fit or somebody suffering from an obsessive compulsive neurosis did not perform compulsive acts, or at least, not as frequently as previously.

Reports are documents which may be referred to at a later stage, particularly if a query or a problem arises. It is important therefore that they should be legibly written and carefully stored. Different hospitals have their own rules about how long records should be kept, but in any case it is unlikely to be less than two years.

7.14 Accidents

Efficient management of the ward and the hospital environment can do much to prevent accidents. Old people are more prone to accidents than younger people, they are more likely to slip and fall over; highly polished floors should always be avoided. They are more likely to fall out of bed or to set fire to themselves whilst smoking. Efficient management and sharp observation can obviously do much to prevent such things happening, but despite this some accidents may still happen.

When an accident happens it must be reported immediately to the doctor and the nursing administration. Accidents are later reported to the general administration, and to the management committee of the hospital. Many hospitals have special forms for the purpose of reporting accidents and you should become familiar with the local practice. In any case, the facts should be written to avoid mistakes in recall of memory at a later time.

It should be remembered that accident reports may be the subject of litigation and a nurse may be called as a witness. This may appear to be a frightening prospect, but it need not be if a nurse has developed the facility to report accurately; she will be asked for the facts and generally will not be asked for an opinion. The nurse should also bear in mind that for a claim for damages against the hospital to be successful, it has to be proved that there was some negligence on the part of the hospital. A combination of efficient management and a high level of professional knowledge and competence, blended together to produce a high standard of nursing practice, provides a good indemnity should litigation arise. This should be backed up by membership of an appropriate professional organization, to give the nurse security in the practice of her art. A high standard of nursing will also give the sick person confidence in the nurses and thus provide security which is, of course, a basic psychological need.

7.15 Abscondence and absence without leave

In the not too distant past mental hospitals had little to offer in the way of treatment and therefore their principal function was to provide custodial care. In such an atmosphere abscondence and absence without leave was important, but today the majority of people enter hospital informally so this aspect is less important. There are still a number of instances when it is important, for example, in the case of an old person who may have been admitted informally and is confused. If such a person wanders, he or she may get lost and suffer from exposure if not found in time. In the case of persons detained under the terms of any of the sections of the 1959 Mental Health Act, the hospital has an obligation to detain such patients until they are discharged.

When it is discovered that someone is missing a search should be made. If a thorough local search produces no results then the matter should be reported. In the case of cumpulsorily detained people, the police are informed. This is normally done by a nursing officer and it is important to find out the local procedure. When reporting the matter to the police, an accurate description is required and this is where the nurse's observation comes in very useful. The person's general appearance, height, weight, colour of hair and eyes are required and so are details of the clothes worn. Any distinguishing feature or peculiar characteristic is also helpful.

When the person is found, he or she may be returned to the hospital by the police or the nurse may be sent by hospital transport or taxi to escort the person back. For escort purposes it is better to use some form of private transport because the person may make a scene on a bus or train which may be difficult to control. Moreover the sympathy of the public is likely to be with the patient rather than the nurses. It scarcely needs to be said that many people will object to returning to hospital and may resist. It is important to have enough nurses to cope with such resistance should it arise.

7.16 Management of emergencies—psychiatric first aid

Whatever problems arise the nurse is most likely to be the first to encounter them. She is in the front line as it were. Many problems are in the realm of the doctor's field of duty, but often the doctor may be busy somewhere and it may take time for him to get to the patient. In the meantime help must be given and the nurse will need to be competent to deal with a variety of problems ranging from aggression and agitation, to delirium and suicide. The initial methods of dealing with these problems are in the field of psychiatric first aid. Like first aid generally, there are a number of principles to help the psychiatric first-aider and these are:

A. A nurse must always remain cool, calm and collected and in control of herself as well as the emergency.

B. No matter how busy she is, time must be made available to cope with an emergency and the person should be made to feel that the nurse has all the time in the world for him and that only his problem matters.

C. Attentive listening is vital and is something which a nurse should develop.

D. When the problem has been heard out, and not until then, attempts at reassurance should be made.

E. When the person has settled, some form of activity such as occupational or recreational may be necessary to provide a means of diversion from the problem. The different aspects of psychiatric first aid will now be considered.

7.17 Listening

A sympathetic ear is an invaluable tool in psychiatric nursing and the nurse should develop the art of listening. The person should be allowed to talk freely and without interruption. The nurse may have to give a cue here and there to make occasional encouraging gestures, but if the conversation is flowing free these should be kept to a minimum. If the train of talk tends to wander there is no need to try to direct it in any particular direction, a passive but interested role will serve the nurse best. A spontaneous unloading of problems allowing the person 'to get it off his chest', brings great relief.

7.18 Understanding

Some people with psychiatric illness feel that nobody understands them. The person in the depths of depression may say 'but you don't know what it's like nurse'. Similarly somebody with a troublesome phobia may think that no one appreciates the degree of terror which he experiences, or in the case of a person with obsessive compulsions, the private hell he goes through by being compelled to carry out what he knows to be absurd and pointless rituals. A nurse must show that she understands the person's problem not by a show of effusive mawkish sentimentality, which does more harm than good, but by a show of genuine sympathy, professional competence and a display of a sincere wish to help. Understanding involves getting on the same wavelength, not irritating and saying the wrong thing at the wrong time. But it means more; the ability to gauge when a little give-and-take and a little humour may be introduced. A sense of humour, kept in perspective, is a priceless attribute in a nurse and can make a valuable contribution towards promoting understanding.

7.19 Reassuring

When the person has been heard out and when an understanding has been established, then the nurse may try reassurance. Some people may be so overwhelmed by their problem that they may not be able to see any solution and therefore feel helpless and unable to cope. Reassuring means giving support, and therefore security, to help the person to cope. Reassurance can be likened to the walking stick or crutch used by someone with an orthopaedic condition. It is a form of psychological support which most of us need from time to time, but of course like any other prop, it should be slowly withdrawn when no longer required.

7.20 Counselling

When rapport has been established, the next logical step is that advice may be given and this is counselling. People readily consult nurses and ask for advice. This should be freely given and common sense should be used. There is good backing for recommending the common sense approach, for Lord Chesterfield (1694–1773) in letters to his son in 1748 wrote: 'Common sense, which in truth is very uncommon, is the best sense I know of'.

The nurse should be careful so as not to find herself making decisions for the person. Advising or counselling is not synonymous to deciding. As we have said before, the object must be to help the person to find his own solutions; ready-made solutions are of no use. A nurse should develop the technique of looking at both sides of the argument clearly and fairly and evaluating the pros and cons of each. If the problem is looked at in this way it may be that a nurse might introduce some aspects which the person had not thought of before. This may help the person to decide and it may also help to improve the quality of the decision taken.

There are pitfalls associated with counselling which a nurse should be aware of. Some people may try to manipulate the nurse and other people, through the advice given. Then there is the question of the doctor/patient relationship; nothing must be done to undermine this. In the early days of treatment, the person may have difficulty in establishing rapport with the doctor, or he may not like the doctor's approach. For these reasons and the fact that a nurse is more frequently available and therefore more accessible, the person may approach a nurse in the hope that he can get her on his side. A nurse has a loyalty to the doctor and also to the sick person. To maintain this she will need to tread a neutral path, for she certainly must not take sides.

Another thing a nurse must avoid doing is making moral judgements. The person's behaviour may be unpleasant and considered by some to be morally wrong, but however bad this may appear to be, no attempt should be made to moralize. People should be accepted as they really are and not as we ideally think they should be.

7.21 Suggesting

It may be sometimes necessary to suggest a course of action or a line of approach to someone. Most people are susceptible to suggestion to some extent from their social circle, the mass media or public opinion. The success of advertising rests in the ability of the advertiser to suggest that his product is better than any other on the market. If suggestion is used it is often necessary to wait a while for results. Many people react to a suggestion by rejecting it initially, later they consider it and perhaps then adopt it as if it were an original idea. It should be remembered that some people are exceptionally suggestible and it is important to remember that the suggestions made are in the person's best interest.

Suggestion depends on three things. First, the personality of the nurse, her relationship with the person and the degree of rapport with him. Second, the actions and behaviour of the nurse; the example set by the nurse is very important and is an indirect form of suggestion which may be more effective than direct or verbal suggestion. Third, there is the suggestion of the subject. Some people are more suggestible than others.

7.22 Persuading

Persuasion is not used in psychiatry or psychiatric nursing as often as is popularly thought because the person should be helped to find his own solutions and should not be provided with ready-made ones.

There are also the ethical considerations. It is all too easy to think that one's own ideas are best. The person who is doing the suggesting is placing herself/himself in the role of an arbiter and this is not a good thing.

Persuasion is different from suggestion. The technique of suggestion is to put forward an idea, a course of action or a possible solution. The suggestion may or may not be accepted, but in any case a little time must be allowed to elapse for the suggestion to germinate. Persuasion depends on the presentation of a logical reason for carrying out a particular action.

There are a number of occasions when gentle persuasion is appropriate. For example in the case of the confused, disorientated person who wants to go home late in the evening and is neither well enough to go nor has made any previous arrangements for his discharge. Somebody who is depressed may need encouragement to eat. Someone who is being treated for alcohol or drug dependence and who is finding it difficult to carry on with his course of treatment, may be persuaded and encouraged to persevere. Likewise someone who has been given a job as part of his occupational therapy/industrial therapy which is not exactly to his liking, but is considered useful in the re-establishment of the work habit, will also need to be encouraged.

Persuasion should always be tempered with encouragement and a nurse should not try to dominate and impose her will on the person. Persuasion requires a gentle touch, a friendly and an encouraging approach.

7.23 Aggression

Aggressive outbursts are something which the nurse will have to deal with, though modern methods of treatment and management have contributed much to reducing these. These are most likely to occur in young fit people, that is, in the people who are most difficult to control. A general rule for dealing with aggressive people is that there should be enough nurses to cope. This sometimes presents problems; the person may be breaking up valuable property or more seriously may be attacking or injuring someone who is unable to defend himself. If one nurse intercedes he/she is unlikely to be able to control the aggression alone and may be injured in the attempt. If at all possible it is better to fetch adequate help. Contrary to the opinion of some of the public, psychiatric nurses are not taught the techniques of self defence but rely on common sense. This means, apart from having adequate help, approaching the patient from behind when possible and then standing as close to him as possible so as to limit the effects of his blows. Rough handling does not help and the minimum of force required to immobilize the person should be used. Physical restraints of any sort are not used. If the person continues to be aggressive, it is tempting to put the person in a side-room and to close the doors, but this must not be done except on the doctor's orders.

Aggressive outbursts, like any other unusual incidents should be reported to the senior nursing staff and the medical staff. If possible the cause should be sought and then measures taken to prevent such incidents in the future. It will not always be possible to find a reason or a cause. For example, in the case of people suffering from schizophrenia, aggressive outbursts are not uncommon in the acute phase of the illness, and afterwards such people are completely bewildered and mystified by their behaviour and are usually at a complete loss for an explanation.

7.24 Coma

Some patients may be aggressive and overactive and by contrast others may be completely inactive and be in a coma. The state of coma resembles a deep sleep in many ways but differs in one important point; it is not possible to rouse the person. The person in a coma is therefore unconscious and the nurse should be acutely aware of the threat to life which unconsciousness presents. Many of the functions of the nervous system are either not possible or impaired and the fact that irritability is one of these functions highlights the seriousness of this condition.

We shall return to this subject later in the section on physical diseases of the nervous system. At this stage we shall bear in mind the threat to life which a coma, due to any cause, presents and thus the necessity for prompt and efficient action.

7.25 Death

Death is a normal and inevitable event in the biological cycle. Just as there is much joy and happiness surrounding a birth, there is usually much sadness associated with death.

A nurse should be prepared to cope with the dying and death, and there are a number of points to bear in mind. There is the question of whether to tell the person he is dying. Some people fully realize that they are about to die and accept the fact, they may even welcome death as a relief from suffering. Others are afraid of dying and will ask questions to find out whether they are. It is the doctor's job and not the nurse's to answer such questions and the policy varies. However, it is a nurse who is likely to be asked most of the questions. A nurse may try to be as helpful and straightforward as possible, but at the same time she must not assume the function of the doctor. She must also be on the look out for the indirect question or she may find herself in an awkward position.

There are relatives who will need help. They will need help in the period before the person dies and more help once death has occurred. There is likely to be an emotional release. Dealing with this is a highly personal thing and depends on the personality of the nurse and the personalities of the relatives. It is better to let the tears flow freely rather than encourage the person to stifle them. Some people like to be alone for a while, others like to have someone near but not to talk and others need to talk and talk. A nurse must use her judgement as to what kind of reaction she is dealing with and modify her approach accordingly. She should also observe how experienced nurses deal with the problem. Some nurses have the knack of saying the right thing at the right time.

Next there is the problem of the other patients. Death nearly always causes an 'atmosphere'; it is often like a heavy black cloud descending over the ward. A nurse must not be surprised if other patients start demanding her attention at a time when she is apparently very busy. She should remember that such behaviour stems from fear and personal insecurity and should try to make a little time available for everyone. The value of a cup of tea in such circumstances, both for the relatives and the other patients, should not be overlooked.

There are the nurse's own reactions to consider. Nurses experience the same range of emotions as any other group of people. In a stressful situation such as death produces, the onus is on the nurse to remain as objective as possible, for the relatives and patients will look to her for a lead. The ability to be objective is something which takes time and personal discipline; this is part of a professional training. One way of achieving this is by thinking of the needs of others rather than one's own needs and feelings.

If death is imminent, the appropriate religious minister should be sent for, if requested, and a nurse should know how to contact these. This is of particular importance to people of the Roman Catholic

Church as the Sacrament of Anointing the Sick has a special significance.

7.26 Destructiveness

Some patients are destructive towards their surroundings. This may be the case in children and young people with delinquent traits. A destructive tendency may be found in people with subnormal intelligence, in those with personality disorders and also among confused aged people. Hospital property should be treated as if it were your own, for in fact, everyone who pays taxes contributes to the upkeep of the hospitals. Destruction of property cannot be allowed and of course the best thing to do is to prevent it from happening by providing an interesting programme and by avoiding conditions which produce boredom. It can also be prevented by continuous and vigilant observation which will detect early changes in the person's behaviour pattern and so allow preventative measures to be taken.

7.27 Discipline

For many people the term discipline is synonymous with restrictive and possibly punitive measures, but this need not be so. Any collection of people living closely together need to have a set of rules to organize their community if chaos is not to result. Discipline in this context will be seen to be necessary; it is the type of discipline and how it is applied that is sometimes open to question. There are three types of discipline:

a. Autocratic. In the autocratic type of discipline the rules and standards are prescribed by one person, the head of the organisation. The discipline may be punitive and repressive or benignly benevolent according to the personality of the leader. Some leaders can by outstanding ability and the force of their personality provide inspiration. The less able leader who is unable to inspire, will have to rely on the insistence that rules are obeyed, with stiff penalties when they are not.

b. Democratic. This form of discipline implies that the leaders as well as the led, jointly contribute to the formulation of disciplinary policy. When one has contributed to a policy and has been consulted, it is much easier to support such a policy. The leader does not have to play such a dominant role and there is likely to be a greater spirit of co-operation. This is the type of discipline to be found in therapeutic communities. Discussion and consultation forms its basis and free communication with feedback are the lubricants on which it works.

c. Laissez-faire. This type of discipline literally means to let the people do as they think best, that is, non interference. Very little help or guidance is given by the leader and discussion is lacking; it is a sort of free-for-all.

Each type of discipline has its merits. The autocratic discipline gives security and people know where they stand. On the other hand it does not allow much initiative to be used and requires a forceful or 'bossy' personality if it is to be successful. In the absence of the leader the system does not work so well, in other words, loyalty may not be so marked.

Democratic discipline seems to have a lot to commend it and is the type most organizations, including hospitals, would profess to use. It certainly gives more job satisfaction and evokes more loyalty. Sometimes people who are accustomed to autocratic discipline have difficulty at first in accepting this approach. On the other hand democratic discipline is not leader centred and is therefore not so dependent on the presence of the leader for its working, in fact it should work just as well when he is away as when he is there.

Laissez-faire discipline is usually unacceptable in an organization such as a hospital. It creates an uncertain and aimless atmosphere and gives rise to unrest and lack of purpose.

A nurse, whether she be a junior pupil or a student responsible for a few patients or a chief nursing officer responsible for a group of hospitals, is automatically cast in the role of a leader and must therefore be able to maintain discipline. The type of discipline which is possible will depend on the general policy of the hospital and the personality of the nurse. If most people had a choice they would choose the democratic type.

7.28 Management of people

Here a nurse has a dual function. She is responsible for meeting the needs of the individuals in her care and she is also responsible for the group as a whole. Care of psychological (already mentioned) as well as physical and social needs of the individual is necessary.

In order to meet the needs of the group it is necessary to consider some aspects of living in a group. It is a self evident fact that experiences from the environment affect behaviour and that these experiences involve other people. In a group, relationships are formed and these are based on past experience. Members of the group are accorded a position within it, and this position, which is technically called status, is judged in terms of responsibility. A ward sister, or charge nurse, carries a good deal of responsibility and therefore has a high status within that area. A standard of behaviour is expected from the members of the group and this is related to status. The onus is on the leader to set a standard of behaviour which is an example and a model for others. Role is the term given to the behaviour appropriate to any person's status.

If the relationships are good, status fairly accorded and roles well defined, then the members will get satisfaction from being a member of the group, they will contribute constructively towards it and will defend it if criticized. This is a good or high morale and is related largely to the personalities involved. It is true that pleasant surroundings, tastefully decorated and nicely furnished, help morale, but it is possible to have palatial surroundings and a poor 'atmosphere'. The nurse should be aware of the effects of good morale and do everything she can to achieve it. There is some evidence to suggest that people recover more quickly from illness when the morale is good.

As well as the factors already mentioned, *communication* is an essential ingredient for good morale. This should be a two-way system with feedback. There are two types of communication.

a. Superficial. This is the common form of communication involving language.

b. Copying. The copying of other people is a primitive form of communication and it may take the form of copying actions, *imitation*, copying thinking, *suggestion* and copying feeling, *sympathy*. We all know that a world of meaning may be conveyed in a single expression or gesture. The junior nurse is only one link in the long chain of communication, but she should ensure that hers is a strong and effective link.

In order to manage people effectively the nurse must be able to meet the needs of the individual and the group, watch out for incompatibilities and resolve differences without taking sides. She must, in fact, have some of the qualities of a diplomat. The nurse is largely responsible for creating and maintaining a cheerful, friendly and optimistic atmosphere in which people may be restored to health. Such conditions are sometimes referred to as the *therapeutic environment.*

7.29 Management of the hospital day

A little planning is necessary if the best use is to be made of the time. The time of rising in the morning varies from hospital to hospital, but the tendency is for this to be as late as possible. In some hospitals the night staff call the patients and start off the routine tasks. In others, patients are not called until the day staff come on duty at 7 or 7.30 a.m.

Patients are encouraged to make their own beds and where possible to wash themselves. Some may need help with these activities, others may need to be dressed. It is often quicker for a nurse to dress a person who is having difficulty rather than help the person to do it himself. This must be resisted and the person should be given as much independence as possible.

If there is a group of people who need a good deal of supervision in matters of hygiene and dress, as is likely in the case of senile people, and if a habit-training programme is in operation, it is a good idea to have a nurse responsible for a small group of say 5 or 6. This is *case assignment*. It gives the patients, who are likely to be confused and disorientated, security, by having contact with only one nurse for the majority of their needs.

Breakfast should not be too late so as to allow time to get to the hospital activities. The difference between a good and a bad hotel is judged mainly by the quality of service and particularly the service of food. In hospitals it is never possible to reach the standards of home-cooking because of the quantities and thus the extra time involved. But it is possible to have a high standard of service with appropriate extras for each meal and a display of flowers where possible.

The prescribed drugs and medicines are given after breakfast and after other meals and the patients go to the occupational/industrial therapy or other work places. Some people will need to be escorted to these activities, others will need help and encouragement. In all cases it is a good idea to have some form of check and an attendance register is usually kept at the main places of employment. It is better for the nurse to go with the patients and stay with them whilst they work, unless there are definite reasons for remaining behind. The nurses should be participating members of the group, helping and encouraging where necessary, withdrawing to the background and taking part in what is happening, but always observing.

A purely supervising role can be boring for the nurse and can invoke the 'they' complex in the patient.

The dining arrangements vary and lunch may be taken in the ward or alternatively in a communal dining room. If a central dining room is used, it is a good idea to have some nurses present with responsibility for their own groups so that individual needs are known and catered for.

A variety of activities are arranged for the afternoon. For some it will be work as usual whilst others, on a rota basis, will take part in some sport or recreational activity. These activities might include field sports such as football, cricket, hockey, bowls, tennis or athletics. They could include a walk, a shopping expedition or a coach outing. More leisurely activities could include playreading, art, sculpture, pottery, musical appreciation and psychodrama. It is essential to have the programme well planned so that everybody gets an opportunity to take part in the activity of his choice.

The afternoon's activity finishes with tea and there is usually a short period which patients have to themselves and the time of the evening meal varies. There are usually a variety of activities in the evening, there are dances, cinema shows and games, such as bingo.

Some of the important events in the hospital day are the meals; these should be as enjoyable as possible. The hobby or recreational session is important and something should be provided to cater for all tastes. Letters provide an important link with the outside and these should be distributed promptly. Visitors are also a vital link with the world outside and they should be courteously received and given privacy.

The time of lights-out will vary. Older people like to turn in early and the converse is true for young people. In a therapeutic community, matters such as this are usually decided by the community. In any case a common-sense approach should be adopted.

In certain circumstances, the hospital may need to be modified. For example if people are going out to work as part of their rehabilitation, such people will need to be called earlier and special arrangements must be made for breakfast and the evening meal. If electroconvulsive treatment is given on the wards, then the programme will need to be altered accordingly. If the ward is for older people the programme needs to be no less dynamic, but many items will need to be excluded as they would be inappropriate.

In the interests of hygiene a daily bath is desirable, but in many wards there are only one or two baths available thus making a daily bath impossible. In order to allow fair access to bath for everyone, it may be necessary to have some sort of rota system. Again, this is an example of something which could be solved by the patients at a ward meeting.

7.30 Management of the ward

Any big store has a great variety of items on display and has a stock to meet the demand for any one item. Yet despite the great diversity of items it is possible to find any object fairly quickly. One is left to conclude that the best possible use is made of the available resources; this is what is meant by management.

The same principles can and should be used in relation to ward management. It is true that many of our hospitals are not purpose-built and therefore present us with difficulties, but these are the available resources and they must be used to the best advantage.

Washing up is an ever present chore and domestic help is difficult to find. It may be necessary to have a washing up rota with everyone playing their part. This is a normal family activity and if the ward is considered to be an enlarged family with everyone sharing the chores, then such chores become less of a burden.

A similar arrangement may be necessary for cleaning. Modern floor-coverings and the increased availability of vacuum cleaners, have eased the problem of cleaning. Moreover some hospitals use contract cleaners, but nevertheless some cleaning has to be organized at ward level. The question of what to use when cleaning baths, toilets, woodwork, metalwork or floors is a local matter and you should find out what the practice is. A procedure book, if available, should give guidance on these points. Cleaning materials and disinfectants should be used sparingly.

Nurses should not expect domestic work to form a regular part of their day's work, but they should expect, because of domestic staff shortages or other exigencies, to be involved from time to time. In any case some practical experience is desirable so as to have first hand knowledge of something which they may have to supervise later on.

A considerable amount of ordering is necessary to ensure that the ward has the supplies of every sort which it needs. The required number of meals and special diets must be ordered from the Catering Officer. Groceries, cleaning materials and daily supplies of bread and milk are usually ordered from the stores and so are items of stationery and crockery to replace breakages. In order to spread the work-load, specific days are allocated for the issue of certain materials. A list is usually circulated and it helps everybody if this is followed.

Drugs, medicines and disinfectants are ordered from the pharmacy. Drugs are ordered as prescribed by the doctor and the practice of keeping a stock of commonly used drugs is generally discouraged. Certain disinfectants, lotions and surgical equipment may be ordered in the ward stock book by the ward sister or charge nurse. All drugs and similar substances should be stored in secure cupboards. This is particularly important when potentially suicidal patients are present.

The appropriate number of dressing packs and instruments, if there is a full C.S.S.D. (Central Sterile Supply Department), have to be ordered daily from the C.S.S.D. as well as the required number of needles and syringes.

The ward and the equipment should be maintained in good condition. Frequent and regular checks should be made to see that everything is in order. It is a general rule that help is sought from the appropriate tradesmen to put things right. A do-it-yourself approach is not usually encouraged. This applies particularly to electrical fittings and apparatus. Most hospitals have rules that simple things such as changing plugs and fuses, which you would automatically do at home, should be left to the electrician. This might seem unduly careful, but there is no doubt that electricity is potentially dangerous in the hands of the amateur. It can cause shocks and burns, which may be fatal to the operator and poor workmanship could result in a serious fire. Electrical work is therefore left to the experts.

7.31 Fire precautions

Fires can have tragic results and fires in hospital are a particular problem with so many people living closely together. Every nurse should be familiar with the procedure in the event of fire and should act quickly though without panic. She should be familiar with the local system of raising the alarm, this usually means breaking the glass on the fire alarm point, followed by telephoning the hospital switchboard to report the site of the fire. Some hospitals have an alarm system incorporated in the telephone system and the alarm rings when the number is dialled; this number varies but it is often 333. The nurse should be proficient in rescuing people from danger, particularly elderly and seriously ill people if stairs are involved. Normally the fire-officer or members of the local fire brigade come to the hospital regularly to demonstrate and to allow for the practice of these techniques.

If there is an outbreak of fire there are a number of things the nurse must do:

1. Raise the alarm.
2. Remove the patients.
3. Fight the fire.

7.32 Rehabilitation

We have considered the various aspects of psychiatric nursing and we have seen that these are varied, and that there are many technical skills involved. The ultimate desired effect of the use of all these skills is to rehabilitate the person into the community, and rehabilitation means restoring the person to the highest level of physical, psychological, social, vocational and economic activity possible. In many cases this is a return to the person's previous position in society, but in other cases illness may have blunted abilities and the sights may need to be lowered.

There are a number of problems in rehabilitating the mentally ill. First, mental illness generally operates on a longer time scale than other forms of illness, and thus the longer the person has been away from society the more difficult it is to return. Second, there is the problem of finding living accommodation if the person has no home. It will not help the person if it is known that he has been in a psychiatric hospital. Third, there is the problem of employment. Some employers are still not very sympathetic about employing anybody with a psychiatric history. Fourth, there is the question of making friends and establishing relationships with the neighbours, and such contacts are a vital part of community existence.

The person will need a lot of help, support and guidance if he is not to be daunted by these problems. Rehabilitation can be eased if links with the outside world are maintained during the illness. The work habit must be maintained and hence the need for adequate occupational therapy/industrial therapy facilities. Some people find it helpful to go to work from the hospital for a start and appreciate being able to return to the secure environment of the hospital at night. This also means that the person has an opportunity to save some money and this provides a degree of financial security when ultimately discharged.

There are other ways of helping rehabilitation such as half-way houses. These are hostels where the people can live with the minimum of supervision. Some hospitals operate a boarding-out system. Patients are placed as paying guests in the homes of people willing to accept them. This is arranged by the hospital and the rent is guaranteed. There is supervision by the community nurse or social worker who will try to smooth out any problems which may arise, and if there is great incompatibility, there is an understanding that the person will be found alternative accommodation or will return to hospital.

A number of people with psychiatric illness are in the elderly age range and need to be rehabilitated from the accommodation rather than the work aspect. Some hospitals with strong links with the community have introduced an 'adopt-an-old-person' scheme. Considerable care must obviously be taken to match up both sides and the method has not been widely adopted, but where it has, many placements have been very successful.

Rehabilitation is the ultimate goal of treatment and is often the biggest hurdle which has to be overcome in the path from illness to normality. Long term planning, a dynamic programme coupled with nursing, medical and other support makes this goal more attainable.

7.33 Follow-up and after-care

Rehabilitation does not end at the hospital gates, for if it is to be successful there must be adequate follow-up and after-care. Ideally there should be medical, social and nursing follow-up. On discharge the person will be given an appointment to see his doctor who will keep an eye on the medical aspects of his condition and prescribe drugs as appropriate. When a person is discharged the mental health department of the local authority should be notified, so that the mental welfare officer can arrange to visit. This is very important in the early days because this is the time when help is most needed. The Mental Welfare Officer can bring the benefits of the statutory social services to the person and can at the same time contact the various voluntary organizations which offer help.

A nurse has an important role in follow-up and after-care because of the uniqueness of her relationship with the patient. She, above everybody, is likely to be on the same wavelength and though she does not prescribe she can listen, understand, reassure or counsel as necessary. A firmly based nurse-patient relationship can provide a good deal of security when the person is taking his first few faltering steps in a complex and often bewildering world.

7.34 The nurse in the community

Despite the fact that the majority of people live in the community, and even those with long term illnesses spend more time in the community than in hospital, this is relatively new territory for nurses. Yet the terms of the 1959 Mental Health Act shifted the emphasis of psychiatric care from the hospital to the community. In some areas, this aspect of nursing is being developed and it is likely to increase in the future.

There is much the nurse can do in the community. By entering people's homes she can gain a better picture of the person's social setting than by reading reports, however graphically written. As already mentioned she has a special relationship with the patient and she can draw on this to encourage the patient to keep appointments. She can check that medication is being taken and by virtue of her clinical knowledge she can observe whether the symptoms, if any, are controlled. Not taking medication has always been a problem in discharged psychiatric patients. If they experience a long symptom-free period there is a natural tendency to stop taking the drugs. Gradually the symptoms recur and often the person has insufficient insight to restart taking the drugs and eventually re-admission to hospital is required. Long acting phenothiazine drugs in the form of 'Moditen' and 'Modecate' have been introduced to overcome this problem. In the case of Moditen an injection is required about every two weeks, and in the case of Modecate an injection is required every three to four weeks. Mutually convenient arrangements can be made for the nurse to give these injections in the person's home. These should not be simply 'Moditen rounds'; the nurse should take the opportunity to observe the person's overall behaviour.

In addition to visiting the person's home, the nurse may also visit his place of work or a convalescent home or a half-way house, or anybody directly or indirectly involved with the patient. She can listen to any problems that may be arising and simply by being a good listener can be very helpful. She can introduce a professional and therefore a more objective dimension to the problem and she can give advice and make suggestions if appropriate. A good deal of tact and diplomacy will be needed. She must remember that people may feel 'threatened' by her presence and for this reason in particular, she must not rush her fences. There is also the question of professional demarcation. Some doctors and social workers may not understand or accept the role of the nurse in the community. It is therefore important that she should not trespass in their territory.

The nurse in the community has an important preventive role. *Prevention* has three aspects:

a. Primary. Primary prevention is concerned with the modification of contributory factors in individual or community life which may increase the likelihood of mental illness.

b. Secondary. Secondary prevention is concerned with the early detection of illness, so that the symptoms may be relieved as quickly as possible thus ensuring minimum upset and long term effects.

c. Tertiary. Tertiary prevention is concerned with the prevention of the disability which may have been caused by an illness.

A full preventative role will include consideration of the primary, secondary and tertiary aspects of prevention, but the nurse is most likely to be involved in tertiary prevention, at least initially. The nurse's clinical experience and skill can be utilized in secondary prevention. Primary prevention involves a multi-disciplinary approach and includes health education. Nurses of the future are likely to be increasingly concerned with mental health as well as with mental illness.

7.35 Summary

Psychiatric nursing involves considerable professional knowledge, varied technical and managerial skills, expertise in human relations and an aptitude for diplomacy, patience, perseverance, kindness and above all humanity. There are many problems to be solved, many questions without answers, and many frustrations, but there are equally as many challenges. Who can side-step a challenge? 'Problems are made to be overcome,' wrote Florence Nightingale. This seems a very good motto.

8

Sexual deviation

8.0 Introduction

Sex is one of the basic drives, sometimes called the *libido*, and is essential for the continuation of the species. A person's sex is determined by the nature of the genetic material in the fusing gametes. The female contribution is referred to as X and in the diploid state contains XX. The male contribution may be Y or X, because the diploid (46 chromosomes) male cell has both. But at fertilization the gametes are in the haploid (23 chromosomes) state and thus the female always contributes an X and the male X or Y.

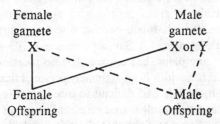

Female gamete X   Male gamete X or Y

Female Offspring   Male Offspring

There is some debate as to whether infants and young children are sexually aware and therefore capable of perceiving sexual stimuli, but there is no doubt that there is a strong awareness from puberty onwards. Physiological changes take place in the female which include the menses, a deposition of fat giving rise to the smooth feminine curves, development of the breasts and a feminine distribution of hair. Physiological changes in the male include a 'breaking of the voice', the development of rugged male contours, the growth of hair on the face and sometimes there is an associated facial acne. Puberty in both sexes is usually associated with a spurt in the growth rate and youngsters simply 'shoot-up' at this age.

There are also psychological changes. Boys and girls become conscious of their manhood or womanhood and may feel embarrassed unless adequately prepared. There may be self-consciousness in social situations and this is heightened by the fact that due to the increase in growth there is physical clumsiness and a tendency to drop things, This sometimes gives rise to a feeling of inadequacy, moodiness, bad temper and even depression.

Sometimes at about this stage, the young person may have a 'crush' on someone of the same sex. It may be a teacher, or someone in the world of sport, films or television. This hero-worship is quite normal, there is usually no contact between the people concerned and the phase passes. Dating begins with members of the opposite sex. Many of these affairs are short lived and provide both members with opportunities to gain experience of relationships in a new dimension. Later on more lasting relationships are established and courtship and marriage follows. According to Kinsey (1948), nearly 90 per cent of the population get married.

The accepted pattern in our society is that the majority of people get married. Again Kinsey found that about 5 per cent or so of the population have such low sex drives that they are capable of living happy and contented lives without sex. We said in Chapter 2 that adjustment to the single state is possible. There are others such as priests and certain religious people who are required to remain celibate, though there is much current discussion about celibacy. But this is nothing new, for Samuel Johnson (1709–1784) wrote: 'Marriage has many pains, but celibacy has no pleasures'.

Sex and sexual behaviour is an extremely personal thing and some-thing which many people find difficult to discuss. Of late people are not so reticent and the result is that much information has come to light. It has also come to light that there is much deviation from what is considered normal sexual behaviour.

8.1 Homosexuality (*G. home* = same)

Homosexuality means sexual relations between members of the same sex, either men or women. A female homosexual is called a *lesbian*, but there is no special word for the male homosexual.

Homosexuality has a long history and there is reference to it in Egypt at about 1580 B.C. and in Babylon at about 957 B.C. At first the Jews had a liberal or permissive attitude towards it, but later they prohibited sex outside marriage, made masturbation punishable by death and prohibited homosexual activity. Many of the early Christians were Jews, and consequently they carried over these ideas about sex from the Jewish culture. Religion had almost complete control of sexual matters for a long time. In England the Magna Carta was signed in 1215 and this was the first step in diminishing the power of the Church and transferring that power to the State. But it took nearly a century for the State to wrest control from the Church, and even the State did not modify the existing church laws.

Homosexuality was first made a crime against the State by the

Labouchere Amendment of 1885. This made homosexual acts between males, in public or in private, a criminal offence. Women were not included in the Act. The story goes that Queen Victoria refused to believe that women engaged in homosexual acts and had the part dealing with them changed so that they were excluded from the legislation. Another story is that the law officer responsible was too embarrassed to explain it to the Queen and had it omitted. In any case women were excluded from the terms of the Act. The law remained basically unchanged until quite recently. The Wolfenden Report published in 1957 caused the subject to be discussed more freely and it was suggested by many that the law should be reformed. This reform was undertaken by Mr. Leo Abse M.P. who introduced a private Members bill. This was the subject of much debate both inside and outside of Parliament, and contrasts with the Labouchere Amendment of 1885 which was accepted as a Bill without debate or discussion. The outcome was that the Sexual Offences Act 1967 came into effect on the 27th July of that year. The chief provision is to make a homosexual act between men no longer a crime provided it involves not more than two consenting adults and is performed in private. If more than two are present, or if either is under 21 years of age, then it remains a crime with a maximum prison sentence of 10 years.

The incidence of homosexuality in the community is high and there are approximately equal numbers of males and females involved. Bryan Magee (1966 and 1968) gave his book on the subject the title 'One in Twenty'. This means that 5 per cent or about 2,500,000 in the community are homosexuals.

The cause or causes of homosexuality are not clear, but there seems to be no hereditary factor. It is said that homosexuals are not born but made. Often there is a pattern where there is a close relationship with the mother and a poor relationship with the father who tends to play a recessive role. Many homosexuals would like to have relations with the opposite sex, that is *heterosexual* relations, but are unable to do so.

8.2 Male homosexuality

Some male homosexuals have an effeminate appearance and are usually referred to as 'queers' or 'pansies', but many have no such outward characteristics and in fact may have typically masculine appearances. In the past the lot of the male homosexual was an unhappy one. He was a social outcast and often ridiculed by society; he was open to blackmail and subject to the rigours of the law. Because of these factors ordinary social contact of homosexual persons was a particular hazard.

Homosexual acts occur in a number of circumstances. When a lot of boys and men are in close contact and when there are no females as happens in boys' schools, prisons, the armed forces or prisoner of war camps, then homosexual acts are likely to take place involving those with a strong libido. The majority of such men become heterosexual in the company of women and are said to be *bisexual*. Some boys and men are ambivalent in their feelings and indulge in homosexuality only to find it unsatisfactory and abandon the practice. Others are confirmed homosexuals and indulge only in homosexual acts. It is not unusual for a married man with children to have homosexual affairs; Oscar Wilde is a notable example.

Homosexual pick-ups and homosexual acts often take place in public lavatories and for this reason there are usually 'no loitering' notices in such places. Other relationships are more lasting and it is not unusual for two men to set up home together and have strong emotional bonds. Sexual acts, such as sex play, mutual masturbation and less commonly sodomy—the insertion of the penis into the anus—form only part of the total relationship.

8.3 Female homosexuality (lesbianism)

As a sexual deviant the lesbian has not been involved with the law, but she has been subjected to great social pressure. She has the same problems as her male counterpart in making contacts. Lesbianism is practised in all-female institutions just as homosexuality is practised by men in similar circumstances, but less so because the female libido is generally less strong.

Some lesbians can be recognized by their manly appearance, they dress like men, have men-like hairstyles and a deep man-like voice. But this type accounts for but a small portion, for many are as feminine as heterosexual women.

Like the male homosexual they form some fleeting relationships, but many set up home together. If one of the partners is a masculine type of lesbian, then she is likely to assume a 'husband-like' role, but it may happen that neither partner is of this type. Sexual acts between the partners consist of sex play, mutual masturbation using the hands, or heterosexual intercourse may be simulated. Very rarely a substitute penis may be used. Like the male counterparts there is usually strong emotional involvement and sex only forms a small part of the total relationship.

8.4 Psychiatric aspects of homosexuality

For a century the law of the state dealt severely with the male homosexual and still does except in certain specified conditions, though the sending of a homosexual to jail has been likened to sending an alcoholic to a distillery to be cured. The Church and society have disapproved of homosexuality and have brought pressures to bear. When these factors are combined with personal guilt, loneliness, particularly in old age, and no prospect of having children, it is not surprising that the incidence of psychiatric illness in this group is higher than average. Many turn to alcohol.

Many homosexuals seek psychiatric help because of the problems arising out of their homosexuality. Depression may be the associated problem and this is treated in the usual way. Others may seek treatment for their homosexuality. Practices vary but the psychoanalytical approach involving psychoanalysis, individual and group psychotherapy may be used, or alternatively use may be made of the behaviourist approach usually in some form of aversion.

8.5 Homosexuals and the nurse

With a quoted incidence of 1 in 20 (Magee) in the community, any nurse is likely to have contacts with homosexuals of both sexes. The nurse may personally find the subject unpleasant, unsavoury or even disgusting, but she must be objective in dealing with such people and put her own feelings on one side. As we have mentioned before, the nurse must not set herself up as a judge or a moralist. If it is remembered that the majority of homosexuals are unhappy to be as they are and if they had a choice they would prefer to be heterosexual, then it may be easier to understand their plight.

Homosexuality is numerically the most common form of sexual deviation, but there are a number of others which will be described in the following sections.

8.6 Masturbation

This is self-stimulation of the sex organs in order to cause sexual arousal, a practice common to both males and females. It is not a form of sexual deviation for it is commonly practised particularly during adolescence, but it was at one time considered to be a sin and there are still very profound guilt feelings associated with the practice. The accepted view is that masturbation does the person no physical harm whatever. It does however give rise to psychological reactions and it would seem there is room for more or better sex education.

8.7 Fetishism

Most heterosexual men are sexually aroused when they observe an attractive woman. Sometimes such arousal can be achieved by an object removed from the body such as stockings or underwear and this reaction is called fetishism. This sometimes accounts for the purposeless theft of underwear from clothes lines. If treatment is sought, which is not often, aversion techniques are likely to be employed.

8.8 Sadism

This term is derived from the Marquis de Sade (1740–1814). He was a French writer of obscene novels and his main theme was lust and cruelty. Sadism does not include the horseplay which normally accompanies love-making. In sadism, pleasure is obtained through inflicting pain. Sexual assaults and lust murders, which are rare, are extreme forms of sadism.

8.9 Masochism

Like sadism this word is also derived from the world of literature. It was Leopold Von Sacher-Masoch (1836–1895), an Austrian novelist, who described men being dominated by women. Pleasure is derived from having pain inflicted. The subject is frequently a male and the pain is inflicted by the partner usually, but not always, a member of the opposite sex. The sadist may progress to serious injury or even murder, but the masochist does not proceed further than suffering pain and humiliation.

8.10 Transvestism

A transvestite is a person who prefers to wear clothing belonging to the opposite sex and has a desire to assume the role of that sex. The subject who is often, but not always a man, may also seek hormone treatment or even surgical operations in an attempt to change sex. Transvestism may arise because these people dislike their own sex, it may occur because a homosexual wants to assume the feminine role in a relationship or it may result from masochistic tendencies, for traditionally the female assumes a passive role.

8.11 Paedophilia

This is the desire of an adult to engage in sexual activity with children of either sex. Such people unconsciously feel that they are so immature sexually, that they are incapable of having normal sexual relations with partners of their own age. It is against people like this that children must be warned, for such an experience can be shattering for a child. In hospital such people present a problem because the current policy is to give people as much freedom as possible, but people such as this make further attempts when on leave and thus incur the wrath of the community for the whole patient population.

8.12 Exhibitionism

This is the derivation of sexual pleasure and gratification from exposure of the male genitals to females. Exhibitionism is almost wholly confined to males, but strip-tease shows by females are in a similar vein. The male exhibitionist may be of low intelligence who is unable to approach girls normally and this behaviour is a form of courtship. It also occurs in people with presenile or senile dementia, particularly that due to cerebral arteriosclerosis. Others may be of good intelligence with an apparently normal sex life but are overcome with a compulsion to expose themselves.

8.13 Voyeurism

This is the 'Peeping Tom' phenomenon and sexual pleasure is derived by witnessing sexual acts or through observing naked bodies. It is confined almost exclusively to men. Some voyeurs run risks by perching themselves precariously on high buildings in order to have a vantage point to view bedroom scenes, others use binoculars from a bedroom window or from a point overlooking a 'lover's lane'.

8.14 Pornography

We have already mentioned pornography in relation to the mental mechanisms and we saw that it is an indirect means of expressing an experience. It includes obscene words, graffitae (drawings or writing scratched on lavatory walls and similar places), bawdy songs and obscene literature. Like voyeurism, pornography is almost exclusively a male domain.

8.15 Problems in heterosexual relations

So far we have considered various forms of sexual deviation. There are, however, a number of problems which are associated with heterosexual relationships. One of these is the difference in libido. Men generally have a stronger libido than women and for a successful relationship adjustments must be made. This is only possible if an attempt is made to understand the feelings of the other person. For the woman there is the risk of pregnancy and if pregnancy does occur the pattern of sexual relations alters. The advice given by obstetricians varies but ranges from complete abstinence from sexual intercourse during the period of pregnancy to, at the most, very limited relations. The female also has the problem of premenstrual tension and its associated discomfort and this calls for understanding on the part of the male partner. Then there is the question of sexual intercourse during the menstrual period. There are various ethnic and religious codes as well as personal attitudes about this subject. Couples should discuss these aspects of their relationships and try to come to an arrangement satisfactory to both.

The menopause or 'change of life' occurs from the end of the fourth decade onwards in women and marks the end of the child-bearing period. There are marked physiological changes and many of these have psychological counterparts and sometimes an accompanying depression. Sometimes the onset of the menopause is taken as the signal to cease having sexual intercourse. This need not be so and partners can have intercourse until late in life. Menopause for men does not come until the sixth decade or later and though it does not have the same physiological changes it has similar psychological counterparts.

8.16 Impotence and premature ejaculation

These are problems encountered by men concerning their sexual relationships. Impotence occurs where the person cannot achieve or sustain an erection. Rarely it is due to a physical cause, but most frequently it is due to psychological factors associated with sexual inadequacy. The discharge of seminal fluid just before or at the point of intercourse is called premature ejaculation. Although the male reaches orgasm it is very unsatisfactory but it is more unsatisfactory for the female because she is never likely to reach orgasm in such circumstances. Premature ejaculation like impotence has a big underlying anxiety factor. Very often this can be relieved by reassurance and advice about love-making and sexual techniques.

8.17 Frigidity

This is a female problem and is based on an underlying anxiety due to fears of sex generally or of pregnancy in particular. As a result there is a failure of the vaginal secretion and muscular relaxation which makes intercourse painful. This pain increases the fear and thus a vicious circle is established. The approach to treatment is the same as that for impotence and premature ejaculation.

8.18 Infertility

This is the inability of a married couple to have children. It occurs fairly commonly and about 10 to 15 per cent of marriages are infertile. There are many reasons for this; for example, it may be due to a disease such as diabetes mellitus which can affect either partner. On the other hand the reason may be specific to one of the partners. In the case of the man there may be an anatomical defect, the production of spermatozoa (*spermatogenesis*) may be insufficient or absent, or the love-making technique may be faulty. The woman may also have an anatomical defect such as stenosis of the vagina; she may have a disease such as fibroids, the fallopian tubes may be blocked or the ovaries may be diseased thus affecting ovulation.

Infertility is a severe blow for a couple who greatly desire a family and considerable maturity on the part of both partners is needed in order to adjust to the fact. It is easy to resort to mutual blame and recrimination. There are some solutions to the problem. If the woman is fertile there is the possibility of artificial insemination. On ethical and religious grounds this solution is unacceptable to many. The other solution is adoption and this is very successful in the majority of cases.

8.19 Prostitution

A prostitute is a woman who offers herself to men for sexual intercourse, usually for hire. This is an ancient practice which has flourished in all areas and in all times. The reasons for prostitution are many. Some of the practitioners have personality disorders (psychopaths), some have limited intelligence and others have been lured into it as part of a white slave traffic by ruthless operators or protectors. Prostitutes do not work on their own but are usually part of an organized system. The protector or 'pimp' provides the accommodation in return for more than a fair share of the earnings. The prostitutes are often cruelly treated by these protectors but often seem incapable of breaking loose.

The prostitutes' clients vary from sailors and long distance lorry drivers, to the young who may be experimenting and others seeking excitement. There is usually little excitement to be had for the prostitute feels no love and may in fact hate her clients.

Prostitution is illegal and there is much legislation concerning the subject. For example, the Street Offences Act 1959 which makes it an offence for a common prostitute to loiter or solicit in a street or public place for the purpose of prostitution.

8.20 Summary

Sex is one of the basic drives and is essential for the continuance of the species, but it is also one of the most intensely private areas of a person's life. Unfortunately it is the subject of many jokes and people are reluctant to state their problems for fear of being laughed at. There is little doubt that many people bottle up their problems for these reasons. A more frank and open approach would be much healthier. The nurse should always be aware of the delicate nature of the subject. At the same time she must not be surprised to hear of perverse, degraded and degrading practices.

9

Disordered intelligence

9.0 Introduction

We have previously considered the distribution of intelligence in the community and the means by which it is measured. Now we shall consider disorders of intelligence, and as always, we shall see that many other facets of the person's life are affected by a disorder of one attribute.

Intelligence is affected at the two extremes of life. In early life a variety of factors, which we shall consider later, affect the normal development of intelligence and result in *mental subnormality*. At the other end of life the ageing process, and other factors, affect the intelligence of previously intelligent people and result in *senile dementia*. In the in-between-years a number of disease processes involving the brain affect intelligence and result in *presenile dementia*.

MENTAL SUBNORMALITY

9.1 Subnormality

The Mental Health Act 1959 (Section 4) includes a definition of subnormality as: 'a state of arrested or incomplete development of the mind which includes subnormality of intelligence and is of a nature or degree which requires or is susceptible to medical treatment or other special care or training of the patient'. There is a separate definition for severe subnormality which runs as follows: 'a state of arrested or incomplete development of mind which includes subnormality of intelligence and is of such a nature or degree that the patient is incapable of living an independent life or of guarding himself against serious exploitation, or will be so incapable when of an age to do so'.

The World Health Organisation has produced an International Classification of Diseases, Injuries and Causes of Death (I.C.D.), but its classification of mental disorders and mental subnormality is not considered satisfactory. The Registrar General's Advisory Committee on Medical Nomenclature and Statistics have produced 'A Glossary of Mental Disorders (No. 22)' and classifies subnormality as follows:

310 Borderline mental retardation—I.Q. 68–85
311 Mild mental retardation   —I.Q. 52–67

312   Moderate mental retardation —I.Q. 36–51
313   Severe mental retardation   —I.Q. 20–35
314   Profound mental retardation —I.Q. under 20
315   Unspecified mental retardation

9.2 Incidence

The responsibility for the subnormal rests with two government departments, the Department of Education and Science and the Department of Health and Social Security.

The Department of Education and Science is governed by the terms of the 1944 Education Act which provides for the education of the *educationally subnormal*. It does this by providing special or remedial classes in ordinary schools or by providing special schools. The number attending such special schools was nearly 19,000 in 1970. In the past the Department of Health and Social Security was involved in the education of the subnormal, but on 1st April 1971 responsibility for the entire educational function was transferred to the Department of Education and Science.

One in every hundred children born is mentally subnormal to some degree. According to the 1963 census, there were 7,000 severely mentally subnormal and psychotic children receiving institutional care in Britain. The overall incidence of mental subnormality in the community is 250,000 and at any time about 63,000 of these are in hospitals for the subnormal.

The Department of Health and Social Security has the overall responsibility for caring for the mentally subnormal, apart from those educated by the Department of Education and Science. It is directly responsible for the hospitals and it is indirectly responsible for the local authority services. There are 55 local authority hostels in England and Wales with accommodation for over 1,000 children and 110 for adults with nearly 2,300 places.

9.3 Causes

There are many causes of mental subnormality, but a large group is genetically determined and another large group is due to environmental influences. The quality of the inherited genes may be poor, or normal genes may undergo changes resulting in defects. Infection, injury, poisons and placental insufficiency are some of the environmental hazards which can give rise to subnormality.

There are causes related to the period of life in the uterus before the child is born and these are called *prenatal*. These are causes associated with the time of birth and these are called *perinatal*. Factors contributing to subnormality in the early formative years after birth are called *post natal*.

9.4 Prenatal

A. GENETIC. There are two types of genetic defects and these are dominant and recessive and can be explained as follows. Each chromosome is made up of two strands which make up a pair. Genes for each character appear at a particular point, called a locus, on both strands of the chromosome. If we consider two characteristics for a particular locus *A* and *a* we see that there are three possible combinations.

1. *AA*. these are of the same type one said to be *homozygous*.
2. *aa*. these are also homozygous.
3. *A.a*. there is one of each and one said to be *heterozygous*.

If a heterozygous person presents only the hereditary characteristic determined by gene *A* while the effect of gene *a* is not apparent, then gene *A* is said to be dominant and gene *a* is said to be recessive —Gregor Johann Mendel (1822–1884), an Austrian monk, is considered to be the father of the science of genetics. He grew peas in a monastery garden at Brünn and conducted many experiments. From these experiments he was able to account for the transmission of characteristics from one generation to another.

Dominant Defects

1. *Tuberous sclerosis* (*epiloia*). This form of subnormality has three components:
   a. There is a nodular rash with a butterfly-like distribution on the nose and cheeks.
   b. There may be tumours affecting various organs of the body including the lungs or the kidneys.
   c. There are tumours of the nervous system including the eye and the brain. These brain tumours give rise to a severe form of epilepsy which is difficult to control. If the lesions are in the temporal lobe, the epilepsy is of the temporal lobe type which is associated with disturbances of behaviour.
   Severe subnormality nearly always occurs in this condition, though some sufferers may be borderline cases.

2. *Neurofibromatosis* (*Von Recklinghausen's disease*). The skin

and the nervous system are involved. There are areas of pigmentation in the skin varying in size from freckles to large diffuse areas. Fibroma occur (neurofibroma) along the nerve tracts and may give rise to compression. If these fibroma occur in the brain then subnormality occurs, but this happens in only about one third of the cases and the degree of subnormality is not severe.

3. *Haemangiomatosis.* An haemangioma is an innocent tumour composed of dilated blood vessels and is otherwise known as a birthmark or naevus. The Sturge-Weber syndrome is an example of an haemangioma giving rise to mental subnormality. In this condition the underlying brain tissue is involved and there may be calcification which is recognizable on X-rays. There is likely to be epilepsy, paralysis of limbs and impairment of intellectual function, which may be severe.

4. *Rud's syndrome.* This is called the fish-skin disease (ichthyosis) and is characterized by generalized dryness, harshness and scaling of the skin. There is often an associated epilepsy, mental subnormality and occasionally spasticity.

5. *Cranio-facial dysostoses.* Dysostosis means defective formation of the bone. In this condition the bones of the head and face are involved and mental subnormality occurs due to the mechanical effects of the defective bone formation.

6. *Marfan's syndrome* (*dystrophiameso dermalis*). This is a disorder of the connective tissue and is characterized by exceptionally long extremities, including the fingers and toes. The fingers are described as spider-like. Mental subnormality is frequently part of this syndrome, but it is rarely of the severe variety.

7. *Acrocephaly.* This is a deformity of the head, also called oxycephaly, in which the crown rises to a blunt point. Sometimes there is a protrusion of the eyeballs (exophthalmos) from small orbits or there may be wide separation of the eyes (hypertelorism) and webbing of the fingers (syndactly). The associated mental defect is often severe.

8. *Sjogren's syndrome.* In this condition the cerebellum is involved giving rise to spino-cerebellar ataxia. There may be cataracts and there is severe mental subnormality.

Recessive defects

From the explanation given earlier one would expect that the chances of a dominant genetic defect occurring are greater than a recessive one and this is true, yet nearly 20 per cent of those with severe subnormality have recessive defects. For a recessive defect to occur, the person must inherit the same abnormal gene on the same locus from each parent. This is an important argument against marriage between blood relations. It considerably increases the risk of recessive defects occurring.

1. *Phenylketonuria.* In this condition there is an enzyme missing and the result is that phenylalanine cannot be metabolized to tyrosine. The absence of tyrosine means that there are few pigments in the skin and many sufferers are blonde. It has also been found that there is a lack of pigmentation in the substantia nigra. There is severe mental subnormality and there may be an accompanying epilepsy.

The phenylalanine is changed into phenylpyruvic acid, instead of to tyrosine, and is excreted in the urine. Fortunately there is a quick urine test available and all new-born babies' urine is now tested for this substance. If the condition is present, the emphasis is on early diagnosis for it is possible to give a child a phenylalanine-free diet and thus prevent any serious damage to the nervous system.

2. *Maple syrup urine.* In this condition there is a loss of amino acids in the urine, particularly leucine, isoleucine and valine, and this causes the urine to smell like maple syrup. Because of the loss of the important amino acids, the child fails to thrive and is severely subnormal. The life expectancy of such a child is usually short.

3. *Galactosaemia.* As in phenylketonuria, there is an enzyme missing in galactosaemia, with the result that galactose cannot be converted to glucose and consequently galactose accumulates in the bloodstream and tissues. A child with this condition naturally fails to thrive, its abdomen becomes distended and occasionally there is jaundice. If the condition is not controlled, subnormality follows. The condition can be diagnosed by testing the urine and treatment involves the exclusion of milk or galactose containing foods from the diet.

4. *Fructose intolerance.* In this condition there is a defect in the metabolism of fructose and hypoglycaemia results. The accumulation of metabolites in the bloodstream and the frequent attacks of hypoglycaemia cause mental subnormality. The condition is diagnosed by a history of fructose intolerance and confirmed by a fructose-tolerance test. A small quantity of fructose is given and this causes the subject to vomit, the blood pressure is lowered and the skin is

sweaty. The subject may be revived by giving intravenous glucose. The treatment is to exclude fructose from the diet.

5. *Hartnup disease.* As in maple syrup urine there is a considerable increase, up to 10 times the normal, in the amount of amino acids lost in the urine, and a corresponding decrease in the blood plasma amino acids. There are two reasons for this. First the absorption of tryptophan and other amino acids from the small intestine is defective. Second their reabsorption by the proximal renal tubules is inefficient and hence the heavy loss in the urine. Again the loss of the all important amino acids results in mental subnormality. Nicotinamide improves the condition generally, but unfortunately it does not affect the mental condition.

6. *Tay-Sachs disease* (*amaurotic family idiocy*). This condition is characterized by an accumulation of fats in the body, a failure to develop mentally and sometimes blindness and paralysis. It is always fatal and death occurs about two years from the onset, which is usually in early infancy. The condition was first described by Tay (1881) and Sachs (1887) and is common in the children of Jews from Eastern Europe.

7. *Laurence-Moon-Biedel syndrome.* This syndrome consists of pigmentation of the retina with visual defects, webbing of the hands and feet (polydactyly), diabetes insipidus and mental subnormality which is usually not severe.

8. *Hepato-lenticular degeneration* (*Wilson's disease*). In this condition copper is not properly metabolized and this in turn causes interference with the oxidation enzyme in the body and results in lesions in the brain and liver. There is cirrhosis of the liver and degeneration of the lentiform nucleus, hence the name hepato-lenticular. The condition, which usually occurs in adolescence and gives rise to choreo-athetosis, mental impairment and behaviour disorders, responds to anti-metallic drugs such as BAL (British Anti Lewisite) and penicillamine.

9. *Gargoylism* (*Hurler's syndrome*). The skeletal system and the metabolism of carbohydrates are involved in this condition. The bones of the head and face are malformed and give rise to a protruding forward and a broad nose and jaw thus accounting for the term gargoylism. Polysaccharide metabolism is defective and this gives rise to fat deposits in the brain similar to that in Tay-Sachs disease. There is severe subnormality.

B. CHROMOSOMAL DEFECTS. In the previous section we considered defects due to genes. These genes are of course sited on the chromosomes, but in the conditions mentioned, though individual genes were defective, the chromosomes as a whole appeared normal. We shall now consider conditions which result from defects in the larger unit, the chromosome.

It will be recalled that there are 46 chromosomes or 23 pairs in the cells of the human species. The obvious things which can go wrong are that there may be too few or conversely too many chromosomes, they may either be too big or too small, or there may be an additional piece. The normal complement is referred to as *eusomy*, the loss of a chromosome from a pair is called *monosomy* and is nearly always fatal, but the gain of a chromosome called *trisomy*, which whilst it is likely to cause trouble, is not fatal.

1. *Down's syndrome (Trisomy 21)*. This syndrome, which used to be called *mongolism*, is the most common condition found in subnormal hospitals. Penrose has estimated the risk at about 1 per 1,000 live births. It accounts for up to 15 per cent of subnormal population and is due to an extra chromosome at pair 21, hence the name trisomy 21. The condition often occurs in the last born of mothers approaching the menopause or in the first born of elderly parents and germinal exhaustion has been suggested. On the other hand it can arise in the first born of young parents or between two unaffected children. In these cases acceptable explanations are more difficult to find.

A child with Down's syndrome is small in stature with a small rounded skull, sparse hair, dry skin, slanted eyes (hence term mongol) which may have squints and are frequently infected. The tongue is too large for the mouth and is often cracked and fissured. The neck is shorter than normal and breathing is often noisy. There is a large abdomen and sometimes an umbilical hernia. The limbs are short and stumpy and there may be one crease across the palm of the hand, the Simian line, instead of the usual two. There may be lesions in any part of the body, but the heart is most commonly affected resulting in poor circulation.

Mentally such children are severely subnormal, but are generally cheerful, friendly and have a capacity for imitation, a sense of rhythm and music. Because of their loving natures many parents look after such children at home with support from the local authority. Many attend occupation centres and can be trained to a high level of efficiency in some skills, but few are capable of an independent existence.

2. *Trisomy* (*the XXX syndrome*). It will be recalled that the sex chromosomes in the female are referred to as XX (eusomy). In this condition there is an extra sex chromosome resulting in XXX. From studies done so far it is estimated that this state is found in about 1 per cent of subnormal females. The severity of the subnormality varies.

3. *Trisomy-XY* (*XXY Klinefelter's syndrome*). Again it will be recalled that the sex chromosomes in the male are referred to as XY (eusomy). In Klinefelter's syndrome there is an extra X chromosome giving rise to an XXY arrangement. It will be readily deduced that such a person will be more female than male, and this is what happens. The subject is infertile with small genitalia, he may have breasts (gynaecomastia) and is mentally subnormal.

4. *The Cat Cry syndrome.* Unlike the syndromes just mentioned, which are due to an extra piece of chromosome, this one is due to a piece being missing. A piece of chromosome 5 is missing and the clinical effects are an unusual mewing cat-like cry, hence the name, and severe mental subnormality.

C. INTRA-UTERINE HAZARDS. Nature provides an ideal environment for the developing embryo. Within the uterus it is well protected from temperature changes, physical injury and other environmental stresses. The nutritional requirements are brought via the umbilical cord and placenta and the waste products are removed by the same route. There are however a number of intra-uterine hazards which can interfere with the development, particularly in the first three months.

1. *Nutritional problems.* Anaemia in the mother may severely deprive the developing embryo or foetus of vital nutrients and lead to permanent damage. Nature sees that the needs of the child are met, even at the expense of the mother's health.

2. *Inadequate oxygen.* The brain either in the intra-uterine stage or afterwards, has a high oxygen demand. Any condition that interferes with the supply of oxygen to this infant may result in permanent brain damage. Experiments have been carried out to increase the oxygen supply to the developing embryo with the object of improving the infant's intelligence, but the results so far are not conclusive.

3. *Circulatory failure.* The developing infant may have a circulatory problem which deprives the brain of an adequate blood supply. For example a blood clot can result in serious brain damage.

4. *Drugs and poisons.* Rapidly growing cells, as in the case of the embryo in the first twelve weeks, are particularly vulnerable to the effects of drugs and poisons. For this reason mothers are advised not to take any form of medication during pregnancy, especially in the early days. The thalidomide tragedy is an example of what can happen.

5. *Infections.* Like drugs and poisons infections can have equally tragic results. The following are some of the infections which can occur:

a. Rubella (German measles). In ordinary circumstances this virus injection is relatively mild, but in a pregnant mother it can have disastrous effects on the infant. If a mother develops this infection during pregnancy there is a 50–50 chance that the infant will have one or more deformities which may include congenital heart defects, deafness, deaf-mutism as well as mental subnormality.

b. Syphilis. This infection passes from the mother through the placental circulation and may affect various parts of the embryo or may concentrate in the brain and meninges. There are recognizable stigmata associated with congenital syphilis which include a saddle-back nose, Hutchinson's teeth and scabbard-like tibia. The subject may be blind or deaf or both. The degree of mental subnormality varies.

c. Toxoplasmosis. This is a pathogenic protozoa carried by birds, rodents, dogs and cats. It is transmitted to the embryo by the infected mother and affects the brain causing calcification resulting in epilepsy, and sometimes hydro or microcephaly. The degree of mental subnormality may be severe.

d. Erythroblastosis foetalis (kernicterus). This condition is caused by rhesus incompatibility on the part of the parents. About 85 per cent of the population are described as Rh-positive and the remaining 15 per cent are Rh-negative. If a Rh-negative woman marries a Rh-positive father, there is a strong possibility that Rh-agglutinins will develop in her blood during the pregnancy and these may enter the foetal bloodstream, via the placenta. A child so affected is born with very severe jaundice due to the wholesale destruction of its red blood corpuscles. The brain and basal ganglia are usually heavily stained by bile pigments and this gives rise to lesions of the nervous system and severe mental subnormality. The serious effects of this condition can be averted by its early recognition and then by carrying out an exchange transfusion of blood.

9.5 Perinatal

There are a number of things which can occur at the time of birth and can affect the intellect of the child.

1. *Prematurity.* Mental subnormality is often, though not always, associated with prematurity and the risk is greater for an infant of seven months gestation than one of eight months.

2. *Caesarian section.* Some babies cannot be born in the ordinary way; there are many reasons for this and one may be that the mother has an exceptionally small pelvis. When the baby is removed by means of an operation, the operation is called a caesarian section. There is a risk that children brought into the world this way may be mentally subnormal.

3. *Forceps delivery.* It sometimes happens that whilst a caesarian section may not be necessary, the mother may need help with the birth of her baby. Using instruments to provide such help is called a forceps delivery. The instruments are applied to the baby's head and whilst great care is taken to avoid injury there is obviously a risk of brain damage. Such damage could result in cerebral palsy.

4. *Anoxia.* Anoxia means without oxygen and it is a serious state which may be due to a twisted umbilical cord, anaesthesia or a protracted labour. It results in serious brain damage which may be manifested by cerebral palsy or epilepsy as well as severe mental subnormality. It has been observed that the degree of mental handicap is out of proportion to the physical one.

9.6 Post natal

A child may be born with a normal intellect, but if subjected to certain hazards in the period after birth, the post natal period, mental subnormality may occur. The principal post natal hazards are:

1. *Infections.*

a. Encephalitis. This is a general inflammation of the brain which may be caused by a variety of micro-organisms, either bacteria or viruses. Some forms of encephalitis respond to antibiotics and leave no after effects. Others give rise to encephalitis lethargica which is accompanied by a form of Parkinson's disease. There is also mental subnormality which is more severe in the younger child.

b. Meningitis. This is an inflammation of the meninges which may be caused by a variety of organisms, but most commonly it is caused by meningococcus or mycobacterium tuberculosis. A child with meningitis usually has severe cerebral irritation and the associated meningeal cry is very distressing. The efficacy of antibiotic treatment means that meningitis rarely causes serious after effects now, but when it does there is likely to be hydrocephalus and very severe mental subnormality.

2. *Poisons.* Infants are susceptible to poisons in intra-uterine life and they are equally susceptible once they are born. Lead is particularly damaging to brain tissue and is found in paints and lead toy soldiers. The effect takes some time to show itself because it is dependent on the accumulation of large quantities in the bloodstream. As mentioned earlier there is treatment available, but the best thing to do is not to buy paint containing lead or lead soldiers, for children will insist on putting things in their mouths.

3. *Endocrine disorders.* The baby inherits from its mother supplies of some of its requirements for the first six months of life, and this includes a supply of hormones. In the meantime the baby's own glands should begin to supplement such stores and later take over the function completely. If for some reason the baby's thyroid gland fails to function, there will be a lack of the thyroid hormone, necessary for growth, in the bloodstream resulting in physical and mental stunting. This condition is called cretinism.

Cretinism or hypothyroidism is endemic in certain parts of the world such as in Derbyshire, Switzerland and in the Rocky Mountain areas of North America. The overall appearance of a cretin is one of stunted growth, rough dry hair and skin, a large tongue and frequently nose or eye infections. The overall expression is one of dullness. The abdomen may be distended and there may be an umbilical hernia. There is severe mental subnormality and in addition some cretins are deaf and dumb.

The treatment for this condition is replacement of the thyroid hormone usually in the form of thyroid extract. If the condition is diagnosed in the first months of life, and before the sixth, then the outlook is excellent and subnormality does not occur. Treatment must be continued for life.

4. *Demyelinating diseases.* The most common demyelinating disease is multiple or disseminated sclerosis, which affects adults, but there is a pathologically similar disease, called Schilder's disease, and this produces mental subnormality.

5. *Leukodystrophy.* This condition, which is thought to be hereditary, causes degeneration of the white matter of the brain. The onset

of the disease begins at about 18 months or 2 years and is accompanied by epilepsy and severe mental subnormality.

6. *Injury.* A brain injury occurring in the post natal period can affect the intelligence and result in subnormality.

9.7 Observation of the subnormal

1. *Appearance.* Many of the mentally subnormal are recognizably so. They have dull vacant looks and many have anatomical defects such as a big or a very small head. Their dress is likely to be dirty and untidy. High grade subnormals may have nothing about their appearance to indicate subnormality.

2. *Conversation.* The conversation of high grade subnormals may be normal but limited. In others it is likely to be childish, self-centred and incoherent. The severely subnormal are unable to communicate.

3. *Mood.* Some subnormal people are quite happy and cheerful, those with Down's syndrome are an example, but very often the prevailing mood is one of apathy.

4. *Attitude.* Behaviour disorders do occur but many subnormals are co-operative and dependent. Some are totally withdrawn.

5. *Intellect.* The intellect is always impaired. Insight, judgement and reasoning are either defective or non-existent. On the other hand memory is sometimes good.

6. *Eating.* The eating habits are often poor and there may be indifference towards food, or alternatively there may be excessive eating.

7. *Sleep.* Sleep may be normal or it may be restless and noisy.

8. *Physical state.* Physical deformity is often present and growth is usually stunted. The skin and hair is often coarse and the hair may be sparse. The severely subnormal are usually incontinent of urine and faeces, though the high grade may be completely continent.

9. *Group activities.* High grade subnormal people will readily participate in group activities and appear to enjoy them. As the degree of subnormality increases in severity, there is a corresponding decrease in activity. Many tasks in the occupational/industrial therapy are suitable for the moderately retarded as well as the high grade.

10. *Response to treatment.* Treatment is aimed at making the most of the available intellectual function and consists of cultivating

an acceptable level of social behaviour and developing a work habit. The more severely handicapped often have poor muscular co-ordination so that the main effort is concentrated on gaining and maintaining bowel and bladder control by habit training.

9.8 Helping parents

'Will my baby be all right?' is a question which frequently crosses the minds of expectant mothers, and perhaps fathers too. When it is discovered that the baby is subnormal, this comes as a profound shock. The doctor is responsible for telling the parents, but there is much that the nurse can do. This calls for psychiatric first aid of a very high order, but the approach used will depend on the circumstances of each individual case. The initial reaction is one of outright rejection, but later the subnormal child is often accepted and more care may be given to him than a normal child.

9.9 Home care

From the numbers given earlier it will be seen that many subnormal people are cared for at home. This is the best arrangement, for institutions, however well run, tend to have undesirable effects on their residents. For home care to be successful there must be adequate social, welfare and voluntary help for the parents. However well motivated, caring for a subnormal child can be a demanding and tiring job and parents should be relieved occasionally for holidays. This can be achieved by arranging for short-term admissions to hostel or hospital.

Subnormal children grow up and become adults, but with a mind of a child. This poses problems, for parents may find it difficult to control the aggressive and destructive behaviour which occurs. The other problem is that the physical effort involved may affect the parents' health and so make them incapable of carrying out the task of caring, thus making admission to hospital inevitable.

9.10 Education and training

Borderline subnormal people can read and write and generally find their way in the world, though their judgements and reasoning are likely to be faulty and thus they are vulnerable to exploitation. Those with a more severe mental handicap are unlikely to be able to read and write, or only in a very limited fashion. Education for them includes exercises to enable them to tell the time and to use money.

At this level of training it is more appropriate to develop any aptitude or skill which may exist.

9.11 Residential care

Local authorities provide residential care in hostels when home care is not possible. This may be on a short term basis to ease the burdens on parents or it may be on a more permanent basis. If home care is not possible it seems that hostel care is the second best thing.

9.12 Hospital care

Admission to hospital in many cases is inevitable because of parental rejection, inadequate hostel facilities and severe physical disabilities or behaviour disorders which cannot be treated elsewhere. Long periods spent in hospital often result in institutionalization. For this reason it is important to have as purposeful and as dynamic a programme as possible for the mentally subnormal.

9.13 Legal aspects

There are a number of Acts of Parliament concerned with the mentally subnormal. The 1944 Education Act is concerned with the educational aspects. The Children's Act 1948 and subsequent Amendments makes provisions for children, is operated by the Children's Officer at a practical level, and sometimes includes Guardianship. The majority of the mentally subnormal are admitted to hospital informally, 95 per cent or more are admitted in this way. The remaining minority are admitted under the terms of the appropriate section of the 1959 Mental Health Act. (There is also the Children and Young Persons Act 1969.)

9.14 The mentally subnormal and marriage

Society does not look favourably on marriages between subnormal persons for the obvious risk of increasing the subnormal population. Moreover they are generally not good citizens, they are sexually promiscuous and would have more children than they could support. Their work record is not good and some engage in criminal activities. Because of their lack of stability there is a high incidence of broken marriages. Poor husbandry affects the children and increases the work of the Children's Department of the local authority. Despite this, the marriages of some subnormal people are successful.

9.15 Prevention

We have seen that genetic and chromosomal factors are major contributors in the causation of mental subnormality. The state of genetic knowledge is such that it can be fairly accurately forecast what the chances are of a subnormal child being born to prospective parents. This is very important to parents with one subnormal child who are contemplating having another child. Advice on these matters, usually called Genetic Counselling, is increasingly available to those who seek it and is likely to make an important contribution in this field of health education.

9.16 Summary of subnormality

Mental subnormality is a big problem with infinite clinical variations, enormous social ramifications and considerable human suffering and misery, especially on the part of parents. But the picture is not wholly black, for many subnormal people have a loving nature and form rewarding relationships with their parents and nurses. Many have an aptitude for a particular job and can be trained to a high level of efficiency. The increasing knowledge of genetics and the development of genetic counselling are likely to make important contributions in reducing this problem in the future.

DEMENTIA

9.17 Our senior citizens

We have more senior citizens in our society than ever before and this is due to the fact that more people are living their full life span. This is the effect of improved medical and welfare services and not to any increase in the life span.

9.18 Number of elderly people

There are a considerable number of elderly people in the community. It has been estimated that 1 in 7 of the population or about 15 per cent, are over 65 years. In round figures this is something of the order of 7,000,000. Many of course are completely self sufficient and require little or nothing from the health and welfare services. Others receive help in the following ways. There are about 1,500 local old people's welfare committees in the country with the object of assisting the work of statutory authorities and voluntary organizations in caring

for old people. There are 100 voluntary homes with about 5,500
beds and many are occupied by the elderly. 1,200 registered nursing
homes provide 18,700 beds and again many are occupied by the
elderly. The National Health Service provide over 60,000 geriatric
beds in purpose-built geriatric units or in the geriatric wards attached
to general hospitals. It is estimated that about 200,000 of the elderly
suffer from dementia and approximately 40,000 of these are receiving
in-patients' treatment in psychiatric hospitals at any time.

9.19 Dementia

The intellectual powers often, but not always, fail in the elderly.
A certain amount of forgetfulness is accepted, but when there is an
exceptional degree of forgetfulness resulting in confusion and wandering, then the person is considered to have dementia. We shall now
consider presenile dementia.

9.20 Presenile dementia

There are a number of conditions of the brain which affect intellectual
function in the adult years and before the ageing process begins.

1. *Alzheimer's disease.* In this condition, which occurs in the fifth
decade, there is a wasting (atrophy) of the brain in the frontal and
parietal regions, though the whole brain may be affected. The
furrows (sulci) between the convolutions are considerably widened
and degenerative plaques are found in the affected areas. The disease
which was described by Alzheimer in 1907 is more common in
males than the female: male ratio is about 2:1. The onset of the
disease is gradual, but in the later stages there is a severe degree
of dementia.

2. *Pick's disease.* This disease was originally described by Arnold
Pick (1851–1924) in 1892. As in Alzheimer's disease there is atrophy
of the brain which is more localized and is found in the frontal or
temporal lobes. In the later stages of the disease there is a considerable degree of dementia.

3. *Huntington's chorea.* This is a degenerative disease of the nervous system which is due to a dominant genetic defect. Its main
features are choreiform movements and dementia. There is atrophy
of the brain, particularly in the frontal ridges (gyria) and the ventricles of the brain are usually enlarged. Degeneration of the basal
ganglia occurs and this accounts for the unco-ordinated movements.

The onset of the disease, usually in the third or fourth decade, is slow and may be characterized by choreiform movements or mental changes. Later on, both features are present and the dementia is severe.

The treatment is symptomatic. Chlorpromazine reduces the choreiform movements and controls mental symptoms as well, but of course it does not affect the dementia.

4. *Arteriosclerosis.* In some people, as they grow older the blood vessels, including the blood vessels of the brain, become steadily narrower due to the presence of atheromatous plaques. The reason for these plaques is not fully explained but their presence is always associated with an above normal concentration of cholesterol in the bloodstream and raised blood pressure or both. The blood vessels thus affected with arteriosclerosis lose their elasticity and become rigid. It follows that the tissues supplied by these blood vessels will receive less nutrients and less oxygen. Thus function is impaired and there may be a loss of cells.

There is a wide age distribution for arteriosclerosis and a number of cases have been known in the late 30s and 40s, but the more usual age of onset is 55 years and afterwards. As would be expected, the highest incidence for this condition occurs in the 70 to 80 age group.

Cerebral arteriosclerosis can be diagnosed by examining the blood vessels of the fundi of the eyes. Instead of the normal red appearance the fundal blood vessels appear like strands of white thread. Cerebral arteriosclerosis accounts for a number of the cases of presenile dementia.

5. *Infections.* We have seen earlier that infections can cause mental subnormality, but they can also affect the intellect of the older person and cause dementia.

a. Ear infections. In the days before antibiotics, it was not unusual for a middle-ear infection to spread to the mastoid process and from here to the brain giving rise to a brain abscess. Brain damage followed which often gave rise to epilepsy and dementia. Fortunately this sequence of events is now rare.

b. Encephalitis and meningitis. These infections can cause brain damage in the adult and thus presenile dementia, but with improved treatment and management this rarely happens.

c. Syphilis. This is an infection caused by a spirochaete called the treponema pallidum which is transmitted at sexual intercourse. We have already mentioned how an infected mother can pass on the disease to her child. As a result the child is mentally subnormal. The infection, if untreated, follows a predictable course in adults. Primary and secondary lesions occur but they cause little constitutional upset and quickly clear up. The tertiary syphilis may not appear for up to ten years. Tertiary syphilis may affect any system of the body, but when it affects the brain it is called General Paralysis of the Insane (G.P.I.). In G.P.I. the weight of the brain is much less than usual. The meninges are thickened and there is atrophy of the cerebral convolutions, particularly in the frontal and parietal regions.

There are a number of physical signs including slurred speech, characteristic pupils known as Argyll Robertson pupils, muscular inco-ordination and sometimes convulsions.

On the mental side there is gross memory disturbance, the mood is often grandiose and euphoric and the person may believe, when actually penniless, that he has unbounded wealth, is related to Royalty or is a world famous general or politician. Such beliefs when obviously false are called delusions and because of their expansive nature these particular ones are called delusions of grandeur.

Syphilitic infections respond well to antibiotics such as penicillin, but any brain damage caused cannot be reversed.

6. *Poisons.* These can have two effects on the brain. First they may produce immediate and florid physical and mental symptoms or secondly they may have long term effects which take some time to appear. Alcohol comes into both categories. In the long term it produces the condition known as Korsakoff's syndrome. This was first described in 1887 by the Russian psychiatrist Sergei Korsakoff (1854–1900). It is due to chronic alcoholism and its main features are disorientation, unusual suggestibility, confabulation and polyneuritis. There is usually a considerable degree of presenile dementia.

7. *Head injury.* This can cause presenile dementia depending on the degree of injury. Very often epilepsy follows injury and if the frontal lobe is involved there may be muscular clumsiness and unco-ordination of voluntary movement. People with moderate frontal lobe damage have no control over their temper and fly into a rage at the slightest provocation. Severe injury of the frontal lobe results in complete apathy and inactivity.

8. *Brain tumours.* Primary lesions of the brain are not common, though it is often affected with secondary ones. Mental changes may be the first sign of a tumour. There may be vague symptoms, forgetfulness and poor concentration. Hallucinations, other than

auditory ones, may be present. Some such tumours respond to surgery and thus the mental deterioration is halted. Others do not and the dementia is steadily progressive.

9.21 Senile dementia

Two principal factors operate in this condition. We mentioned earlier that the highest incidence of arteriosclerosis is found in the 70–80 year group and this contributes to the deterioration of intellectual function. Secondly there is the ageing process. There are two principal aspects to this process. First there is the loss of cells which is continuous and whose effect obviously increases with the years. This is the quantitative aspect, but there is also the qualitative one. The cells no longer function as well as they might. The combination of these, and other factors, has the effect of slowing down psychomotor activity and there is impairment of short term memory. The result is that such people cannot recognize once familiar objects or people and become disorientated for time, place and person. Dreams are not separated from the waking state and the person lives in a dream world in which dreams are mixed with reality. The sleep rhythm is upset and there may be delusions and hallucinations as well as confusion. The mood is often variable and there may be depression and tears. Behaviour is also affected and there may be aggression stemming from the great insecurity and bewilderment. Standards of hygiene and eating habits become poor.

9.22 Observation of the senile

1. *Appearance.* The general appearance of the senile person is a vacant and dreamy one often with a suspicious outlook on life. The dress is likely to be dirty and untidy. Shoes and socks may be mismatched and there may be absence of a tie in men. Women may also neglect their dress and not use make-up.

2. *Conversation.* This is scanty and may be childish. It is very self-centred and may be incoherent. It is sometimes abusive and may be accusative or may reflect delusions and hallucinations.

3. *Mood.* The mood may vary between inappropriate sadness and happiness, but there is frequent apathy.

4. *Attitude.* The prevailing attitude may vary from a suspicious and demanding one, to one of withdrawal or dependency.

5. *Intellect.* Intellectual function is always impaired and the mental

reactions are slow. There is usually little or no insight and judgement and reasoning are defective. Memory for recent events is extremely poor, but facts of childhood and youth are vividly remembered so that the person's conversation is several decades out of date. Orientation is poor or non-existent so that the person cannot appreciate time, place or person and this leads to bewilderment.

6. *Eating habits.* The appetite may be very poor or the person may have an enormous appetite and consequent overweight. Accepted table manners are often non-existent and the senile person may clear the plates of his neighbours as well as his own. There is often muscular inco-ordination with the result that food and drink is likely to be spilled on the table, the clothing and the floor. It is extremely important to see that such people have an adequate intake of nutrients and fluid. Old people's cells break down more quickly than those of younger people, therefore the elderly have an increased need for protein foods because more wear and tear takes place.

7. *Sleep.* This is often disturbed, but the disturbance varies with the degree of dementia. Very demented people may sleep for up to 16 of the 24 hours. Others, who may appear not too demented during the day, become restless and noisy at night and sometimes get up and wander off. Such people have a disturbing influence on the ward at night and mild hypnotics may be needed.

8. *Physical state.* The physical state may vary from emaciation due to malnutrition and neglect, to over-weight from excessive eating. The elderly often present with multiple symptoms:

a. Nervous system. In addition to insomnia there may be headaches, deafness, visual and sensory defects. The sense of taste is also less acute and many old people complain that food, milk, beer and the like do not taste as they used to.

b. Cardiovascular system. The blood pressure is often raised and the extra strain on the heart often causes it to fail. This results in breathlessness (dyspnoea) and blueness of the skin (cyanosis). Exercise tolerance is low and the person is unlikely to climb a flight of stairs without a rest or rests. Fluid collects in the tissues and causes swelling at the ankles and sometimes the buttocks—oedema. Because of the oedema the skin breaks easily and heals slowly. The heart failure responds to drugs such as Digitalis and the oedema to diuretics such as Mersalyl or Lasix.

c. Respiratory system. Bronchitis and emphysema are common in the elderly and give most trouble in the winter months. Pneumonia is also a common condition in the elderly.

d. Digestive system. Digestive upsets are common in the elderly. The appetite may be poor or excessive and the absorption of nutrients may be defective. There is also difficulty in eliminating waste products from the bowel so that constipation occurs. On the other hand there may be uncontrolled elimination of the stools—incontinence.

e. Urinary system. If there is heart failure, the output of urine is likely to be less than normal. A careful record must be kept so that the output does not drop below an unacceptably low level without being noticed. If there is incontinence of stools, there is often an accompanying infection of the bladder—cystitis. If the infection travels upwards and affects the pelvis of the kidney it causes pyelitis and if the whole of the kidney is involved the result is pyelonephritis. In such infections the urine smells 'fishy', there may be nausea and vomiting and the body temperature is raised. In pyelonephritis the raised temperature may cause shivering which, in severe cases may resemble a convulsion and is called a rigor. In many men the prostate gland enlarges and obstructs the outflow of urine and thus causes retention of urine which usually needs surgery to correct it. In both sexes the bladder sphincter muscles become inefficient and urine passes out uncontrolled—urinary incontinence.

f. Musculo-skeletal system. There is a high incidence of osteo-arthritis and rheumatoid arthritis among the elderly and this causes them much pain and also impedes locomotion. The bones may become softer than usual (osteomalacia) or less dense (osteoporosis). Because of these changes in the bone and because the elderly tend to be unsteady on their feet, there is a high risk of fractured bones.

g. Temperature control. In recent years it has been observed that many old people have abnormally low body temperatures—hypothermia. In the management of old people two things should be borne in mind in relation to temperature. There should always be thermometers available for recording temperatures well below the normal range. The lower point on a centrigrade clinical thermometer is 34·8 °C, but if such a reading is obtained it should be checked with a subnormal thermometer graduated to record temperature of 30 °C or below. Extra clothes should be provided and the heating arrangements should be adequate.

h. New growths. The incidence of new growths, both benign and malignant, is high among the elderly and this should be borne in mind by anyone caring for them. A persistent cough, a chest infection

8

which fails to clear up, weight loss, appetite loss, alteration of the bowel habit, blood in the urine must all be looked upon with suspicion and should be reported to the doctor immediately.

9.23 Home care

Most people prefer to end their days in the familiar surroundings of their own home and where possible this should be the aim. If the old person is living alone, then much help will be needed to achieve this aim. Support will be needed from the statutory social and welfare services and help will also be needed from voluntary bodies. Home helps, meals-on-wheels and voluntary visitors all contribute towards making the old person's life livable.

9.24 Purpose built flats

Some local authorities provide purpose built flats and maisonettes for elderly people. These are designed with the daily living needs of old people in mind.

9.25 Hostel care

This is also provided for those unable to manage a house of their own, but who are able to manage with a minimum of supervision and require little or no nursing care. Such hostels are made to look as much like homes and as little like hospitals as possible. Residents are encouraged to keep personal belongings and treasures.

9.26 Hospital care

The degree of dementia may in many cases make admission to hospital inevitable. When this happens the tendency is to allow the person to keep as many familiar objects as possible, though it must be recognized that some may be lost or misplaced.

A settled but varied routine in hospital gives the older person security. The tendency is to encourage these people to get up and about, for prolonged bed rest gives rise to muscular weakness, and increased risk of circulatory thrombosis and chest infections, and also an increased risk of fractures of the bones occurring due to the excessive losses of calcium from the bones.

Incontinence is often a problem and this can be solved or improved by a vigorous habit-training programme. There are many ways of approaching this and one is to have one nurse responsible for a small group of patients and meeting the group's needs. If a regular pattern of taking the person to the lavatory is established and maintained, then people who have previously been continuously incontinent show much improvement.

Dentures are a continual problem in geriatric work. They are frequently lost or mislaid and bearing this in mind, a system of marking by which they can be identified is essential. It is better to have a system of marking the dentures themselves rather than marking containers which are likely to become mixed up.

The overall programme for the elderly should be a fairly dynamic one. Apart from habit training there should be occupational therapy suited to the individual's needs and capabilities. There should be short walks, suitable recreational activities and social events like dances and tea parties.

9.27 Prevention

The march of time cannot be halted, therefore there is no way of preventing old age, though things like monkey glands and a substance called H.3. have been said to have an effect on the ageing process; their efficacy have yet to be proved. What can be modified are the effects of ageing and this is done by preparation for retirement. It is often the case that when someone whose whole life has been his job retires, the person becomes apathetic, careless and aimless. Conversely when people with many interests and hobbies outside work retire, they continue to function well intellectually and physically and generally enjoy life.

Preparation for retirement should begin about ten years beforehand and before it is too late to develop new interests. Such preparation can take place as part of the employer's welfare service for employees. Alternatively many of the courses run by evening institutes and similar places are suitable for this purpose. A big problem in any such programme of health education is to establish where the need lies, but when this is established the problem of motivating those in most need remains.

9.28 Summary of old age

Dementia presents a sizable problem with physical, mental and social dimensions, but it is merely part of the larger problem of old age. Planned programmes for retirement and efficient management of their potential resources can add fullness and meaning to the waning years of our senior citizens.

10

Fear and anxiety

10.0 Introduction

This chapter could be called 'The Neuroses' or 'Neurotic Reactions', but the present one has been chosen to keep in front of the reader's eye the fact that fear and anxiety is the central factor in the conditions under consideration. Fear is something which must have been felt at one time or another and it is also a subject on which many people have expounded. Edmund Burke (1729–1749) wrote: 'No passion so effectively robs the mind of all its powers of acting and reasoning as fear'. Approaching the subject from another viewpoint Franklin D. Roosevelt (1882–1945), the American President during World War II, in 1941 included the freedom from fear as one of the four essential freedoms.

10.1 Incidence

Fear and anxiety is the most common mental disorder, though it is not possible to give precise numbers. It has been estimated that about 5 per cent of the population or over 2,500,000 people suffer illnesses involving fear and anxiety. Most of such people are treated at home or as outpatients and the number is hospital at any one time is about 5,000.

10.2 The nature of fear and anxiety

Anxiety is a universal and an unpleasant experience which occurs in response to a stimulus which threatens the integrity of the person and involves the physical and psychological sides of life. There are two principal sources of such stimuli. First there are those arising outside the person (*exogenous*) and include things such as examinations, interviews, financial difficulties and bereavement. All these factors act as stresses and these stresses set up a state of tension in the person. Other exogenous factors are frustration which may arise from an inferiority complex, expecting too much from oneself, being unsuited to a job or failure. These enter consciousness in a similar manner to a drive and give rise to free-floating anxiety.

The second source of stimuli is the person's unconscious mind. When we considered the mental mechanisms we saw that some experiences are banished from consciousness but may still continue to affect behaviour. Unpleasant childhood experiences and guilt feelings particularly about sexual matters, are often repressed. Stresses arising in this way from within are said to be *endogenous* and cause a state of conflict. Fear and anxiety are always associated with states of conflict.

An anxiety reaction depends on two things. It depends on the nature of the stress and the nature of the material tested. We mentioned earlier that some people can withstand considerable pain whilst others have a low pain tolerance. A similar state of affairs exists with anxiety and there is great variety in individual tolerance. When an anxiety reaction occurs it may be of the passive or active variety. In passive anxiety the person becomes 'frozen' or 'paralysed' with fear and breathing temporarily slows or stops and the heart rate is slowed (tachycardia). Active anxiety reactions result in the fight/flight reactions and large quantities of adrenaline are released. There is panic and the muscular tension is increased, the heart and respiratory rates are also increased and sweating occurs. The person in a state of mental tension is unable to relax, worries and frets over small things and tends to turn mole-hills into mountains. Memory is impaired, concentration is poor, the thinking process is upset (cannot think straight), the mind goes round in circles and there is insomnia.

Everything about fear and anxiety is not on the debit side, for there is no doubt that it serves a useful protective function by preventing reckless behaviour. The fear of failure at examinations stimulates the intense revision which usually takes place before such events. In competitive games the tension built up before an important race, has the effect of mobilizing the body's resources beforehand and thus adds to the performance. It seems a reasonable thing to fear present dangers and to take avoiding action, and it seems an intelligent thing to be concerned or to worry over possible future dangers. It is when fear and anxiety about the present or worry about the future gets out of proportion and dominate the person's whole life that mental health is threatened. We shall now consider some of the principal fear and anxiety reactions.

10. Anxiety neurosis

This is often a free-floating type of anxiety though sometimes it may be of a fixed nature. Mentally the person has what is generally called an anxious personality and is tense, timid, self-doubting and worries a lot. Such a person sets very high standards and there is usually a gap between expectation and achievement. This achievement gap gives rise to insecurity and a sense of inferiority. Concentration is poor and there is absentmindedness and insomnia and an exceptional degree of fatigue.

On the physical side the symptoms are often varied and many. There may be dizziness, headaches, a feeling that one's head is about to burst open, muscular weakness, tremors, blurring of the vision and ringing in the ears (tinnitus). The heart is often involved and there may be heart pains, palpitations and a fear that the heart is about to stop. There may be respiratory difficulty and the person cannot get a full breath and pants for air. The digestive system is often affected and there may be nausea, water-brash, constipation or diarrhoea. There may be frequency of urine or stress incontinence. It will readily be seen that these free-floating anxieties have diffuse physical and psychological effects.

The causes of anxiety neurosis and fear and anxiety reactions generally are many, but it seems a big number fall within one of three categories, though the picture is often a mixed one:

1. *Heredity*. There is often an inherited predisposition towards such reactions.

2. *Morbid family environment*. This means an unhappy home during the person's period of development. There may be rows and quarrels between the parents, or, there may be separation because of employment circumstances or because of a marital rift and thus a broken home. The home conditions may be such that the family lives on its nerves and staggers from one crisis to another. Members may over respond to stresses, the so-called 'flap-responses'.

3. *Predisposing factors*. These are any of the everyday stresses which we have mentioned before such as domestic unhappiness, poor social adjustment, employment or financial difficulties. Difficulties of sexual matters also contribute and there is a high incidence of mental illness, including anxiety reactions, among sexual deviants.

10.4 Hysterical neurosis

This type of neurosis has two principal components:

1. Dissociative states.
2. Conversion phenomena.

1. DISSOCIATIVE STATES. In these states there is, in the absence of organic brain disease, narrowing of the field of consciousness

which may be limited to one area of experience. The resulting behaviour may appear consistent and is often directed to a goal within that area. Wandering away from home and acting in an automatic fashion and then coming to with a complete loss of memory for the wandering period is a common dissociative reaction and is called a fugue. Other examples of such states are amnesia, multiple personality, sleepwalking and the Ganser syndrome. Amnesia though nearly always associated with a fugue, may however occur on its own. The person loses completely his identity and cannot tell his name or give similar information. We have already referred to the multiple personality phenomenon and 'The Three Faces of Eve' depicted the condition well. Sleep-walking is a fugue-state found in children though it is sometimes found in adults.

The Ganser syndrome was first described by Joseph Maria Ganser (1853–1931) in 1898 and is otherwise known as 'prison psychosis' or the 'syndrome of approximate answers'. This condition has been seen in prisoners awaiting trial. There are reasoning defects and the subject usually claims that he cannot remember. Answers to simple arithmetical questions like adding $2+2$ are always wrong but never very wrong, hence the term 'syndrome of approximate answers'. Common household objects are misidentified, a spoon may be called a knife and so on.

2. CONVERSION PHENOMENA. This means a stress of psychological origin which causes a disturbance of function of an organ or organs of the body. In other words a psychological conflict which may be difficult to express adequately in words, is converted into physical symptoms involving one or more organs of the body. This phenomenon has been observed for a long time and it did not pass the notice of Shakespeare, that astute observer of the human condition for he wrote:

'His flight was madness: when our actions do not
Our fears do make us traitors.'

Macbeth IV iii 22.

Take the plight of the soldier going into battle. If he goes forward into battle he risks being maimed or killed. His state of fear may be such as to make him run away, but then he risks being labelled a coward or possibly shot for desertion. His mind is in a state of conflict based on fear. (Unconsciously) he converts his conflict into physical symptoms by going blind and thus finds a solution to his problem. Conversions may also take the form of paralysis, disturbances of gait, tremors, deafness, epileptiform—seizures and fainting (*syncope*). The mechanism is always unconscious; if it were conscious it would be *malingering*, and it always serves a purpose.

Unlike anxiety neurosis, the anxiety in hysterical neurosis is not free-floating but is much more specific. There are also other differences; the person with hysteria is not obviously worried and may deny worries. On the contrary there may be a distinct air of indifference. The term La belle indifference has been used to describe this typical mental attitude because it has been found in women. The person with a hysterical reaction personality is usually self centred and likes to attract attention. Feelings are shallow; there are no deep emotions and in the case of women there is frigidity in sexual relations. Such people are highly suggestible, but this is a general feature of fear and anxiety reactions.

10.5 Phobic neurosis

The word phobia comes from the Greek phobos and means flight, panic-fear or terror. The ancient Greeks honoured Phobos as a God who could induce fear or panic in their enemies. The condition was also familiar to Shakespeare for in the 'Merchant of Venice' he wrote:

'Some men there are love not a gaping pig;
Some, that are mad if they behold a cat.'

A phobia is. an abnormally intense dread in the presence of an object or situation often amounting to panic. American workers have listed over a hundred phobias and common objects and situations are cited such as cats (ailurophobia) confined spaces (claustrophobia), heights (acrophobia), night (noctophobia), Number 13 (triskaidekaphobia), work (ergophobia) and fear of fear itself (phobophobia).

Sometimes there is a specific phobia, but there may also be free-floating anxiety as well. The person may not seek help or even confess to a phobia, help being sought because of a depression caused by the phobic condition. The tension caused by the phobia is intense and often unbearable and for this reason such people often turn to alcohol and drugs for relief. Cases have been known where the person has had to take alcohol before leaving for work in the morning, further alcohol being needed at ever decreasing intervals to make life livable. Needless to say in such conditions alcohol dependency soon occurs. Phobias can be quite crippling, even to the point of preventing the sufferers from going outside the house let alone going to work. The degree of panic and terror by a person in a phobic situation has such dimensions that it cannot be readily understood by the onlooker.

10.6 Obsessive compulsive neurosis

When we considered the mental mechanism we saw that compulsions serve a useful purpose biologically. Compulsions are a means of controlling anxiety through the repetition of thoughts and acts. The process is of course an unconscious one and occurs in two forms:

1. Obsessional thoughts or ruminations.
2. Obsessional acts (compulsions).

1. OBSESSIONAL THOUGHTS OR RUMINATIONS. When there are obsessional thoughts or ruminations it is usually impossible to reach a decision over the simplest of matters because there is persistent doubting and the problem has to be considered from so many aspects. For example a simple decision to see a friend a short distance away may involve consideration of whether it is safe to leave the house as it might be burgled. There are dangers in travelling, the bus might not run or there may be an accident and there is danger in crossing a busy road. The distance may be considered too long to walk and anyway it might rain. Their friend may not be in, may be busy, may have other visitors or may want to go out. Coming home also presents problems, the street lights may fail and so it goes on. Other doubts may revolve around whether the gas taps have been turned off, or the doors locked or whether an appointment has been forgotten. These ruminations make life very difficult if not impossible. For people in managerial or executive positions whose functions are to make decisions they can be crippling.

2. OBSESSIONAL ACTS (COMPULSIONS). These vary a great deal from the normally accepted fidgeting in the dentist's waiting room to very elaborate rituals. These rituals include repeated washing which is thought to be due to repressed guilt feelings. The subject has to wash repeatedly and finds, after spending considerable time over the exercise, a speck of dirt in the wash-basin or bath. Now these objects have to be cleaned and the whole ritual has to be repeated. The house-

wife may have to do the washing-up several times or makes the beds many times over before being satisfied with the result. Considerable time is wasted and the housewife becomes more and more behind with the work, she also becomes fatigued from the needless repetition of such acts and plays the role of wife and mother very inefficiently and thus the problems increase.

The majority of people with obsessive compulsions are intelligent people who fully realize the absurdity of their actions. Many try to resist doing these compulsive rituals but find that the effort required to resist is greater and more exhausting than that used in the rituals. This should be borne in mind when nursing such people, for stating the obvious does not help much and only adds to a sensitive person's problem.

Obsessive compulsions may occur as a separate clinical entity but such compulsions may be found in other conditions such as endogenous depression, schizophrenia and mental disorders arising out of physical lesions such as encephalitis.

10.7 Depressive neurosis (reactive depression)

When there is a state of prolonged and profound sadness of such a degree as to make the person ill, this is said to be depression. In this condition the person's mood is primarily involved and this will be considered in a later chapter. There is one type of depression, *depressive neurosis* which is sometimes known as reactive depression, which is considered as a fear and anxiety reaction. In a depressive neurosis there is always an external (exogenous) precipitating factor to which the person reacts. As usual in fear and anxiety reactions there are two principal factors involved. These are the nature of the stress and the strength of the material tested, that is, the nature of the personality. A family bereavement may be a precipitating factor in some cases, though others will react to much more minor stresses.

Depressive neurosis is more common in women than in men and tears are common. Such people have a great feeling of inadequacy and suffer from insomnia and hypochondriasis.

10.8 Neurasthenia

The use of this term has largely been abandoned, for the features associated with it in the past such as lassitude, easy fatiguability irritability, headache and disturbed sleep are also features of other reactions such as depression. The term was commonly used to describe the state of a person following an infection or other physical disease.

10.9 Depersonalization syndrome

This condition is characterized by an unpleasant change in awareness of the external world which takes on a strange or an unreal quality. There may also be feelings of unreality in relation to the person's body and bodily functions may be experienced as automatic or robot-like actions.

This syndrome is most likely to occur in intelligent subjects in the adolescent or early adult period. The onset is often sudden, though there may be a history of poor parent-child relationships. A complete recovery can happen spontaneously and without treatment, apart from supportive treatment. Repeated episodes are likely.

10.10 Hypochondrial neurosis

When a person is convinced that he has a disease, usually a physical one, and when there is no evidence whatever of such a disease, then the person is said to be hypochondriacal. Hypochondriasis is found in many psychiatric illnesses such as depression and schizophrenia. A hypochondriacal neurosis is said to exist when there is a persistent anxious pre-occupation with concern over health in the absence of any other psychiatric illness or syndrome. The condition is frequently formed in the elderly, particularly elderly men, and the person may think that he has a specific illness such as syphilis or cancer or he may present with many and varied symptoms.

10.11 Other neuroses

We shall now mention a few of the more rare neuroses which you may meet in practice.

1. COMPENSATION NEUROSIS. In this condition, as its name suggests, there is a pre-occupation with compensation arising out of accidents.

2. THE COUVADE SYNDROME. This is a rare form of neurosis in which a husband suffers from a variety of symptoms during his wife's pregnancy, including morning sickness, labour pains and actual swelling of the abdomen. The condition usually clears up at the end of the pregnancy.

3. THE MUNCHAUSEN SYNDROME. This is also a relatively rare condition where the subject repeatedly presents himself to hospitals with a convincing set of signs and symptoms with a view to having a surgical operation. Such people, though investigations prove negative, are given the benefit of the doubt by surgeons who carry out operations rather than risk missing a real lesion. The wish for mutilation by surgery is the principal feature of this syndrome. One such person had 13 abdominal operations over 28 years and in the same period she had at least 126 hospital admissions.

10.12 Course of fear and anxiety reactions

This varies a great deal and as mentioned before depends on the nature of the stresses present in the subject's life and the strength of the material tested. It is possible to have a single neurotic reaction in the course of a life-time which is quickly cured and never returns. It is also possible to have repeated episodes at various stages during the person's life-time, but many neurotic reactions last a life-time.

Many of the long lasting neuroses follow a set pattern. The subject is usually suggestible and laps up advice from any source. Because of the mental make up of the subjects any advice given does not stand the test of time and advisers, including medical advisers, are frequently changed. A new adviser is often hailed as the answer to all the subject's problems, but all too soon disenchantment sets in. When the resources of orthodox medical science have been exhausted, then there is recourse to quacks, charlatans and faith healers.

There are a great number, with appropriate support and treatment, who live a fairly full and productive life with only a minimum of inconvenience. In phobic neurosis for example, the person may be able to lead a full life apart from the aspects concerning the phobia. Likewise neurotic depressions quickly respond to treatment.

10.13 Principles of treatment

There are a number of approaches available and the one chosen will depend on the needs of the individual and the training and experience of the particular doctor. For example, if the doctor is Freudian oriented then he is likely to use the psychoanalytic approach and conversely if the emphasis was on the behaviourist approach, then he is more likely to adopt this technique. As already mentioned many adopt appropriate aspects of each method and thus have an eclectic approach:

A. PSYCHOLOGICAL.
  a. Based on psychoanalytic theory.
    1. Psychoanalysis.
    2. Individual psychotherapy.
    3. Group psychotherapy.
  b. Based on behaviourist theory.
    1. Desensitization.
    2. Aversion.
  c. Based on social interpretation of behaviour.
    1. Therapeutic community.

B. CHEMICAL.
  a. Sedatives.
  b. Hypnotics.
  c. Anxiolytic drugs.
    1. Meprobamate.
    2. Chlordiazepoxide (Librium).
    3. Diazepam (Valium).

C. SURGICAL.
  a. Leucotomy.

D. ELECTRICAL.
  a. Electroconvulsive therapy.

E. OCCUPATIONAL.
  a. Occupational/Industrial therapy.
  b. Music, drama or art therapy.

Psychological methods of treatment are likely to be used in all cases and group psychotherapy is perhaps most commonly used. Behaviour therapy is used in the form of desensitization for phobias and in the form of aversions for sexual deviants and various forms of addiction.

Chemicals in the form of drugs are used for most forms of fear and anxiety reactions. There is a danger of dependency arising, particularly dependency on barbiturates.

The use of surgery is limited to cases of obsessional compulsive neurosis which do not respond to the other forms of treatment.

In pure fear and anxiety reactions, electroconvulsive therapy is not indicated but frequently the clinical picture is a mixed one and some doctors may prescribe this form of treatment in such cases.

Some form of occupational or recreational therapy is invaluable in the treatment and rehabilitation of people with neurotic conditions. As always the activity must be carefully chosen to meet the individual's needs.

We have seen that while the incidence of fear and anxiety reactions in the community is high, the number in hospital at any one time is not great. This is a good practice, for such people readily become dependent on hospitals and similar institutions where they have their needs met and are spared the task of having to make decisions. The aim is to treat such people as outpatients or in Day Hospitals in some cases and so keep them circulating in the community. Admission to hospital is reserved for acute crises which cannot be managed any other way and should be as short as possible. Voluntary organizations such as Neurotics Anonymous give much help and play a useful role in supporting the person in the community.

10.14 Observation

1. APPEARANCE. Except in the case of hysterical neurosis, the facial expression is one of fear which may amount to terror in acute form of this illness. Many people with fear and anxiety reactions are meticulous and fastidious about their dress, though in depressive neurosis this is not likely to be so.

2. CONVERSATION. The conversation is often precise and guarded. It may also tend to be monotonous as there is a tendency to repeat what is said so that the hearer does not misunderstand. There is little or no humour in the conversation and this coupled with the pedantic concern over detail makes it heavy going.

3. MOOD. The prevailing mood is that of anxiety and often there is sadness leading to depression. In hysteria of course there is often an air of indifference.

4. ATTITUDE. The person generally wants to be helpful and is often submissive, apologetic and may be withdrawn.

5. INTELLECT. Generally speaking such people are intelligent and have insight, though not necessarily insight in relation to their symptoms. Intense fear and anxiety temporarily impairs intellectual function.

6. EATING. The effect on the appetite varies. When anxious some people over-eat and no doubt this is a factor in some cases of obesity. In others there is a loss of appetite and consequent weight loss.

7. SLEEP. Sleep is often disturbed. There is often difficulty in getting to sleep. When sleep does occur it may be disturbed and often the person wakes up unrefreshed. Hypnotics are often needed.

8. PHYSICAL STATE. The physical state is affected in many ways. There may be weight loss, there may be excessive sweating or there may be nausea, vomiting or diarrhoea. The heart rate may be increased and there may be urinary incontinence or stress incontinence. The menstrual cycle may also be upset.

10.15 Nursing care

The nurse's attitude in relation to fear and anxiety reactions is all important. Many such people are intelligent and sensitive and quickly become attuned to the atmosphere. Much damage can be done by the 'he is only a neurotic attitude'. For the panic and terror experienced by such people is very great indeed and their suffering is certainly no less than that in any other form of illness. An understanding of how such people feel should help to mould the right attitude.

To say 'don't worry' is to add fuel to the fire and almost amounts to an admission of failure on the part of the nurse, for the subject knows full well that it is absurd to worry but is powerless to stop. In order to divert the person from his worries, the nurse should gently alter the course of the conversation to an area of interest outside them. Depending on the person's aptitudes and interests this can often be best done when participating in some occupational or recreational activity.

The nurse will be involved in the patient's treatment, though her position in relation to some of these vary with local practices and have been mentioned in an earlier chapter (6). Particular mention must be made to the question of group dynamics. Many of the people are very sophisticated and this may give rise to a sense of inadequacy in an inexperienced nurse. It is therefore important that all nurses should have a good grounding in group dynamics before becoming involved in group therapy.

Fear and anxiety reactions often produce panic and terror and thus psychiatric first aid situations, with which the nurse may have to cope. Human contact alone can be very helpful in these situations. The nurse should accept that the subject feels great terror and should not try to minimize it or dwell on it. From the first aid point of view it is better to talk around the subject or adopt a diversionary approach: the analysis or the underlying factors must be left to the therapist. The nurse who is faced with such first aid situations should bear in mind the suggestible nature of the subjects and should exercise care in matters of counselling and suggestion so that what are intended as first aid measures are not interpreted as long-term solutions.

10.16 Prevention

This seems a daunting task because of fear and anxiety reactions are a common feature of everyday life and because there are many unanswered questions such as: what are the precise mental mechanisms which produce anxiety and how can they be held in check? Has neurosis a purpose? What is the best child-rearing technique to prevent neuroses in adulthood? Answers to these, and many other such questions, will be found through research and only then will it be possible to adopt a solidly based preventative approach.

10.17 Summary

Fear and anxiety reactions are the most common of mental disorders. They cause considerable distress from illogical and unrelenting emotional tension and present in a variety of clinical types, ranging from the diffuse anxiety neurosis to hysterical neurosis, phobia, obsessions, depression and the depersonalization syndrome to hypochondriasis. Such reactions may be short lived and occur only once, but many are life-long. There are a variety of treatments available and there is considerable help to be offered to such sufferers. As is often the case there are many questions to be answered and these are in the domain of the research workers.

11

Disordered thought (Schizophrenia)

11.0 Introduction

In this chapter we shall consider schizophrenia which is a common mental disorder and accounts for up to 30 per cent of all admissions to psychiatric hospitals.

11.1 Historical

In 1860 Benedict Augustin Morel (1809–73) introduced the term 'demence praecoce'. Emil Kraeplin (1856–1926), who did much work in classifying mental illness, introduced the term 'dementia praecox' in 1898. The next person to look at the problem was Paul Eugen Bleuler (1857–1939). Bleuler accepted Kraeplin's classification of the condition we now call schizophrenia, but he did not accept that it need progress to dementia. He introduced the term 'schizophrenia' from the Greek schizin = to divide, and phren = mind. Usage has given the term an established position, but it is not an accurate descriptive term for as we shall see 'splitting' does not take place, it is rather a fragmentation of mental function, in particular of thinking. In order to understand schizophrenia, an understanding of thinking is necessary, for it is primarily a thought disorder, though, as usual, nearly all facets of mental life are involved.

11.2 Thinking

The ability to think is the most outstanding feature that distinguishes man from other species. Thinking involves planning, talking about and executing a piece of activity and anticipating the outcome. It involves ideas. An idea is a mental image, form or reperseñtation of anything; a notion, a conception, a supposition, a plan, an intention or design and so on. Ideation is a mental activity which does not depend upon sensory and motor contact with the environment. Ideation may be of two sorts:

1. DREAMS AND DAYDREAMS. In dreams and daydreams the ideational activity is not deliberately controlled in any direction, but the sequence and continuity of ideas and images result from their past association together in the person's experience. Dreams are related to the motives and desires of the person; the content of the dream may be a distorted and symbolic expression of motives which the person does not admit even to himself. As we mentioned earlier dreams are a useful safety valve which operate during the sleeping

hours and the mental mechanisms (see Chapter 3) operate in day-dreams and so contribute to mental health.

2. PURPOSIVE THINKING. Purposive thinking is an ideational activity which is controlled and directed towards goals of discovery and invention.

Let us now consider the 'tools' of thinking. The 'tools' of thinking are *concepts*. *Symbols* are objects, expressions or activities which stand for concepts in the absence of the actual items:

1. LANGUAGE SYMBOLS. These are oral or written expressions used in the first place for communication between persons and secondly for ideational activity. Young children often demonstrate the role of language symbols in thinking by talking aloud as they work on a problem. As they grow up they learn to talk by mouthing and later in the adult fashion without any motor activity. Jean Piaget, a Swiss psychologist, has made a study of the thinking process of children and has written much on the subject. If you are interested in this subject, you must read some of his works.

2. DIAGRAMS, MAPS AND MUSICAL SCORES. These are useful symbols to represent complex situations with multiple relationships between the items. For example it is made easier to explain how to find a particular place by using a simple drawing. This is why oral instructions of how to get there are usually so ineffective. From a first right, second left and bear right at the fork explanation, the traveller has no symbolic grasp of the route and consequently gets lost. Insurance companies nearly always request a sketch map when their clients have been involved in road accidents, for a map symbol is superior to language symbols for such situations.

3. CONCEPTS. Concepts are ideas which refer to objects, events or qualities. They are formed by noticing the similarities and differences among items, and learning a word or symbol for each concept. Thus the concept becomes the meaning of the word. A concept may have a number of aspects:

    a. Generalization. This is the mental process of forming a concept of a class of items on the basis of experience with a certain number of instances.

    b. Differentiation. This is the opposing process of making distinctions among the items of a class; of forming two or more concepts out of one.

    c. Abstraction. This is a related process in which some attribute

or characteristic is considered independently of other characteristics or of the object as a whole.

 d. *Principles*. These are relations between concepts, usually
expressed in the form of a short sentence, statements or mathematical equations.

Purposive thinking is used for *solving problems*. Let us now consider
some aspects of this process. Problem solving occurs in new or difficult
situations where a solution is not obtainable by the habitual methods
of applying concepts and principles derived from past experience
in similar situations:

1. GUIDING IDEAS. These determine what kind of attempts will be
made. For example if it is winter time and the car will not start,
the first line of approach may be to look at the battery, for batteries
become run down in cold weather. This is a guiding idea. If all the
attempts arising from a certain guiding idea are fruitless, it is wise to
try a different guiding idea. For example if the battery is functioning
and the car still will not start, the carburettor should be examined,
for fuel supply problems could also prevent the car from starting
and so on.

2. HYPOTHESIS. This is a principle which is invented and applied in
a problem situation in the form of a question and is the basis
of research work. A hypothesis is tested by figuring out its logical
consequence in the situation, trying it out, and observing whether
the predicted results are obtained.

3. INCUBATION PERIOD. This is an interval of time during which
the problem is laid aside after preliminary attempts to solve it have
failed. It implies that the subconscious mind works on the problem
and this is why the advice to 'sleep on it' often works.

4. RATIONAL THINKING. This is similar to trial-and-check behaviour,
but it differs for it is an ideational rather than a motor approach,
and is a planned attack on the problem.

5. LOGICAL THINKING. This involves a consideration of the relevant
data and leads to a correct conclusion by a proper process of
reasoning.

11.3 Disorders of thinking

If the data presented is insufficient, irrelevant or inconsistent then
clear thinking is obviously impossible. The level of intelligence,

tiredness, fatigue, illness, drugs and alcohol all affect the process of thinking. The principal ways it can be affected are:

1. SPEED. The speed may be greatly increased as in mania or very slow as in depression.

2. CONTENT. Ideas may be held which are not in keeping with the person's background and patterns of belief. Such ideas are called delusions.

3. NATURE. There may be an inability to think in the abstract with the result that the thinking becomes vague and woolly as happens in schizophrenia.

11.4 Schizophrenia

Schizophrenia, in its most typical form, consists in a slow deterioration of the entire personality, which often manifests itself at the period of adolescence. It involves a great part of the mental life and expresses itself in disorder of thought, of feeling, and of conduct, and in an increasing withdrawal of interest in the environment. From the above definition we see that schizophrenia affects thought, feeling and conduct. We shall now consider how these are affected.

A. THOUGHT. The thoughts of someone suffering from schizophrenia are vague and woolly. Conversation wanders and there is excessive attention given to irrelevant details. It is usually impossible to follow such a conversation as it is not linked together at all. Sometimes all one hears is a jumble of meaningless words and this is called a 'word salad'. At other times the person produces words of his own and these are called neologisms, for example 'gligling', 'slamham' and 'ragchuck'. As we have seen the person finds abstract thinking difficult. The opposite of abstract thinking is concrete thinking and in schizophrenia there is said to be a concretization of the thought process. This is demonstrated if the person is asked for the meaning of a well-known proverb. For example the meaning given to the proverb 'a burnt child dreads the fire' may be given as 'if a child has been burned by the fire then it will always be afraid of it' rather than the abstract meaning of experience.

In addition to the above thought disorders there may also be *thought blocking*. The person may feel that his thoughts are 'blocked' or held up in some way. There may be poverty of thought, in an intelligent person, and the person may feel that his head is like a vacuum. There is often a long lapse in the conversation or in responding to a question, but almost always a response is eventually made.

Delusions, which are false beliefs that cannot be corrected by an appeal to the reason of the person and are out of keeping with the person's cultural background, are common in schizophrenia. These delusions are sometimes of a wish-fulfilment type though sometimes they may be very frightening. Delusions may be described as primary or secondary. A primary delusion is said to be present when the subject apparently in good health suddenly believes that he is someone important like a King. Secondary delusions have no such sudden onset and are often an attempt by the person to explain his abnormal inner feelings. When a person complains that the rays from the television are affecting his thoughts, that electricity is being passed through his body, that his food is poisoned or that there is a plot to kill or abduct him, he is saying that he feels the world is hostile towards him.

Hallucinations also occur in schizophrenia and are often closely related to the delusional system. An hallucination is a false perception in the absence of any external stimulus. Hallucinations have also been described as inner feelings which are projected and experienced as if they were external perceptions and like delusions they may be wish-fulfilling or frightening. Any of the senses may be involved, but auditory hallucinations (hearing voices) are the most common. The person hears voices which do not belong to anyone about him. These voices are often unkind and may say unpleasant things about the person. Sometimes the person may feel that his thoughts are echoed aloud. At other times the voices may direct or command the person to do something and this accounts for some schizophrenic. behaviour. Visual hallucinations may take the form of distorted and frightening scenes of animals and monsters. A man may appear as half man, half monkey or it may appear that worms are coming out of a subject's eyes. Tactile (touch) hallucinations may occur and take the form of 'creepy-crawlies' crawling all over the body. Gustatory (taste) hallucinations are nearly always unpleasant when they occur. Sometimes visual hallucinations may be very pleasant with a 'bring on the dancing girls' flavour. This is true in some cases of hallucinations induced by drugs such as L.S.D.

B. FEELING (AFFECT). The person suffering from schizophrenia is generally a cold, aloof person with whom it is extremely difficult to make contact and it is often impossible to establish rapport with him. It has been said 'that such people are of us, but not with us'. The capacity for emotional response is greatly reduced and the term 'emotional blunting' is sometimes used to describe the emotional state, for there is neither elation nor depression and the outward appearance is one of indifference or apathy. The person may have lost the capacity to react emotionally, but he may show signs of distress and anxiety, even depression, which are not wholly appropriate. There is thus disharmony between mood and thought and this is sometimes described as incongruity of affect. Sometimes people with schizophrenia have a 'far-away look' which may be due to blunted emotions, but it may also be due to day dreams or hallucinations.

C. CONDUCT. The person's conduct may be affected in several ways:

a. Volition (will-power). This is frequently affected and is sometimes the presenting feature. An example of disordered volition is that the person will not get out of bed and relatives have been known to care for such people often for years on the grounds of 'delicacy'. Drive is greatly diminished and though the person may make many plans, these rarely come to fruition. There is loss of concentration for the job in hand so that the person is likely to be sacked or take on a less demanding job. This contributes to the social drift which we mentioned in the introduction.

b. Passivity. Passivity is the term given to the condition when the person feels that he is no longer in control of his thoughts and actions and that these are controlled by some external force or agency. Televisions rays, atomic rays, radar, rare gases, electricity or the rays of the sun are some of the things which may be cited. An extreme example of passivity is seen in the catatonic variety of schizophrenia. Such people adopt a wax-like flexibility, which is sometimes called flexibilitas cerea, and will maintain the limbs in any position they are placed for long periods of time without any apparent fatigue.

c. Negativism. This is a strong resistance to suggestion and can show itself in stubborn behaviour or complete refusal to do anything. The person may refuse to eat, to empty the bladder or bowels and thus become physically ill.

d. Impulsive movements. In contrast to poor or no will power and negativism, people with schizophrenia may also act impulsively and run about in a state of extreme agitation or frenzy. To 'go berserk' or to 'run amok' would be extreme examples of this form of behaviour.

e. Repetition. The repetition of actions (echopraxia) and sounds (echolalia) sometimes occurs in the catatonic variety and with flexibilitas cerea are facets of automatic obedience.

f. Posture. People with schizophrenia sometimes adopt unusual postures such as the crucified position or the curled up 'intra-uterine' position. The person may also point to or touch objects or may have mannerisms, tics, grimaces and may purse the lips. These features are called stereotypes of posture and movement.

g. Withdrawal. This occurs for a number of reasons. The description of the normal thought processes means that the person lives in a world of fantasy and this world is so fantastic that it has no place for the ordinary person. Then there is the loss of affect which makes social contact difficult if not impossible. In these circumstances withdrawal is inevitable.

11.5 Incidence

About one person in every hundred born suffers from schizophrenia. There are about 500,000 in the community who suffer from this condition and about 80,000 of these are in hospital at any one time.

11.6 Causes

The precise cause of schizophrenia is not known, but a number of avenues have been and are being explored and we shall now consider some of these:

A. SOCIAL. Schizophrenia knows no frontiers of age, sex, social class, intelligence or special training. A higher incidence of the condition is however found among the lower social classes and the admission rate from the slum areas of bigger cities is greater than from the wealthier surrounding suburbs. This has been explained by the phenomenon of 'social drift'. People with schizophrenia are poor mixers and like to be alone. It has often been said that the loneliest place in the world, despite its dense population, is a big city. Whether true or not these people find their way to the cities, and usually the poorer parts. The higher incidence among the lower classes can be explained by the fact that people with schizophrenia take on less demanding jobs as the disease progresses. In such instances a uni-versity graduate may be found washing dishes or in some similar occupation. Finally such people become unemployed and vagrants. Note has been made of the family background of people with schizophrenia. It is often found that the mother is a bossy and domineering type with a forceful personality who makes all the decisions and by contrast the father is quiet, timid and unassuming. Such mothers have been described as 'schizophrenogenic mothers'.

B. GENETIC. The role of genetic influences in the causation of schizophrenia is the subject of debate and so far no clear cut conclusion has emerged. Kallman (1953) reported that if a monozyous twin became schizophrenic then it was likely that the other would as well. This happened in 67–86 per cent of the samples examined. Slater (1953) found that the figure was 76 per cent. These reports put the genetic factor on firm ground for a while, but these works have been challenged. At the present state of the discussion it is not possible to say just what part genetic influences play in the causation of schizophrenia.

C. BODY BUILD. The person most likely to develop a schizophrenic illness is the tall, thin, angular type with a narrow chest and poor muscles. Such people were given the description of asthenic by Kretschemer (1925) and ectomorphic by Sheldon (1940). Nearly 70 per cent of people with schizophrenia have such a body build, but it is unlikely to be an important factor.

D. PERSONALITY. People with an ectomorphic body build are frequently shy, aloof and reserved. They tend to be introspective and may be a little eccentric and are thinkers rather than doers, preferring lone pursuits to group activities. Such people are said to have a schizothymic personality and should such people develop a mental illness it is most likely to be schizophrenia. The doctor usually takes pains to determine the type of pre-morbid personality a person had and this can be useful in the formulation of a diagnosis.

E. ENDOCRINE. Many studies of the endocrine glands have been made but there is no conclusive evidence that endocrine disorders are a major causative factor in schizophrenia.

F. BIOCHEMICAL. A number of investigations have or are being made and these include various enzyme systems, the electrolytes, water metabolism and the nitrogen balance. The most recent investigation revolved around an amine found in the urines of many schizophrenics called dimethyloxyphenylethamine (D.M.P.E.) which produced 'the pink spot test'. It was found there was no connection between the appearance of the pink spot and schizophrenia.

G. NEUROPHYSIOLOGICAL. E.E.G. changes have been found in a small number of people with schizophrenia, but there is no pattern which is exclusive to this condition.

H. PATHOLOGICAL. Extensive pathological and histopathological studies have provided no evidence of any pathological changes in the brain.

I. PRECIPITATING FACTORS. These are many and include physical conditions such as fever and surgical operations. Paradoxically these conditions can also bring about an improvement in established schizophrenia. On the psychological side separation from home such as joining the forces or going to university can precipitate schizophrenia in some people.

11.7 Clinical varieties

We have previously defined schizophrenia and discussed some of the general features of the condition. It is now time to consider some of the clinical varieties which are met in practice.

11.8 Simple type

The onset of this type of schizophrenia occurs during adolescence. Often the first signs are a falling off in school performance, excessive daydreaming, secretiveness and a steady withdrawal from the environment. The condition develops slowly and delusions or hallucinations are not always present and when they are, they are not of a very disturbing variety. The subject has difficulty in concentrating and may leave school at the first opportunity and also change jobs on the slightest pretext. Some leave home and may drift into vagrancy, prostitution and petty crime. Others get married and with the support of an understanding wife may hold down an unskilled job, but the majority of people with simple schizophrenia lead an idle and an aimless existence.

11.9 Hebephrenic type

The hebephrenic variety of schizophrenia also begins during adolescence and first shows itself by a steady withdrawal from the environment, as in the simple type, but the deterioration of the personality is more rapid and more extensive. Affective change is prominent. The affect may be humorous, fantastic and full of conceit and is expressed by meaningless giggling or by a self-satisfied and self-absorbed smile. Such people have a lofty manner and are likely to have mannerisms and grimaces. Thought-blocking occurs and there are delusions and hallucinations. The hallucinations are nearly always auditory ones and the delusions are fleeting. Rapport is very difficult to establish and the person tends towards a solitary existence.

The course of the illness varies. There may be one acute episode with a complete remission, but more often the condition persists in a subacute or chronic form. In the chronic form there may be exacerbations and remission, but the periods of remission become shorter and shorter so that the subject is more or less continuously disturbed. Later the symptoms appear to give little trouble and the subject becomes mute and apathetic.

11.10 Catatonic type

The main features of the catatonic type of schizophrenia are disorders of volition resulting in contrasting forms of behaviour. On the one hand there may be extreme passivity with automatic obedience and waxy flexibility (flexibilitas cerea). The person becomes totally unresponsive to external stimuli, although not unconscious. Such a condition is described as a stupor. The person may change from a stuporose condition to one of wild and violent excitement and the change may occur quite suddenly. Such outbursts are difficult to control and plenty of help is needed. Because of more effective methods of treatment, these two extremes are fortunately rarely seen these days.

11.11 Paranoid type

The paranoid type of schizophrenia begins later in life than the other types and usually after the age of 30 years. Delusions and hallucinations are common and the delusions are often of a persecutory nature, though there may also be delusions of grandeur and the person may believe that he is the Messiah. Thought disorders and passivity feelings are less in evidence and there is thus less deterioration of the personality. The delusions often follow a definite system and are called systematized. People with paranoid schizophrenia make numerous complaints to people in authority such as the police and town hall officials. Others may indulge in letter writing as part of the delusional system. Sometimes a person forming part of the subject's delusional world, and thus a persecutor, may be attacked and occasionally homicide takes place. Because the person is often intelligent and because the intellect is more or less unimpaired, very careful, elaborate and detailed planning goes into such homicide acts.

The course of paranoid schizophrenia is variable. Many remain fairly static for years, others have occasional acute episodes and periods of remission and others become severely and chronically disabled by the condition.

11.12 Acute schizophrenic episode

This is characterized by acute onset of schizophrenic symptoms, often presenting as a dream-like state with slight clouding of consciousness and perplexity. It may occur in a healthy person with a schizoid personality who has been subjected to a great stress. It may clear up in a few weeks or months, but sometimes it develops into the chronic form of schizophrenia.

11.13 Latent schizophrenia

This term has been used to designate states in which, in the absence of obvious schizophrenic symptoms, the suspicion is so strong that the condition is schizophrenia.

11.14 Residual schizophrenia

These are chronic residual states in which fragments of faded schizophrenic symptoms occur. Hallucinations, delusions, thought disorder and emotional blunting may have been present and have left slight evidence of their existence. Residual schizophrenia may be a sequel to one or more schizophrenic illnesses and is often compatible with an ordinary life in the community.

11.15 Schizo-affective type

This condition includes cases showing typical manic or depressive and schizophrenic features, with a tendency to remission with no marked effect. Such a diagnosis is only possible when both affective and schizophrenic symptoms are pronounced.

11.16 Childhood schizophrenia

This term is used for psychological disturbances occurring in childhood which approximate to adult schizophrenia. Delusions and hallucinations in childhood are much simpler than those in adulthood

9

and the main features of childhood schizophrenia are abnormal behaviour and a consistent lack of emotional rapport.

11.17 Autism

This condition was first described by Kanner in 1943 and consists of an inability to respond to the environment. In the past autistic children were either considered to have childhood schizophrenia or to be subnormal. In fact many found their way into subnormal hospitals. More recently it has been recognized as a clinical entity in its own right and operant conditioning may prove to be an effective form of treatment.

11.18 Principles of treatment

An eclectic approach involving the use of several methods of treatment is used in schizophrenia for there is no specific treatment for this condition. The available treatments aim at relieving the symptoms produced:

A. PSYCHOLOGICAL.

   a. Individual psychotherapy. This form of treatment is sometimes used and the response is variable.
   b. Group psychotherapy. This is used more commonly than individual psychotherapy. Careful selection is necessary for this form of treatment for it may not always be appropriate.
   c. Social. Social therapy in the form of a therapeutic community is being used increasingly. This helps to prevent the withdrawal from the environment which occurs by providing social contacts.

B. CHEMICAL. Drugs are the most common form of treatment used in the treatment of schizophrenia and drugs from the phenothiazine group are most commonly used. These include chlorpromazine and trifluoperazine. Long acting drugs such as Moditen or Modecate are particularly useful for treatment in the community. Haloperidol may also be used to control very disturbed behaviour. Some of the drugs used cause a drug-induced Parkinsonism and for this reason an anti-Parkinson drug such as orphenadrine is given at the same time.

C. ELECTRICAL. Electroconvulsive therapy is indicated when the delusions and the hallucinations are disturbing and are giving rise to restlessness, overactivity or aggressiveness. It sometimes proves useful in the treatment of catatonic stupor, but is of less value in the simple and paranoid types of schizophrenia.

D. OCCUPATIONAL. Occupational methods are invaluable in the treatment of such people. First they provide a diversion from the person's delusions and hallucinations and they also provide social contact. Second they provide an outlet for energy and this is particularly important where able-bodied people are concerned for it may otherwise be directed towards aggression. Activities such as art, music and drama give such people an opportunity to express themselves. The artistic work produced by people with schizophrenia is often abstract and sometimes bizarre. There are some who believe that such work has a symbolic representation and try to interpret it but many do not attempt such analysis.

E. SURGICAL. In the past the operation of leucotomy has been used in the treatment of schizophrenia, but it was not very successful and is now seldom, if ever, used.

11.19 Observation

1. APPEARANCE. The general appearance of those with schizophrenia is untidiness. Their clothes are often dirty and the various pieces may not match. The facial expression may be one of fear and there may be tics or grimaces. Many appear suspicious. People with paranoid schizophrenia usually take care over their dress but appear more than usually suspicious.

2. CONVERSATION. The conversation is usually retarded and childish or it may be non-existent. There is usually evidence of delusions and hallucinations. In the case of paranoid schizophrenia, the conversation may be very self-centred and often pompous.

3. MOOD. The mood is often one of apathy, though there may be evidence of fear or aggression. Sometimes the subject may appear happy but it is nearly always inappropriate or incongruous.

4. ATTITUDE. This varies with the type of schizophrenia. The simple and hebephrenic types are likely to be reserved and withdrawn. The catatonic type may be negative or impulsive depending on the stage of the illness. The paranoid type whilst suspicious may be quite

plausible and co-operative or conversely may be resentful and demanding.

5. INTELLECT. Schizophrenia is no respecter of intelligence and the levels found may range from the subnormal to the genius level. The performance may give little guide to the true underlying intellect for there is thought-blocking, and reasoning and judgement are impaired and frequently, though not always, insight may be absent.

6. EATING. In the majority of cases the eating habits are normal. In others, particularly young subjects, there may be an insatiable desire for food—bulimia. Others may refuse food and drink as part of the delusional system.

7. SLEEP. A great number sleep normally. Others may have disturbed sleep and be noisy and restless.

8. PHYSICAL STATE. People with schizophrenia are most often physically fit. A great number have a slim build and many probably due to inactivity, have a poor circulation to the extremities so that the skin of these areas often has a bluish tinge (cyanosis). In cases of extreme negativism it is possible to find incontinence of urine and faeces.

11.20 Nursing care

The nursing care of those suffering from schizophrenia is varied and a challenging task. On the one hand the behaviour may be extremely disturbed and there may be violence and aggression. On the other hand there may be complete withdrawal and apathy. The delusional system may be varied and may involve the nursing staff who may be attacked. Then there is the element of unpredictability, a quite mute and apathetic person may suddenly become active and aggressive and may start breaking up his surroundings. There is also the nature of the illness. There is often a degree of coldness, aloofness and withdrawal so that it is difficult to establish rapport. It is virtually impossible to get on the same 'wavelength'.

All the facets of the illness present their own problems. Aggression and violence will, initially at least, need physical restraint and as mentioned before this should be sufficient to prevent damage or injury to himself, to other people or to property and there should be sufficient help. Bed rest and seclusion may be necessary, but the rules regarding seclusion, which must be ordered by a doctor, should be carefully observed. On the opposite side of the coin, it is possible to have a person who is doubly incontinent and who requires to be washed and fed. In less severe states of withdrawal the person will sit around talking or giggling to himself. He will neglect his personal hygiene and will not participate in any activities. He thus loses all volition and becomes dependent on the institution, that is, institutionalized. The control of aggression, the care of the severely withdrawn and the mute and the prevention of institutionalization are important aspects in the nursing care of those with schizophrenia, but they must be recognized as largely negative approaches. A positive approach aims at advancement and progress rather than maintaining the status quo.

A positive approach requires a dynamic programme and this is largely in the province of the nursing staff. The doctor prescribes the appropriate treatment and generally supervises the management of those in his care, but it is mostly the nurses who execute his prescriptions. Drugs, E.C.T. or psychological treatment are of little value in isolation; it is the quality of the total programme and the supporting care that contributes so much to success or failure. An essential ingredient is to know those in your care. Know about their peculiarities and idiosyncrasies their delusional systems and their hallucinations, their interests, likes and dislikes. With these facts the person's needs will be more adequately met. The ward atmosphere should be buoyant and optimistic and this is largely determined by the personality of the nurses. The day's programme should be organized to give a good balance between work, rest and recreation. Activities outside the hospital such as visits to the seaside, the cinema or theatre, visits to museums and art galleries and country walks should be organized. These will help to maintain contact with the outside world, but they also help to discover new interests, new talents and new potentials. Every effort should be made to maintain a regular work habit so that the person will always be able to return to a useful role in the community when well enough.

The nurse's attitude, as always, is vitally important. The attitude of 'he's only a schiz and will become chronic' should be avoided like the plague. Optimism breeds optimism and conversely pessimism breeds pessimism. The nurse must believe in what she is doing and convey this belief to those in her care. It is true that in the case of schizophrenia there is no specific cure and that treatment is concerned with the relief of symptoms and the giving of supportive care. But

these given in the right measure and in the right spirit can do much
to relieve human suffering and this is surely a worthy goal.

11.21 Prevention

This can be considered from two points of view. First, if the cause
were known then some action may be able to be taken to prevent
schizophrenic illness in the future, but the causes are not known and
this is likely to prove a fruitful but a difficult area for the research
worker who is likely to be rewarded with a Nobel prize. Second there
is the field of health education. Much work has been done to remove
the stigma which has been associated with mental illness, but much
remains to be done. A kindly and more understanding attitude by
the public, coupled with early diagnosis and treatment should help
very much. At the same time it is essential that the statutory and
voluntary services in the community continue to develop so that there
is adequate follow-up and after-care. The development of out-patient
services, day hospitals and psychiatric units in general hospitals
all contribute to keeping the person functioning in the community
as long as possible. A more dynamic approach by the hospitals with
an increasing emphasis on rehabilitation and after-care in the community should ensure that people with schizophrenic illnesses should
spend less time in hospital in the future.

11.22 Summary

Schizophrenia is a common psychiatric disease and its cause is
unknown. It is primarily a thought disorder though nearly all aspects
of mental life are affected, particularly feeling and conduct. There are
several types of schizophrenia which present with varied and often
contrasting behaviour patterns. Various methods of treatment are
available and all aim at relieving symptoms rather than curing.
Curative treatments depend on the cause being known and this is
still a puzzle which is in the hands of the research workers.

12

Disordered affect

12.0 Introduction

The term 'affect' is used for the emotional and feeling aspect of mental life. Mood is another such term. Mental disorders where a particular affect is involved are called *affective disorders*. The two principal disorders which occur are excessive sadness (depression) and excessive elation (mania). Because both of these states may be seen in the same person at different stages of his life, disorders of affect were given the name of manic depressive psychoses, but this title has largely been abandoned. In Chapter 2 we considered emotions briefly. Now we shall consider them in more detail.

12.1 The nature of emotions

Feelings and emotions must be considered together:

A. FEELINGS. These are conscious states which are of various kinds and intensities. Wilhelm Wundt (1832–1920) classified feelings into three groups of qualities as follows:

    a. Pleasantness—unpleasantness.
    b. Excitement—inertness.
    c. Expectancy—release.

Each feeling has an opposite. We have all had pleasant feelings at some time. For example a family meal where everyone is happy is pleasant, whereas one where there is an atmosphere following a quarrel is unpleasant. There may be excitement over a happy event such as a party, or someone who has failed an examination, for example, may feel unable to do anything (inertness). If a boy has a date with a girl for the first time, there is a state of expectancy. If the person is late, considerable tension is built up, but this is usually released at the sight of the person. There are other aspects to feeling. The tendency to feel the same as the other person is feeling is *sympathy*. This is important in nursing for a little sympathy goes a long way. We have said earlier that nurses must be objective but this does not mean that they must be 'hard'. The tendency to feel what you would feel if you were in the other person's predicament is called *empathy*. To feel empathy it is necessary to have been in the same predicament. This, of course, is not always possible but it adds greatly to understanding. Finally there are the feelings we have for the beautiful things we see—aesthetic enjoyment. We have feelings about the beauties of nature, works of art, architecture or music. Such feelings add to the fulness of life.

B. EMOTIONS. These are 'stirred-up' states of the individual and may be of several types:

1. *Fear*. This is aroused by danger situations, that is by stimuli which the individual has learned to be signs of impending unpleasantness. For example, an unaccustomed noise at night may arouse fear, for it may be associated with an intruder or a burglar; or a ghost if the hearer believes in these!

2. *Anger*. This is aroused by situations in which an activity is held up by some obstacle. Suppose a person sets out for the seaside at the week-end and runs in to a long traffic jam on the way. The person, who wants to be sunbathing on the beach, is uncomfortably hot in the car and is likely to grow angry.

3. *Mirth*. This is the emotional state that goes with smiling and laughing. Babies laugh when played with, older children laugh at practical jokes and adults laugh at stories and jokes.

4. *Joy*. This is different from mirth and is associated with achievement. Passing an examination and winning a race give rise to joy, but the joy of a mother who has given birth to a baby is perhaps the greatest of all.

5. *Ecstasy* (*Gk ekstasis*, derangement). When there is ecstasy, the mind is focused on one idea which gives rise to mental exaltation. The person is oblivious to the environment, adopts a statue-like pose and has a rapturous facial expression. Ecstatic states may be produced through admiring great beauty in art, or music, or in relation to sexual activity.

> Joyous we too launch out on trackless seas
> Fearless for unknown shores on waves of
> ecstasy to sail.
>
> Walt Whitman (1819–1892)
> Passage to India.

6. *Grief*. This emotion is aroused by death. The bereavement permanently deprives the person of an accustomed source of comfort and gratification.

EXPRESSION OF EMOTIONS. Emotions are expressed by smiling, laughing, scowling, sneering, crying, shouting or screaming. In the child 'pure' emotions are seen, but as the child grows he has to control his emotions to conform to the customs of society. In the adult the indicators of the emotional state are the facial expression and the tone of the voice. In Chapter 4 we considered the indirect expression of emotion and the 'organ' language and reference to this chapter should be made for the physical aspects of emotional responses.

THEORY OF EMOTIONS. In 1880 William James (1842–1910) an American psychologist and Carl Georg Lange (1834–1900) a Danish physiologist, put forward a theory that emotional feelings resulted from the sensations coming from the body, especially from the internal organs. This theory has been disproved and it is now accepted that the frontal lobe of the cerebral cortex and the hypothalamus are the controlling centres for emotions. The hypothalamus is also the controlling centre for the autonomic nervous system. All organs supplied by the autonomic nervous system can be affected by psychosomatic conditions, for example, the blood vessels (raised blood pressure), the air passages (asthma), the digestive system (peptic ulceration) and the skin (goose-flesh).

12.2 Disorders of emotion

There is a great range of emotional experience and this has an influence on everyday life. Politicians and social reformers work very hard for their causes often because of a feeling of outrage at present conditions. Artists, dramatists, authors, and playrights often appeal to the emotions. Tennyson's (1809–92) work as a poet had been profoundly affected by the grief he felt over the death of his friend Arthur Hallam and this was shown in 'In Memoriam' in particular.

Shades of emotion add quality and give fullness to life. Emotions may be affected in three ways; there may be undue elation and overactivity; there may be undue sadness and underactivity or there may be absence of emotion-apathy.

It is natural to feel happy and to experience joy over certain events such as passing an examination, getting married, having a baby or getting promotion at work. Such events are occasions for celebrations and rejoicing and after the events the emotional state returns to normal and life carries on in a less hectic fashion. When there is a state of elation which is prolonged and not due to any obvious changes of fortune, this is abnormal. The person, who is said to look at the world through rose-tinted spectacles, is overactive and for him everything seems bright and gay. A mild degree of elation and overactivity is called hypomania and a severe degree is called mania.

At the other end of the scale it is equally appropriate to feel sad about failing an examination, suffering a disappointment or a bereavement. Such events may be associated with tears, inadequacy and self-recrimination. Tears are an excellent way of releasing emotions. There is usually a gradual return to the everyday mode of living, with perhaps occasional lapses. Again if the state of sadness is prolonged or not due to any events in the personal life, this is abnormal. There are degrees of sadness, for example, minor degrees are referred to as a 'touch of the blues' or the 'Monday morning' feeling. More profound states of sadness are called depression.

12.3 Historical

In the past, particularly the distant past, the diagnosis of mental illness was not precise. However a number of notable persons are said to have suffered from affective disorders. Saul (11th Century B.C.) First King of Israel is said to have been a manic depressive with homicidal tendencies. David played to him on the harp and this was partly effective. Martin Luther (1483–1546) suffered from depression and drank heavily. Johann Wolfgang von Goethe (1749–1832) had a manic-depressive illness and also drank heavily. P. I. Tchaikovsky (1840–93) suffered a great deal from depression which was probably associated with his homosexuality. Nearer our own time Charles Dickens (1812–70) was the victim of a manic-depressive illness and often suffered from depression.

In the second half of the 19th century several people were interested in the condition but it was left to Kraepelin to produce a classification which was to pass into common usage. In 1896 he formulated his conception of the manic-depressive psychosis. In this group he included circular insanity, mania, melancholia and some states of confusion or delirium. He considered that these were facets of one illness. As we mentioned in the introduction to this chapter the term manic-depressive psychosis has been replaced by the term affective disorders.

DEPRESSION

12.4 Depression

In Chapter 10 we considered the condition depressive neurosis (reactive depression). We shall now consider the other types of depression. The main features associated with a depressive illness are prolonged misery without adequate cause, slowness, tiredness, agitation, loss of interest and libido, poor concentration, sleep disturbances, particularly early waking and delusions of guilt. There is usually loss of weight and physiological alterations such as lowered blood pressure, a slow pulse rate, a lowered metabolic rate and constipation.

12.5 Incidence

It is estimated that there are 150,000 people in the community suffering from depression and about 50,000 of these are in hospital at any one time.

12.6 Causes

There are no specific causes, but there are a number of contributory factors some of which are found in any case.

1. GENETIC. For a long time it was thought that there was a firm genetic basis for the so-called manic depressive psychoses, but now this is not thought to be so. It has been pointed out that the familial incidence of the condition may be as much related to the cultural as to genetic factors.

2. BODY BUILD AND PERSONALITY. Many people with affective disorders have what Kretschmer described as a 'pyknic' build (endomorphic). With this build goes the cyclothymic personality. This means that a person with this type of personality may have periods or normal mood, may sometimes feel low and sad (leading towards depression) and may at other times feel high or elated (leading towards hypomania); hence our term cyclothymia = a cycle of moods.

3. BIOCHEMICAL. In depression the serum electrolytes are often unbalanced and as a result it is found that the body offers increased resistance to the passage of electricity. The significance of these biochemical changes has yet to be fully worked out.

4. ENDOCRINE. The functioning of the endocrine glands particularly the thyroid gland, affects mental function. Depression is associated

with myxoedema and states of excitement or even mania occur with thyrotoxicosis. Apart from these conditions, it is thought that endocrine malfunction is not a major contributory factor in affective disorders.

5. PRECIPITATING FACTORS. Infections such as influenza, surgical operations or an accident can act as precipitating factors. Psychological upsets such as a bereavement, a broken love affair or other disappointment is most likely to give rise to a depressive neurosis, but there is sometimes a history of some such an event before the onset of an affective disorder.

12.7 Types

There are a number of different types of depression which differ slightly from each other and the following types will be considered now:

Involutional melancholia, manic depressive psychosis, depressed type. Depressive neurosis (reactive depression) was considered in Chapter 10.

12.8 Involutional melancholia

This type of depression occurs between the ages of 45–64 and in women it is often associated with the menopause. In addition to being depressed, such people are usually very suspicious and even paranoid. They have feelings of unworthiness and guilt. Such depression is accompanied by anxiety, tension and restlessness—which gives rise to agitation. This is characterized by constant rubbing or clasping of the hands, and idle movements of the tongue and lips. There is often a pre-occupation with bodily function and a person may say 'my insides are rotting' or 'I have no brain,' and there is preoccupation with death (Nihilistic delusions). There is a strong risk of suicide.

12.9 Manic depressive psychosis, depressed type

This type of depression is sometimes described as endogenous depression, though the use of this term has been abandoned by many. It comes on out of the blue and is characterized by misery, gloom and a slowing down of actions and of thinking. Delusions of a self-reproachful nature are present but not the hypochondriacal type which are associated with involutional melancholia. Sleep is upset and there is early morning waking. There is loss of weight, loss of appetite and loss of libido. In some cases the retardation is so great as to border on stupor. The depression is often, though not always, at its worst in the mornings and there is a danger of suicide.

12.10 Suicide

We have already mentioned suicide in relation to the mental mechanisms and we saw that it was an example of extreme hostility towards oneself. Suicide and attempted suicide have always been frowned upon. From very early times 'Self murder' as it was sometimes called was strongly condemned and the victims' bodies were often buried at the crossroads. This practice was discontinued in 1823. The victims' property was taken over by the Crown. Until 1961 attempted suicide was an offence when the Suicide Act (1961) repealed existing legislation. Now the only official disapproval is a religious one, for the body of a person who has committed suicide may not be buried in consecrated ground unless 'the balance of mind was disturbed' according to the Coroner's inquest.

Over 5,000 people in the United Kingdom kill themselves each year and it is estimated that about 30,000 attempt suicide. The latter figure is not very accurate for it is likely that many attempted suicides are not reported. We can consider suicide in relation to depression because it is frequently, though not exclusively, associated with that condition. People with schizophrenia, for example, also attempt and commit suicide.

People of any age may commit suicide, though it occurs most commonly in the fifties. It is more common in people in classes I and II, that is doctors, dentists and lawyers, according to the Registrar General's classification based on the person's employment. The incidence of suicide is above average for university students.

A variety of methods are used to end life. Domestic gas poisoning and drug overdoses, particularly barbiturates, are those most commonly used. Other methods include jumping from high buildings, bridges or under trains, hanging, drowning, shooting, self-electrocution and cutting of the wrists or throat.

12.11 Principles of treatment

A number of methods are combined to achieve the best results:

A. *Psychological.* Individual and group psychotherapy is used, but these methods are usually impossible and impracticable in the acute stages of a depression.

B. *Electrical*. In many cases a short course of E.C.T. is the quickest way of bringing about a remission in an acute depression. Anything from 6 to 12 treatments may be needed.

C. *Chemical*. Antidepressants such as imipramine hydrochloride (Tofranil), desipramine (Petrofan), amitriptyline (Tryptizol), nortriptyline (Aventil) and mionamine-oxidase inhibitors such as impromiazid (Marsilid) phevelzine (Nardil) and nialamide (Niamid) are available for use. The choice of drug depends on the individual's needs and to some extent the experience of the prescriber with a particular preparation. E.C.T. and drugs complement each other well. The E.C.T. brings about a quick relief of symptoms and the drugs maintain it.

D. *Occupational*. Occupational and recreational activities are important, but activities for the acutely depressed must be very carefully chosen because of the great lack of initiative and interest.

E. *Surgery*. This is seldom if ever indicated in the treatment of depressive illness.

12.12 Observation

The general appearance of the depressed person is one of dejection, despair, despondency and apathy. The facial appearance is one of misery, though one sometimes hears of a 'smiling depression'. The dress is usually untidy and unkempt.

1. CONVERSATION. There is usually very little conversation and the person replies using a minimum of words. From what conversation there is, it is often possible to detect delusions of unworthiness and guilt, or there may be talk of suicide.

2. MOOD. The mood is one of utter and complete sadness. Sometimes this is tinged with suspicion in cases of involutional melancholia.

3. ATTITUDE. The person is withdrawn and is sometimes apologetic. 'I am in everyone's way, I am a nuisance and too much trouble.'

4. INTELLECT. Intellectual function is slowed down and concentration and memory are impaired. There is also a great poverty of thought.

5. EATING. The appetite is usually very poor or non-existent.

6. SLEEP. The main disturbance is early morning waking in the depression of affective disorders. The sleep is unrefreshing and the person wakes in the morning totally unrefreshed and quite unable to face another day. Depression is nearly always at its worst in the morning and the thought of having to struggle through the day is a daunting prospect.

7. PHYSICAL STATE. All physical activities are slowed down. There is loss of weight, the skin becomes coarse and the eyes lose their twinkle. There is alteration of the bowel habit and constipation is common and so is overflow incontinence of urine.

12.13 Nursing care

The nursing care of the depressed person is a very rewarding job. 80 per cent of those with depressive illnesses recover, though there is the possibility of relapses. It is interesting to observe a very sad, tearful and dispirited person, in the depths of despair and contemplating putting an end to it all, become happy and cheerful with a feeling that life is worth living.

It is a rewarding job, but it is also a demanding one. Suicide is an ever present possibility. Some may frequently talk about suicide and others never mention it. It is said that those who talk about suicide never do it. You should not rely on such a generalization for there are always exceptions to every rule and anyway each person should be considered individually.

In all cases of depression sensible precautions should be taken. We have previously mentioned the method used to commit suicide and the precautions should be designed to prevent access to these things. Care should be taken over domestic gas (town gas) and electrical appliances and sharp instruments. Drugs and chemicals, such as disinfectants, are a particular hazard. Care must be taken to see that drugs are not stored: it is probably wise to crush all tablets when giving them. A store is less likely to be gathered in this form. Continuous observation is necessary in order to give help and support as well as preventing suicide. Sometimes when the threat of suicide is great a suicidal caution card may be used as a means of ensuring continuous observation. These cards vary from hospital to hospital and if they are used in your hospital you should become familiar with the type used. It may be that there are no such cards in your hospital for their use has been largely abandoned.

So far much of what we have said about nursing depressed people is of a negative nature. Precautions to prevent suicide have been likened to the fence a farmer puts round his fields, but the farmer's main interest is in growing crops, likewise in nursing; helping the person to return to normal is the prime function. Human contact is an important part of this process. In the early days of a severe depression establishing a relationship often seems a barren prospect. Activity is almost at stupor level and verbal communication is almost confined to words of one syllable. It is likely that the depressed hears and understands what is said, but is unable to respond so that words of encouragement are not wasted. Much can also be conveyed by non-verbal communication using the face and the eyes. Physical nursing care also provides an excellent means of non-verbal communication. Helping to wash and feed and attending to similar physical needs provides an excellent opportunity to establish rapport. Bonds of sympathy and understanding can be built up in this way which make a valuable contribution towards rehabilitation. To make contact is perhaps the most difficult part of the task, but once this is done progress is often steady. As the person's physical and mental processes speed up, the levels of occupational and recreational activities must also be adjusted. The person gradually becomes independent of the nurse's prompting, guidance and suggestions, though encouragement will, as always, still be necessary.

A word of warning is necessary at this stage. Suicide is more often attempted in the period leading up to a depression and in the convalescent period than during the time when it is at its worst. This is due to the fact that during the depths of the depression the subjects do not have enough energy to make the effort. Care must be taken in the convalescent period to avoid such a tragedy.

12.14 Prevention

In order to be able to prevent depressive illnesses much information will be needed about the cause of the illness and this will only come about by research. Many people are interested in this aspect of research including the National Association for Mental Health.

The Samaritans, a voluntary organization founded by an Anglican priest, Rev. Chad Varah, provide a 24-hour telephone service in London and in other centres for people in distress. Any person who is depressed and in need of help can telephone any time, day or night, and there will be someone available to listen sympathetically and to give help and support. The London branch of this service deals with about 100 people a week. The Samaritans make an important contribution to the prevention of suicide.

MANIA

12.15 Mania

The characteristics of mania are a direct contrast to those of depression. In place of sadness there is elation, in place of under-activity there is gross overactivity, in place of little speech there is a torrent of verbiage and in place of a poverty of ideas there are flights of ideas.

You will come across many diagnostic categories associated with mania such as manic attack, hypomania, acute mania, delirious mania and so on, but only those used in 'A Glossary of Mental Disorders', that is, manic depressive psychosis, manic type and manic depressive psychosis, circular type will be described here.

12.16 Causes

As depression and mania are component parts of affective disorders, the contributory factors quoted earlier in relation to depression are equally applicable to mania.

12.17 Manic depressive psychosis, manic type

The person with mania talks incessantly; '...could talk the hind leg off a dog'. The mood is one of gaiety and the 'hail-fellow-well met' approach makes him good company. He seems to have boundless energy and never appears tired. The gay mood may change to one of irritability and anger. There is sometimes an attitude of intolerance towards people who think and act more slowly and there is a tendency to label them as stupid or fools. Punning and rhyming are very common. Often the verses produced, whilst they may have rhyme of a sort, have no reason. This is because the 'flights of ideas' cause a whole lot of unrelated ideas to come into the mind at once so that the resulting verses are not related except from having similar sounding words: this is called a 'clang association'.

People with mania have ideas of self importance (delusions of grandeur) and have been known to spend money recklessly, believing themselves to be wealthy and finish up bankrupt. One old gentleman known to the author would write out cheques on lavatory paper for very large sums, ranging from several thousand pounds to a million pounds or more, as presents or for services rendered: he had no assets and his only income was the indigent allowance. Another claimed to be the seventh son of the seventh son and claimed the extraordinary healing powers which are said to have been accorded to such people. Lack of success never dampened his belief in his healing ability.

In contrast to depression, the libido is increased and excessive demands may be made on the marriage partner or promiscuity may occur.

12.18 Manic depressive psychosis, circular type

As the title implies this type follows a circular pattern. Phases of mania or hypomania regularly alternate with phases of depression. There is usually a period of normality in between.

12.19 Principles of treatment

A. *Psychological.* Psychotherapy is not possible or practicable in the acute stage. Even when the acute stage is passed, care has to be taken over the selection of people with manic illnesses for participation in group psychotherapy because sometimes they have a disturbing influence on a group and so gain nothing themselves.

B. *Electrical.* E.C.T. has a useful part to play in controlling the disturbed behaviour and complements drug treatment.

C. *Chemical.* Large doses of tranquillizers such as chlorpromazine (Largactil), trifluoprazine (Stelazine) or Haloperidol (Serenace) are required to control the overactivity. As large doses are used, a particularly careful watch must be kept for the side-effects of these drugs.

D. *Occupational.* With such an abundance of energy some occupational activity is essential, but it must be carefully chosen. The main problem is to get the person to concentrate as there is a tendency to flit from one thing to another like a honey bee.

12.20 Observation

The general appearance is one of gaiety. There is a tendency to wear bright coloured clothes. Men often wear loud ties and buttonholes. Women have more scope with colour and may appear in outrageous outfits with make-up 'plastered on'.

1. CONVERSATION. This is fast and disjointed, the person flits from subject to subject and has a 'flight of ideas'. As we already mentioned there are delusions of a grandiose nature. Hallucinations are not a common feature as in schizophrenia, but sometimes people with manic illness may say that they can hear thunder or the sound of a waterfall in the distance.

2. MOOD. The mood is often a happy and gay one, but if thwarted this can change to one of irritability or aggression. The apparent happiness and gayness is not always experienced by the person. In fact when recovery takes place many will admit to feeling low whilst apparently elated.

3. ATTITUDE. This alters; it may be demanding, impulsive or plausible, depending on the circumstances.

4. INTELLECT. The person often gives the impression of being brighter than previous achievement or tests would suggest, but it is a 'Smart Alec' type of brightness. Memory is exceptionally good and such people can remember incredible detail. Attention is non-existent, but orientation may be correct. Judgement and reason are impaired and there is usually no insight.

5. EATING. If the person can spare the time he is likely to have a voracious appetite. Despite this there is often a weight loss because of the overactivity. In the days when the treatment of people with manic illnesses was less effective, exhaustion from under-eating and overactivity was not uncommon.

6. SLEEP. This is often disturbed and the amount of total sleep obtained is often small.

7. PHYSICAL STATE. There may be weight loss and due to the general overactivity, the pulse rate is increased and the blood pressure may be raised.

12.21 Nursing care
A brief encounter with someone with a manic illness can at once be interesting, stimulating and amusing. Prolonged contact however

can be rather wearing. Such people have a sharper than normal perception and quickly size people up. 'Nurse is in a bad mood, had a bad night dear, got out of the wrong side of bed? never fear . . . . is here'. Rapid fire conversation of this nature is common. Memory is also sharper and details of the nurse's actions when she was new may be repeated to her embarrassment. People with manic illnesses are natural meddlers and will bring forth a variety of solutions for any problem. Such interference is resented and it may provoke irritation or aggression. There is also the fact that it is difficult to keep pace with such energetic people.

The tendency is to nurse everyone out of bed when it is at all possible, but because of the risk of exhaustion and dehydration it is sometimes necessary to nurse such people in bed, at least, until the treatment begins to control the symptoms. A suitable occupation is the main problem when activity is resumed. It is sometimes possible to channel the enormous energy available into helping others or leading group activities, but most often the person cannot concentrate on anything for long or may irritate other people so much as to be unacceptable.

Despite the gaiety, the flamboyance and overactivity, mania is a severe emotional upset. It has been likened to 'feast days' in many cultures when the constraints of the higher centres on behaviour are loosed. The resulting behaviour is uninhibited and pleasure-seeking (hedonistic). Human contact, reassurance and encouragement are, as always, important.

12.22 Prevention

What was said earlier about the prevention of depression is equally applicable to mania, except that the service of the Samaritans does not apply. The drug lithium carbonate has a dual role in relations to mania. It is sometimes used therapeutically, though in severe manic disturbances the drugs mentioned earlier are likely to be more effective, and it is also used for prevention. We mentioned earlier that electrolyte changes occur in depression, this is also true in mania. Lithium carbonate, which is also an electrolyte, acts at this level and is said to be effective in preventing the depressive phases of affective disorders.

12.23 Summary

Disorders of affect involve feelings and emotions. These add quality to life for it is through them we appreciate the beauties around us.

The spectrum of emotion is a wide one, ranging from love to hate and anger to sadness. There are two principal disorders of emotion and these present strongly contrasting pictures. In one there is such a degree of sadness as to make one feel ill (depression) and in the other there is such a degree of elation that it makes one disturbed (mania). The outlook in such conditions is good. In depression, for example, 80 per cent recover though relapses may occur. The fundamental cause and thus the prevention of such conditions is in the hands of the research workers.

13

Disordered personality

13.0 Introduction

In this chapter we shall consider disorders of personality and the principal one is psychopathy.

13.1 Personality

In Chapter 2 we considered aspects of the personality and in Chapter 5 we mentioned some of the methods of measuring these. We shall now reassemble our thoughts on personality before considering personality disorders. Personality, it will be remembered, is the total quality of an individual's behaviour as it is revealed in his characteristic habit of thought and expression, his attitudes and interests, his manner of acting and his general outlook on life. Personality has many facets and qualities and each of these is called a trait.

The factors which contribute to the personality are physique, strength and looks. You probably know people of small stature who compensate for this by being aggressive or even objectionable to others. On the other hand you may know big people who are easy-going and amiable.

The chemical make-up is also important. Drugs alter the personality considerably. A person who is drunk is very different when he is sober. The Dutch courage makes him seem more brave than he really is, and also more irresponsible. A person who is a drug-addict bears no resemblance to what he was like before drug-taking began. Hormones are also important. Take the thyroid hormone for example. The personality associated with excess of this hormone (thyrotoxicosis) and the personality associated with decreased output of this hormone (myxoedema) are poles apart.

Social influences are important too, for we hear of Scotsmen being mean, Englishmen being reserved, Americans being expansive and boastful and Frenchmen being amorous. It is accepted that many of these traditional generalizations are frequently not valid in individual cases, but it must also be accepted that the environment influences personality through its rules, standards of conduct and moral code.

Social roles are an important influence. Scruffy, unkempt and often rebellious students become the clean-cut professionals. A certain code of behaviour is expected from professional people such as doctors and lawyers, and members must conform if they are to continue in practice.

An ideal personality is an integrated personality where all the traits, interests and desires are combined effectively and in harmony. In many mental disorders there is a lack of integration and an extreme example is the multiple personality which we mentioned earlier.

13.2 Types of personality

There are several types of personality and all of these are accepted within the limits of normality.

13.3 Paranoid personality

This type of personality falls into two groups.

A. THE SENSITIVE. Such people are exceptionally sensitive and react to everyday experiences with a sense of subjection and humiliation. These people are 'very touchy', they tend to take things too personally and to blame others.

B. THE AGGRESSIVE. This type is more thrusting and tends to demand 'their rights' and fight for them. In both types of the paranoid personality there is excessive suspiciousness and self-reference.

13.4 Affective personality (cyclothymic)

We have already mentioned this in relation to affective disorders and the personality alters according to the prevailing mood. At one time the outlook may be dismal, gloomy and grim and pessimism may reign supreme. At the other end of the scale it may be bright, gay and optimistic.

13.5 Schizoid personality

The schizoid personality is characterized by aloofness, shyness and reserve. Such people are very introspective and their conduct may be eccentric.

13.6 Explosive personality

As the name suggests people with such a personality have an instability of mood (labile), and are liable to sudden outbursts of irritability, anger, aggression and impulsive behaviour.

13.7 Obsessive compulsive personality (anankastic)

Such people feel insecure because of underlying fears and anxiety and this is shown in extreme caution and excessive conscientiousness. Obsessive people are inflexible and very meticulous, always seeking perfection and never quite attaining it. They set themselves very high ethical standards and are their own severest critics. The principal personality traits are timidity, rigidity and a tendency to doubt.

13.8 Hysterical personality

Such people are attention seekers and are unsteady and unreliable in their personal relationships. They are emotionally shallow and are over-dependent on others.

13.9 Asthenic personality

The main characteristics of this type of personality are a lack of vigour and vitality and a tendency to passiveness and dependency.

13.10 Antisocial personality (personality disorder, sociopathy, psychopathy).

So far we have considered personality types which are variations of the normal. The antisocial type offend against society, therefore, their behaviour is abnormal. Such people show a lack of feeling and they do not learn from experience because they repeatedly commit the same sort of crimes. They are known by a variety of names as indicated above, but *psychopath* is the one most commonly used.

Some people have what has been described as a 'here-and-now philosophy'. They are unprepared to set long term goals and want instant results. They are likely to leave school early to go after big money, but often dead-end jobs. It is likely they will be irresponsible employees and be frequently sacked or leave of their own account. Such people have countless jobs. When money is short, they resort to stealing and have no qualms about injuring an elderly shopkeeper and robbing the till. Despite probation, fines and periods of imprisonment, the crimes continue and often become worse in nature. Such people have whirlwind romances and get married on very short acquaintance, unfortunately, because due to their lack of feeling for others, they are no sooner married than they are separated or divorced. Others drift into prostitution, alcoholism, drug taking and generally become misfits. Such people may be called 'psychopaths'.

13.11 Types of personality disorder

There are three types and these are:

A. AGGRESSIVE PERSON. The aggression may be of a verbal 'stirring up' sort or it may take the form of actual physical fighting. More seriously it could take the form of murder (homicide). At work it could mean adopting ruthless methods to get promotion. Many such people are successful, at least for a time, because of their steam-rolling tactics. Some become super-salesmen and have no qualms whatever about pressurizing people into buying shoddy unwanted articles. Indeed they can adopt a superficial charm which is difficult to resist.

B. INADEQUATE PERSON. These people suffer in various ways. They form very poor relations with others and therefore tend to be lonely and isolated. Their work record is likely to be bad resulting in frequent changes of job and lack of money. In the case of a family man he is likely to be a bad provider and will thus make heavy demands on the welfare or social services.

C. CREATIVE PERSON. It seems a paradox to describe someone as antisocial and creative at the same time, but there are people such as artists who behave in what is not a conventionally acceptable or Bohemian way and yet produce works of artistic distinction. There are a number of people who are said, by some at least, to have been creative psychopaths. Joan of Arc (1412–1431), Lawrence of Arabia (T. E. Lawrence, 1888–1935), and General Orde Wingate (1903–1944) who led the Chindit battalions in Burma in World War II. There are, of course, many who would dispute this assessment of these people.

13.12 Incidence

The estimated number of psychopaths in the community is 500,000 and there are about 5,000 in hospital at any one time.

13.13 Causes

The cause of psychopathy is not definitely known, but many theories have been put forward.

A. GENETIC. Studies have shown many of the mentally subnormal, who behave in an antisocial way, have an abnormal complement of sex chromosomes and this has also been found in studies of the prison population. This is something which needs further investigation.

B. ELECTRICAL ACTIVITY. People with personality disorders produce a characteristic E.E.G. pattern, particularly the aggressive person. The pattern is said to be due to 'immaturity of the brain' and is similar to the pattern found in children. A psychopath is certainly emotionally immature, hence his lack of feeling for other people.

C. FAMILY BACKGROUND. Often there is a history of unhappiness in the home. There may be parental rows, separation or simply lack of love. The child feels rejected and unwanted and loses the ability to love and develops a 'chip on his shoulder'. There is emotional stunting because normal emotional interactions are not possible. Such a person has a grievance against society because of its hostility towards him, so he takes it out on society by repeated antisocial acts of a criminal nature. This pattern will not be found in all cases, but it is found in a fair number.

13.14 Legal aspects

The legal position of a psychopath is unique for it is the only diagnosis which is defined by Act of Parliament. In Section 4 of the Mental Health Act, 1959 it states:

'Psychopathic disorder' means a persistent disorder or disability of mind (whether or not including subnormality of intelligence) which results in abnormally aggressive or seriously irresponsible conduct on the part of the patient and requires and/or is susceptible to treatment.'

Some inadequate psychopaths find their way into psychiatric hospitals in the ordinary manner, but a great number are compulsorily detained on a hospital order Section 60 with perhaps special restrictions on discharge Section 65. More are transferred from prison when Sections 72 to 78 apply. Some find their way to Grendon Underwood Prison, which is a prison hospital specially designed for persistent offenders requiring psychiatric treatment. Others are sent to hospitals with special security arrangements such as Broadmoor for the mentally ill and Rampton for the mentally subnormal.

13.15 Principles of treatment

The main problem in psychopathy is persistently irresponsible antisocial behaviour and there is no treatment for this apart from removing such people from society and detaining them in institutions. Attempts have been made to modify their behaviour notably at the

Institute for the Scientific Treatment of Delinquency (the Portman Clinic), the Henderson Hospital, Belmont and also at Grendon Underwood hospital prison and at Broadmoor special hospital. Henderson Hospital is run on therapeutic community lines and the patients play a major role in running the hospital. The aim is that the behaviour of the group will influence the behaviour of the individual. Authority as such is removed, and authority is a major problem for most psychopaths, so that when a person rebels, he is rebelling against his peers.

Sometimes people present with features of other illnesses such as schizophrenia or depression. In these cases the treatment appropriate to the accompanying condition is treated.

13.16 Observation

Psychopaths do not have characteristics or distinguishing features.

1. *Conversation.* The conversation has no typical features, though an aggressive psychopath may be abusive. Delusions or hallucinations are not present.

2. *Mood.* The mood may be normal or it may be changeable or aggressive.

3. *Attitude.* The attitude may be demanding, impulsive, plausible or resentful.

4. *Intellect.* Intellectual ability ranges from high-grade subnormality to genius level. Intelligence is in no way affected and the more intelligent they are the more problems they are likely to create.

5. *Eating.* Eating habits are unlikely to be affected.

6. *Sleep.* This is also likely to be unaffected.

7. *Physical state.* The physical state is generally unaffected except in the case of alcohol or drug abuse or in those who live rough.

13.17 Nursing care

People with personality disorders present a difficult nursing problem. They are most likely to be compulsorily detained and this coupled with their natural aversion for authority put a strain on the nurse/patient relationship before it starts. There are other factors; they have no consideration for others and will ruthlessly exploit the young, the old and the feeble and may terrorize such poor unfortunates. They have no qualms about stealing. Some, because of their superior intelligence, are adept at 'throwing spanners in the works'. They quickly size up the staff, their weaknesses and their peculiarities and become expert at playing off one shift against the other. It is therefore important to have regular staff conferences where difficulties can be aired and policy discussed. The extreme plausibility of many psychopaths readily ingratiates them with members of the opposite sex. Having won the confidence of the particular member of staff, that person will be manipulated to achieve the psychopath's ends and will be dropped like a hot brick when no longer of use. Then there is the problem of abscondence. Hospitals are obliged to keep such people, but with poor security arrangements and open doors this is difficult if not impossible.

These are but some of the problems associated with the nursing care of those with personality disorders. Such people are often considered 'awkward customers' but it should be remembered that they do not enjoy behaving in this way; they do so because they are incapable of behaving in any other way. The thing to do is to be aware of the problems and pitfalls so that avoiding action can be taken. Nursing such people need not be a battle of wits, but the nurse needs to keep her wits about her just the same.

13.18 Prevention

Much more will need to be known about this condition, the genetic factors, the cultural, social and psychological aspects before prevention can be contemplated. 'All psychopaths were toddlers.' 'All toddlers do not become psychopaths. Why not?' We must rely on research workers to find the answers to such questions.

13.19 Summary

Psychopathy presents a serious problem to which there is no ready solution. Psychopaths do not respond to the punitive measures of the legal system or to the therapeutic measures, such as they are, of the hospital system. Detention, which is a negative solution, is the only solution available. Fortunately the condition is frequently self-limiting, for from the age of 30 years onwards there is a steady reduction in the number of antisocial acts committed.

14

Alcohol and drug abuse

14.0 Introduction

Humans are complex creatures with delicate and sophisticated nervous systems designed to respond to the environment. For example they are capable of experiencing fear and anxiety; carrying out highly intelligent acts; producing original thoughts; feeling an enormous range of emotions, reproducing the species and of presenting an integrated personality to the world. Factors in the environment of a congenital, traumatic, infective, neoplastic or degenerative nature threaten the physical integrity and cause pain. Absence of security, affection, independence and initiative threaten the psychological integrity and result in a lack of achievement and fulfilment, frustration and aggression. The demands of society, the role, the status and the behaviour related to these and the keeping-up with-the-Joneses attitude, place social pressures on individuals and on groups.

There are a variety of means available for dealing with the trials and tribulations of life such as mental mechanisms, dreams and personal philosophy. A religious faith sustains some people, others seek comfort in literature or music. A considerable number resort to using agents of insensibility or *chemical comforters* when life becomes too much: this means alcohol and drugs. The use of these chemicals allows a temporary escape from reality, but it gives rise to further problems such as dependency. In this chapter we shall focus our attention on the effects of excessive use of these chemicals.

14.1 Drug dependence

The terms drug dependence, drug addiction, drug habit and drug abuse are synonymous, although drug dependence and drug abuse are those most commonly used. Drug dependence is the state which arises from repeated, periodic or continuous administration of a drug resulting in harm to the individual and sometimes to society. There are three aspects of dependence:

A. PSYCHOLOGICAL DEPENDENCE. This is often the first to appear and is due to habit formation. The habit becomes part of the person's every day activities, and if the habit is broken by withdrawal of the drug, then there is emotional distress.

B. PHYSICAL DEPENDENCE. In physical or physiological dependence, the body develops a need for the drugs which is included in the normal metabolic reactions. If the drug is withdrawn there is a physical illness (withdrawal syndrome).

C. TOLERANCE. This is said to have developed when it becomes necessary to increase the dose of the drug to obtain an effect previously obtained with a smaller dose.

These aspects of dependence apply to alcohol as well as to drugs in the ordinary sense, for though not normally considered as such, alcohol is a drug and thus a poison.

14.2 Ethyl alcohol

The alcoholic drinks which are sold contain ethyl alcohol. This substance is obtained by the fermenting of fruit or vegetables and as any amateur wine-maker will know, the choice is limitless: potatoes, cow-slips, parsnips and so on, may be used. Commercially barley is used to make beer, grapes to make wines and apples to make cider.

Alcohol is an excellent social lubricant and enables people to mix better and to converse more freely by removing inhibitions and reducing tensions. It is said to make the eyes and the wit sparkle. It acts by depressing the nervous system and therefore it is not a stimulant as is popularly thought. This effect does not last and there are said to be four stages in alcoholic intoxication:

A. THE DIZZY AND DELIGHTFUL STAGE. In this, first stage, the inhibitions imposed by society are removed and the person may appear happier and more sociable than usual.

B. THE DRUNK AND DISORDERLY STAGE. By now the person's speech is likely to be inarticulate, gait is likely to be unsteady, and control by the higher centres is greatly diminished. There may be aggressive, fighting and irresponsible behaviour such as damage to property.

C. THE DEAD DRUNK STAGE. At this stage the brain is poisoned with alcohol and there is a state of unconsciousness. The cardiac and the respiratory centres in the medulla oblongata continue to function, though maybe more slowly than usual depending on the quantity of alcohol consumed.

D. THE DEAD STAGE. If the entire brain, including the vital cardiac and respiratory centres in the brain stem are put out of action, then the person will die. This sometimes happens, but it also happens during the unconscious stage that the person vomits and inhales this and dies from asphyxia or inhalation pneumonia.

The intake of a very large quantity of alcohol over a short period gives rise to acute alcoholic poisoning, and the intake of a large quantity over a long period gives rise to chronic alcoholic poisoning.

ALCOHOL ABUSE

14.3 The effects of alcoholism

Like most illness alcoholism affects life on three planes, the physical, the mental and the social.

A. THE PHYSICAL. Alcohol is a poison which affects the body in a number of ways. First there is physiological dependence and subsequent withdrawal symptoms. There is often a loss of appetite and sometimes there is inflammation of the lining of the stomach (gastritis) and there may be nausea and vomiting. It is the function of the liver to detoxicate all poisons. If it is overwhelmed by alcohol it reacts by becoming inflamed. This inflammation causes the liver to become rough and irregular in shape (cirrhosis) Vitamin B deficiency occurs in alcoholism and results in peripheral neuritis. Fits (convulsions) may occur, particularly when alcohol is withdrawn.

B. THE MENTAL. Mental life is affected in many ways. Alcohol provokes sexual desire, but it takes away performance so wrote William Shakespeare. This causes problems because the male alcoholic is likely to blame his wife for his plight. He will accuse her of unfaithfulness and become morbidly jealous and suspicious. Intellectual performance is affected in some cases and an alcoholic dementia results. There is a high rate of suicide and attempted suicide among alcoholics.

C. THE SOCIAL. Alcoholism has a disruptive effect on the family and quarrels are a common feature. Financial difficulties are inevitable. Not uncommonly there is break-up of the family, the alcoholic proceeds down 'Skid row' getting deeper and deeper in debt until he finally resorts to living in doss-houses or living rough on bomb sites. It is not unusual for an alcoholic to lose family, friends, jobs and normal social contacts.

A number of alcoholics find their way to prison. There is a relationship between alcohol and road traffic accidents for the peak time for such accidents is the hour after public houses close. The economic effects are likely to be considerable, though they are difficult to calculate. One estimate puts the direct cost of alcoholism to British Industry at £30 million, plus an indirect cost of a further £75 million.

14.4 Alcoholic drinks

The concentration of alcohol in alcoholic drinks varies with the types. Beers contain between 3 and 5 per cent of alcohol and a great deal of solids in the form of starch. A pint of beer contains about 400 calories and for this reason beer drinkers become fat and overweight. Ten pints of beer yield 4,000 calories which is more than most people's daily calorie requirement, but that would not be an unusual amount for an alcoholic to consume. Table wines contain between 8 and 15 per cent alcohol. Fortified wines such as port or sherry contain between 20 and 25 per cent alcohol. Spirits such as whisky and rum are made by distillation and usually contain about 35 per cent alcohol. The strength is usually expressed in terms of 'proof'. The strength of alcohol was once tested by finding the maximum dilution of alcohol and water which would cause a flash when poured on ignited gunpowder. This is said to be the origin of the term proof. In order to work out the percentage of alcohol in a drink the proof, if known, should be halved. Many spirits are described as 70 proof, that is 35 per cent alcohol.

14.5 History of alcoholism

We have mentioned elsewhere that famous people from the past such as Martin Luther and Goethe drank excessively at times. In the middle of the sixteenth century alcoholism was already a problem and taverns were described as 'the common resort of misruled persons'. Towards the end of the seventeenth century spirit drinking became common and this has been described as the 'gin era', because cheap gin became available. The consumption of spirits rose from 500,000 gallons in 1684 to 7,000,000 gallons by 1751. Legislation was introduced in 1729 to deal with the drink problem.

The industrial revolution (1760–1860) brought with it a return of excessive drinking, particularly in the cities. There was a high consumption of alcohol in the nineteenth century which reached its peak in the 1870s.

During the first world war, severe restrictive legislation which prescribed that licensed premises should be open 6 or 7 hours a day instead of 16 to 19 hours caused a fall in the consumption of alcohol.

In 1932 the Royal Commission on Licensing found that there was a tendency towards sobriety particularly among the young.

There has been an increase in alcohol consumption since the second world war, though it is less than it was a century ago.

14.6 Incidence

It is estimated that 400,000 or 1 in every hundred of the adult population is an alcoholic. The figures for 1967 show that 7,500 alcoholics were treated in psychiatric hospitals or in special units.

14.7 Causes

There is no single cause, but there are a number of contributory factors:

A. OCCUPATION. Some occupations such as publicans, salesmen and managers, who conduct business over protracted lunches with liberal amounts of alcohol, run the risk of alcoholism. The armed forces may be stationed in lonely outposts where the only social outlet is the mess. In such conditions there is a danger of alcoholism.

B. SOCIAL. Marital disharmony, domestic pressures and financial difficulties may all contribute. Social contacts are also important. If the person belongs to a club and if the members are heavy drinkers, there is a tendency to join in rather than be the odd man out.

C. CULTURAL. Alcoholism varies in different cultures. Alcohol is widely drunk by Jews, but the incidence of alcoholism is low. This is probably because wine is considered sacred and drunkenness is seen as non-Jewish behaviour.

There is a high incidence of alcoholism among the Irish and a very high rate among Irish-Americans probably associated with problems of adjustment.

D. PERSONALITY. It has been suggested that an underlying personality disorder forms the basis of alcoholism. As we indicated in Chapter 13, people with overt personality disorders readily turn to drink.

14.8 Types

In 1951 the W.H.O. (World Health Organisation) defined alcoholism as 'any form of drinking which in its extent goes beyond the traditional and customary dietary use, or the ordinary compliance with social drinking customs of the whole community concerned, irrespective also of the extent to which such aetiological factors are dependent upon hereditary, constitution or acquired physiopathological and metabolic influences'. This definition was revised in 1952 and says alcoholics are 'those excessive drinkers whose dependence on alcohol has attained such a degree that it shows a noticeable mental disturbance or an interference with their bodily and mental health, their interpersonal relations, and their smooth social and economic functioning, or who show the prodromal signs of such development. They therefore require treatment.'

Complete dependency may take up to 20 years to develop and there are three stages:

A. EXCESSIVE DRINKING. Excessive drinkers are not alcoholics but may become so. In the early days they drink in the same pattern as the social drinker. Drink brings relief of tensions and tolerance to alcohol develops.

B. DEPENDENCY. When dependency occurs alcohol is a necessity. The person drinks to the point of drunkenness, suffers loss of memory and is unable to control his drinking. His interests become narrowed, his work deteriorates, financial and marital problems begin to crop up and the pattern of jealousy and suspicion begins to develop. Drinking now starts early in the morning on the pretext that he has to have 'the hair of the dog' or that he needs a drink to get on his feet.

C. CHRONIC ALCOHOLISM. When this stage is reached no relief is obtained from drinking but the person is compelled to drink just the same. There is likely to be social disintegration, confused thinking and terrifying fears and complications such as cirrhosis of the liver, peripheral neuritis, delirium tremens or alcoholic dementia will be making their appearance.

Alcoholism most commonly develops because of the 'loss-of-control' over drinking, but there is another pattern and this is the 'inability-to-abstain' type. This type drinks continuously and is 'unable to abstain' but may not drink to the point of drunkenness as does the 'out-of-control' type.

14.9 Episodic excessive drinking

This is characterized by occasional bouts of excessive alcohol consumption causing acute intoxication which may last for several days or weeks. These bouts may be associated with physical or mental stress or may be precipitated by cyclical mood changes.

14.10 Habitual excessive drinking

The feature of this pattern of drinking is persistent and frequent intoxication in excess of the social norm.

14.11 Alcoholic addiction

This is a state of physical and psychological dependence on a regular and an ever increasing alcohol consumption. There are marked withdrawal symptoms if alcohol is withheld.

14.12 Withdrawal symptoms

These are very frightening for the person concerned. They include a great deal of anxiety and restlessness, unsteady gait, and there may be fits similar to epileptic fits. Hallucinations may be terrifying and include the traditional pink elephant and insect-like creatures crawling on the skin.

14.13 Delirium tremens

Delirium is a state in which there is clouding of consciousness and occurs in alcoholism, though it can occur in a variety of other toxic conditions. With the clouding of consciousness, the person is not fully aware of what is happening around him. He misinterprets the environment and suffers from delusions and hallucinations of a terrifying nature. In fact all the symptoms of withdrawal are present, but considerably magnified. The person may think he is still at work and therefore goes through the motions of his job (occupational delirium), and he cannot sleep.

14.14 Alcoholic hallucinosis

In this condition the hallucinations associated with delirium tremens are present, but the other features are absent. Consciousness is clear and the person otherwise feels well apart from hearing 'voices'. The voices may say unkind things about the person.

14.15 Alcoholic paranoia

As we have already mentioned this is part and parcel of chronic alcoholism. Paranoid attitudes and delusions of jealousy concerning the fidelity of the spouse develop. At first these may be of a mild nature, but later they may lead to expressions of extreme hostility and physical violence.

14.16 Wernicke's encephalopathy

This is due to a deficiency of thiamine, which is one of the vitamin B group of vitamins, and can result from alcoholism though it can be caused by other conditions and is a feature of beri beri. The onset is slow with anorexia, irritability, emotional liability and a lack of concentration. Later there may be neurological signs such as polyneuritis with paraesthesia and a burning feeling in the feet, particularly at night. The condition was described by Carl Wernicke (1848–1905) in 1881.

14.17 Korsakoff's psychosis

We mentioned this condition earlier as one of the causes of presenile dementia. It results from chronic alcoholism and is characterized by gross disturbances of orientation, extreme suggestibility, a tendency to make up stories about anything if given a lead (confabulation) and polyneuritis. It has many features in common with Wernicke's encephalopathy except that Korsakoff's psychosis is more often due to alcoholism and confabulation is also a characteristic feature.

14.18 Principles of treatment

The treatment varies according to the stage of alcoholism present:

A. UNCONSCIOUSNESS. If the person is unconscious, then the principles of treatment for the care of the unconscious are used.

B. DELIRIUM TREMENS. Drugs are used for the initial treatment of this condition. Chlorpromazine is used provided there is no liver damage. Vitamin B is given by injection. A hypnotic such as amylobarbitone (Sodium Amytal) is given at night. Phenobarbitone is sometimes needed to control fits. Similar drug treatment is required to control the symptoms of withdrawal. Supportive psychotherapy is needed throughout this stage.

If there are complications involving the liver (jaundice) and the heart (cardiomyopathy) the appropriate treatment for these conditions will be needed.

C. REHABILITATION. Alcoholics who have been weaned from alcohol, 'dried out', and free from withdrawal symptoms often need drug treatment for a considerable time. In order to return the person to society and to prevent a return to alcoholism there are a number of approaches available.

a. Psychoanalytic. Group therapy is based on psychoanalytic theory and is a common form of treatment. It is likely to be more successful in the gregarious communicative person who likes people, than in the quiet isolated lone-wolf type. This is the basis of the Alcoholics Anonymous approach.

b. Behaviourist. The behaviourist approach is commonly used in conjunction with certain drugs.

1. *Disulfiram (Antabuse).* This drug, which was produced in Copenhagen, has been available since 1948. It was found that if even a small quantity of alcohol was taken by someone who had previously taken Antabuse, then unpleasant symptoms were experienced. These included intense flushing of the face, palpitations and breathlessness. It was also found that the pulse rate increased and the blood pressure was lowered.

    The treatment begins in hospital and a period of at least three alcohol free days is allowed to elapse before treatment is begun. The prescribed dose of Antabuse is then given, usually 0·5 g daily, for three days. An alcoholic drink of the person's choice is given and the alcohol/Antabuse reaction occurs in controlled conditions. Ascorbic acid given intravenously can stop the reaction if it is too severe or if it looks as if the person is likely to collapse. This may be done once or it may be repeated depending on the policy of the therapist. The person then continues to take Antabuse, often for years, and is adequately warned about the risk of mixing alcohol and Antabuse.

2. *Emetine.* This drug produces vomiting and is used in the treatment of alcoholism. Injections of the drug were given and this was followed by giving the person some of his usual drink. Vomiting occurred and the vomiting was associated with the intake of alcohol. By associating this unpleasant feeling it was hoped that the person would develop an aversion for alcohol.

3. *Apomorphine.* This drug has a similar effect and is used for similar reasons as emetine. Both emetine and apomorphine are used less commonly than Antabuse.

c. Social. The social aspects of rehabilitation are extremely important in the rehabilitation of the alcoholic. Poor after-care in an apparently unfriendly or even hostile world can cause relapses. Help is usually needed with money, accommodation and a job and most important with the right sort of friends. Here the A.A. (Alcoholics Anonymous) serves a very vital function. It provides understanding and friendship at a crucial time. Other voluntary organizations such as the Helping Hand Organization also play an important role.

14.19 Observation

We have already mentioned that the alcoholic may be aggressive, delirious or unconscious on the degree of intoxication. For these observations we shall consider the alcoholic in the non-intoxicated condition.

1. *Appearance.* The appearance may be quite normal, though often it is untidy and unkempt due to living rough.

2. *Conversation.* This may be self-centred, the person may concentrate on past achievements or he may have a 'chip' on his shoulder.

3. *Mood.* The mood may be one of anxiety, suspicion or aggression.

4. *Attitude.* The attitude may be plausible, withdrawn or resentful.

5. *Intellect.* This frequently becomes impaired with a poor memory. Later on this may become severe, for alcholism is a cause of presenile dementia, in which case the person is disorientated and without insight.

6. *Eating.* This is likely to be neglected and malnutrition occurs.

7. *Sleep.* Without the help of alcohol, sleep is frequently difficult and often impossible. Hypnotics of some sort are likely to be needed.

8. *Physical state.* This is often poor and several systems may be involved.

   1. In the nervous system there may be polyneuritis and tremors of the limbs.
   2. There may be heart failure from cardiomyopathy.
   3. There may be repeated infections of the respiratory system.
   4. The digestive system may be affected by vomiting. The liver may be enlarged and there may be jaundice.

14.20 Nursing care

The nursing care of the person suffering from alcoholism is a varied and a challenging task. Physical problems such as neuritis, jaundice, heart disorders or even unconsciousness may be present. On the psychological side there may be suspicion, hallucinations, aggression or dementia. Social ties are often completely severed and the person stands alone and socially isolated.

A nurse's attitude is all important and she must not presume to judge. Many alcoholics are sensitive people and the wrong attitude can drive a person further down rotten row. An understanding and a sympathetic attitude is essential. Great patience and perseverance is also needed, for alcoholics will, despite fervent promises to the contrary, sometimes undo all that has been done. They will go and get drunk when apparently 'cured', they will 'forget' to take their Antabuse and they will drink whilst taking Antabuse. In treating alcoholic excesses a nurse must learn to accept disappointments and to start all over again.

A nurse may or may not be involved in psychotherapy depending on local custom. Following these sessions a nurse will be required to give supportive help and reinforcement. In conjunction with the occupational therapist she will be involved in the occupational and recreational part of the treatment programme.

14.21 Prevention

This presents a big challenge. Alcohol serves a useful social purpose and it is also a big source of revenue. To ban alcohol is no solution, this was clearly shown during the prohibition period in America. What is required is some way of preventing alcoholic use becoming alcoholic abuse. Alcohol presents problems only when used excessively.

Alcoholics Anonymous (A.A.) is a voluntary organization which was founded in 1935 by two alcoholics R. H. Smith and W. Williams. As alcoholics these two founders found that they could help themselves and decided to bring help to others. Membership of the A.A. includes members of all the religions and there are twelve steps laid down and these are:

1. We admitted we were powerless over alcohol—that our lives had become unmanageable.
2. Came to believe that a Power greater than ourselves could restore us to sanity.

3. Made a decision to turn our will and our lives over to the care of God as we understood Him.
4. Made a searching and fearless moral inventory of ourselves.
5. Admitted to God, to ourselves and to another human being the exact nature of our wrongs.
6. Were entirely ready to have God remove all these defects of character.
7. Humbly ask Him to remove our shortcomings.
8. Made a list of all persons we had harmed, and became willing to make amends to them all.
9. Made direct amends to such people wherever possible, except when to do so would injure them or others.
10. Continued to take personal inventory and when we were wrong promptly admitted it.
11. Sought through prayer and meditation to improve our conscious contact with God as we understood Him, praying only for a knowledge of His will for us and the power to carry that out.
12. Having had a spiritual awakening as the result of these steps, we tried to carry this message to alcoholics, and to practise these principles in all our affairs.

14.22 Methyl alcohol

This is the basis of methylated spirits. It is sometimes consumed when ethyl alcohol is found to be too expensive or it may be used to give 'life' to cheap wines. Methyl alcohol is much more poisonous than ethyl alcohol and 'meths' drinkers run the risk of severe confusion, blindness and sudden death.

14.23 Summary

Alcoholism is a disabling condition. It affects physical health by causing jaundice, peripheral neuritis, gastro-intestinal upsets and heart disease. Mental health is affected for there is jealousy, suspicion, paranoia, hallucinations and even dementia. It causes disintegration of social life and leaves the sufferer socially isolated without family, friends or finance. Both sexes are affected though men more commonly than women. All social classes are affected, though there is higher than usual number in social class I and social class V. A large proportion of alcoholics are in the 40s or 50s as it takes up to twenty years of heavy drinking before alcoholism develops. There are, however, many young alcoholics and alcoholism is an increasing problem among the young. There is an obvious need for increased research to provide answers for the many unanswered questions.

DRUG ABUSE

14.24 Drug abuse

In 1964 W.H.O. (World Health Organisation) defined drug dependence as a 'state arising from repeated administration of a drug on a period or continuous basis. Its characteristics will vary with the agent involved and this must be made clear by designating the particular type of drug dependence in each specific case—for example, drug dependence of morphine type, of cocaine type, of cannabis type, of barbiturate type, of amphetamine type and so on.' We shall now consider the abuse of these substances, but first it may be useful to consider reasons for drug use.

14.25 Reasons for drug use

There are at least five reasons why people use drugs and many of these are legitimate medical reasons:

1. To combat fatigue. Drugs such as caffeine, cocaine and those of the amphetamine group act as stimulants and may be used for this purpose.
2. To raise mood. Drugs such as caffeine, cocaine and those of the amphetamine and meprobamate may be used for this.
3. To banish worries. Alcohol, the barbiturates, morphine, or Librium may be used to banish worries.
4. To induce sleep. The barbiturates are most commonly used for this purpose, but chloral hydrate, alcohol or Doriden may also be used.
5. To produce dreams. Morphine, cocaine, marihuana, all cause dreams and so do mescaline and L.S.D. (Lysergic acid).

14.26 Classification of drugs according to effect

Drugs have a wide range of effects as follows:

1. *Analgesic* or relief of pain. Aspirin or codeine are mild analgesics, whilst morphine or pethedine are powerful analgesics.
2. *Sedative.* A sedative is a drug which depresses the central

nervous system especially at its higher levels, so as to allay nervousness, anxiety, fear and excitement, but more normally to the extent of inducing sleep. Barbiturates such as phenobarbitone and Amytal are sedatives.

3. *Hypnotic.* A hypnotic is a drug which is used to produce sleep. It depresses the central nervous system to a greater degree than a sedative does but it has a limited duration of effect. Barbiturates, chloral hydrate and Doriden may be used for this purpose.

4. *Tranquillizer (ataractic).* This is a drug which promotes a sense of calmness and well-being without that degree of depression of the central nervous system which is commonly associated with action of sedatives or hypnotics. Chlorpromazine is the most commonly used tranquillizer.

5. *Stimulant.* A stimulant is a drug which temporarily enhances wakefulness and alertness, it improves mood and lessens the sense of fatigue. Drugs of the amphetamine group are stimulants.

6. *Narcotic.* A narcotic is any drug which brings about a reversible depression of cell metabolism and activity in the central nervous system. Any of the substances mentioned above, with the exception of stimulants, are narcotics, but in common usage the term 'narcotic' is reserved for drugs like opium, pethidine and cocaine. These drugs, which are subject to international control, are also powerful analgesics.

14.27 Causes of drug abuse

The causes of drug abuse are similar to those for alcohol abuse. There is an occupational risk for doctors, nurses and pharmacists who are constantly handling these substances. There is an element of experimentation with young people. They want to try the experience confident that they will not become 'hooked'. Alas, things too often do not work out like that. Young people are also subject to 'gang' pressures. At a party it takes much courage to be the odd-man-out when everyone else is taking drugs. Anyway it is always for 'kicks', it is never serious. Then there is physical illness. Sometimes a person's first experience of narcotics for example, may be to relieve pain associated with physical illness or surgical operation. Legitimate use can proceed to abuse. There is the easy availability of drugs and there are people who illicitly deal in drugs, the so-called 'pushers'. It is likely that the 'pusher' plays an important role in increasing the incidence of drug abuse. In the early stages 'pushers' will give away drugs or sell them very cheaply and when the unfortunate victim is 'hooked' the price rises sharply. As in alcoholism it has been said that those involved in drug abuse have a vulnerable personality and are unable to cope with everyday life without some prop or support: in this case the crutch used is a chemical one.

14.28 Historical aspects

Drug abuse is a fairly new thing, though drugs have been used for centuries. Geoffrey Chaucer (1345–1400), William Shakespeare (1564–1616) and Sir Thomas Browne (1605–82) all mention them. A royal decree in China in 1729 prohibited the sale and smoking of opium.

In the eighteenth and the nineteenth century opium was used in a similar way that aspirin is used today. People who were said to be addicts include Samuel Taylor Coleridge (1722–1834), George Crabbe (1784–1832) and Thomas De Quincey (1785–1859). In 1821 De Quincey produced his book 'Confessions of an English Opium Eater'. Writers were considered to be somewhat eccentric and fortunately not many people followed their example. Sir Walter Scott (1771–1832) and John Keats (1794–1821) used opium enough to affect their writing and George Byron (1788–1824), Charles Lamb (1775–1834) and Percy Shelley (1792–1822) used it as an occasional remedy.

In 1860 as much as 100,000 lb of opium were imported into the United Kingdom without any apparent concern. However, by the turn of the century attitudes were changing and the Indian and Chinese Opium Trade Agreement, which ended the opium trade, came into being in 1908.

At this stage there was considerable international concern and there was a conference in Shanghai in 1909 and another in the Hague in 1912. In 1921 the League of Nations appointed an Advisory Committee to study the drug problem. There followed in 1925 the two Geneva conferences. The second Geneva conference was an important landmark in the international control of drugs. Thirty-six countries attended and some of the control measures are still operative today.

14.29 Current incidence

In 1961 the First Brain Committee commented as follows: 'After

careful consideration of all the data put before us we are of the opinion
that in Great Britain the incidence of addiction to dangerous drugs
is still very small; there is nevertheless in our opinion no cause to
fear that any real increase is at present occurring.' The first teenage
heroin addict was reported in 1960; by 1964 there were 40; by 1967
there were 395 and in 1968 the number had risen to 764. The total
number of addicts to dangerous drugs was 1,729 in 1967. This had
risen to 2,782 in 1968 and the trend continues. The Second Brain
Committee Report in 1964 recognized this development in drug
abuse and commented on the number of young people who took
amphetamine type drugs.

A variety of drugs are used by addicts and we shall consider some
of these now.

14.30 Opiates

Opium as such is seldom if ever used now, instead purified and therefore more powerful derivatives are used and these include morphine
and heroin.

A. MORPHINE. This was the first alkaloid to be isolated from opium
and this was done as early as 1803. It is a powerful analgesic and
15 mg. is the usual dose, and a dose of 60 mg. could kill a normal
person. Dependency quickly develops and so does tolerance: it is
not unusual for an addict to take up to 600 mg in a day. It is sometimes
taken by members of the medical, nursing and pharmaceutical
professions who become dependent. It is known as 'M' or 'Junk'
among addicts.

B. HEROIN (DIAMORPHINE). This is obtained by mixing morphine
and acetic acid. It was discovered in 1874 and was first used in 1898.
It was believed to be a safe non-addictive substitute for morphine,
but it turned out to be even more addictive. It is the drug often used
by addicts as it produces in the beginning at least, a state of well-
being (euphoria). In the language of the street heroin is known
as 'H', 'Horse' or 'Harry'.

The specific treatment for those dependent on either of these
two drugs is gradual withdrawal of the drug accompanied by a
substitute such as methadone (Physeptone) or chlorpromazine
(Largactil).

14.31 Cocaine

This drug is derived from the leaves of a cocoa tree which is found in South American countries such as Peru and Bolivia. Cocaine was isolated in 1860 and its local analgesic properties were discovered in 1886. It stimulates the nervous system and appears to increase physical and mental energy as well as preventing fatigue. If large amounts are taken frequently it may give rise to convulsions or mental disturbance with paranoid ideas. The drug is often taken as snuff 'snow' by 'snowbirds' and ulcers often develop in the nose. People become psychologically dependent on cocaine, but there is no physical dependence or tolerance, so withdrawal symptoms are less of a problem than in opiate dependency. In the street it is known as 'C' or 'Charley'.

14.32 Synthetic analgesics

There are two principal synthetic analgesics in general use.

A. PETHIDINE (DEMEROL). This is a synthetic narcotic which was introduced in 1939. It is a useful analgesic, but not as powerful as morphine. It relaxes visceral muscle and together with atropine it is effective in controlling colicky pain, as in renal colic. At first it was considered to be a non-addictive substitute for morphine, but like heroin, it does cause addiction. Pethidine is sometimes used by professional addicts such as doctors and there is psychological and physical dependence as well as tolerance. The antidote for pethidine, as for morphine, is nalorphine.

B. METHADONE (PHYSEPTONE). This is another synthetic narcotic which was introduced in 1946. It is more reliable when taken orally than morphine. Methadone is an addictive drug, but since withdrawal symptoms are milder and develop more slowly, it is often used as a substitute when other narcotics are withdrawn.

14.33 Barbiturates

This group of drugs, in the form of barbital, was first introduced into medicine in 1903 under the trade name of veronal. In 1912 phenobarbitone (Luminal) was introduced and the number has steadily increased since. There are now about 50 barbiturate preparations on the market and include amylobarbitone (Amytal), amylobarbitone sodium (Sodium Amytal), and butobarbitone (Soneryl). Other examples are methexitone sodium (Brietal Sodium), quinalbarbitone sodium (Seconal), thiopentone sodium (Pentothal) and pentobarbitone sodium (Nembutal).

Barbiturates can produce all degrees of depression of the central nervous system functions, from slight sedation to deep coma. In the case of gross over-dosage, death from depression of the respiratory centre can occur.

For a long time it was thought that barbiturates were not addictive, but recently it has been realized that barbiturates present a far bigger problem than opiate addiction for example. They produce severe psychological and physical dependency and tolerance also develops.

The street names for barbiturates include 'Blue Bombers', 'Yellow Jackets' and 'Red Devils'.

Apart from general care and rehabilitation there are two specific means of treating a barbiturate overdose:

A. By using an antidote such as bemegride (Megimide). This drug neutralizes the action of barbiturates and thus reduces their effect.
B. By using a drug which hastens the excretion of barbiturates from the body. The technique used is called forced diuresis and a substance such as mannitol is used. Mannitol is a diuretic and this means it increases the output of urine by its action on the kidneys. Drugs and their end-products are eliminated from the body in the urine. If the output of urine increases, then the output of drugs in the urine will àlso be increased and the amount of drugs remaining in the body will be lessened. This is the principle of forced diuresis.

14.34 Other hypnotics, sedatives and tranquillizers

There are a great number of other drugs which can cause dependency and we shall mention some of these now.

A. CHLORAL HYDRATE. This drug, which was first used medically in 1869, is derived from chlorinated ethyl alcohol. As alcohol forms its basis, continued use is likely to cause dependency.

B. PARALDEHYDE. This drug has been available since 1829. It has an acetaldehyde basis. Ordinary ethyl alcohol is metabolized to acetaldehyde in the body, but paraldehyde is more potent and more poisonous than ethyl alcohol. Dependency does occur but as paraldehyde is not often prescribed nowadays, it is not a problem.

C. DORIDEN. This is a non-barbiturate hypnotic but dependency can occur.

D. TRANQUILLIZERS. Drugs of the phenothiazine group are the most commonly used as tranquillizers. They give no 'lift' nor is there any conscious change as experienced with alcohol, barbiturates or opium derivatives and therefore do not cause primary dependency. They do, however, control symptoms and there is sometimes a reluctance to give them up for this reason.

14.35 Cannabis sativa (hashish, marihuana)

The use of cannabis has no place in medical treatment, therefore its use is always illegal. It is extracted from hemp plants which are principally found in the Americas, Africa and Asia. Cannabis is taken by great numbers of people all over the world and it may be smoked, chewed, snuffed or swallowed.

Smoking cannabis is said to be a pleasurable experience; it gives a feeling of lightness and causes disorientation of time and space. It gives rise to laughter and lightheartedness and also causes hallucinations. Artists and musicians claim it increases perception, but in reality the quality and the quantity of work performed under the influence of the drug is poor.

Psychological dependence on cannabis is great but physical dependence and tolerance are said to be absent. Because of the last two facts there have been moves to legalize 'pot' (cannabis) in recent years on the grounds that it presents no greater threat to society than alcohol. Others disagree with this view. There are others who claim that cannabis taking can proceed to the use of the more deadly opiate drugs. The outcome is that the possession or use of cannabis is illegal.

14.36 Other psycho-stimulants (amphetamine)

Amphetamine was discovered in 1930 and it occurs in many forms; benzedrine and dexedrine are examples. Before antidepressants became available, amphetamines were regularly used in the treatment of depression.

The amphetamine group of drugs act as a stimulant to the nervous system, they increase alertness and confidence, raise the mood, improve concentration, give rise to euphoria and elation, and they lessen the sense of fatigue. They are sometimes called 'happy pills'.

They are commonly used to reduce weight for they increase the person's energy and reduce the desire for food. Amphetamines may also be used by athletes to improve their performance; in this context they are known as 'pep' pills.

Drinamyl was introduced in 1951 and teenagers began to use it for 'kicks'. By 1965 the Second Brain Committee found the abuse of amphetamine drugs a serious problem. An attempt was made at legal control in 1964 when the Drugs (Prevention of Misuse) Act was introduced. The main provision of this Act was to make possession of amphetamine drugs without authority an offence.

Users become psychologically dependent on amphetamines, but there is no physical dependence. Tolerance does occur. There are no withdrawal symptoms, but an existing psychiatric condition may be aggravated. A toxic type of mental illness may be produced with delusions and hallucinations.

Some of the street names for amphetamines are as follows: Drinamyl ('Purple Hearts', 'French Blues') and Durophet ('Black Bombers').

14.37 Hallucinogens (mescaline and lysergic acid)

These drugs have the ability to induce sharp changes in states of awareness and perception. Their use makes everything seem bigger, better and more beautiful than it really is. There are several drugs of this variety available, but we shall mention only a few.

A. MESCALINE (PEYOTE). This drug is obtained from a cactus plant which grows in certain parts of the United States. Various American Indian tribes chew peyote buttons as part of a religious ritual. Mescaline is used by artists and musicians to increase perception. Aldous Huxley who took mescaline as an experiment describes its action in his little book 'The Doors of Perception': Mescaline has been used to produce a schizophrenic-like reaction as an experiment. One of the dangers of mescaline abuse is that it does produce an acute schizophrenic-like illness in some subjects. Mescaline is said not to cause dependence.

B. LYSERGIC ACID DIETHYLAMIDE (L.S.D.). L.S.D. also produces hallucinations and is said to have a mind-loosening or mind-expanding effect (psychedelic). It was discovered in 1943 by a Swiss research worker who was working on ergot alkaloids. Under the influence of

L.S.D. people develop extraordinary ideas about their abilities. Such people have been known to step out of high windows believing themselves to be able to walk on air. Another person walked on to a busy street in New York, with tragic results, believing he could stop the traffic simply by waving his hands.

C. PSILOCYBIN. This drug is derived from a Mexican fungus and a cult has built up around it. Psilocybin has similar effects to L.S.D.

These hallucinogenic drugs are not used for treatment and are rarely used for experimental work. Possession of such drugs without authority is illegal. The main point against the use of such drugs, apart from the changes in behaviour they produce, is that they permanently damage brain cells.

14.38 Other drugs

There are a variety of other substances which can cause dependency. Chlorodyne is a mixture of morphia and chloroform and is used in the treatment of diarrhoea. Because of its contents people become dependent on it. Petrol sniffing and glue sniffing also occur and cause dependency.

14.39 Tobacco

The use of tobacco is a socially accepted habit, though it is said that if tobacco was being introduced for the first time now it would never be allowed into general use. There seems to be an established link between heavy cigarette smoking and lung cancer, but this is only part of the ill-effects of tobacco. It is said that when tobacco burns nearly two hundred chemical substances interact. The best known of these is nicotine which was first isolated from the tobacco leaf in 1843. Nicotine has a stimulant action at first and then depresses the ganglia of both sides of the autonomic nervous system. Tolerance to nicotine readily develops and so does psychological dependence. It has serious effects on the cardiovascular system, the blood-pressure is raised and there is an increased risk of coronary heart disease. The appetite is less and some people use this as reason for continuing to smoke. In the respiratory system, apart from lung cancer, nicotine causes chronic inflammation of the mucous lining which is accompanied by a cough.

14.40 Principles of treatment

There are two aspects to the treatment of drug dependency:

A. EMERGENCY. Very often such people are seriously ill or unconscious when admitted to hospital. Unconsciousness may be the result of a conscious or an accidental overdosage, above the tolerance level of the drug or combination of drugs. The treatment involves giving the appropriate antidote such as nalorphine in the case of opiates and bemegride in the case of barbiturates. The patient's physical condition is usually poor with multiple infected lesions and perhaps pneumonia. The appropriate antibiotic is required for these. Then there is the general management of an unconscious person including the provision of a clear airway.

B. LONG TERM. The aim of long term treatment is rehabilitation in society. This begins with:

1. *Withdrawal and substitution.* Sudden withdrawal from a drug of dependency gives rise to severe physical symptoms, the so-called 'cold turkey' in the addicts' language. This seldom occurs under medical care as a substitute drug is given. This is also withdrawn later. In the case of opiates, Physeptone is the usual substitute.

2. *Psychotherapy.* This begins as individual psychotherapy and later the person is included in group psychotherapy sessions. These sessions are similar to the group sessions for alcoholics. Sometimes the group is exclusively for people who are dependent on drugs and sometimes they are mixed. Views vary about this. On the one hand it is not thought a good idea to have addicts mix only with addicts. On the other hand many people look upon addicts as no-good layabouts. Condemnatory attitudes are likely to hinder rather than help cure.

3. *Social.* Though the period of time for severe dependency to occur is very much shorter for drug users than alcohol users, it is long enough for a degree of social isolation to develop. Many drug users lose contact with their homes or are given up as hopeless cases by their perplexed parents. They are usually unemployed, without money, accommodation or friends. All these matters must be rectified through the statutory and voluntary bodies if there is to be any hope of success.

14.41 Observation

1. *Appearance.* Assuming that the person is conscious, the general appearance is usually dirty and untidy. The facial expression may

be mask-like and dreamy or miserable depending on the length of time since the last dose.

2. *Conversation.* The conversation may be fast or slow, incoherent or childish depending on the drug used. If the drug is one of the amphetamine group the person is likely to talk quickly.

3. *Mood.* The mood may be one of happiness if amphetamines or L.S.D. are used. If the person is in the withdrawal stage of heroin dependency, then the mood is one of misery.

4. *Attitude.* The attitude may be demanding and resentful or apologetic and dependent. 'So help me I will never get into this mess again, but please give me another "shot", I can't stand it.'

5. *Intellect.* Drugs seriously blunt intellectual function. Memory is poor, judgement and reasoning are defective and in some cases, such as cannabis abuse, orientation is faulty.

6. *Eating.* In dependency of any degree, eating habits are altered and usually less food is taken. This ultimately leads to nutrition problems of varying degrees.

7. *Sleep.* Sleep is always upset. Opiate or narcotic drugs produce sleep and the addict may sleep from one 'fix' (injection) to the next. Very often the sleep is upset by terrifying dreams. When there is a great degree of tolerance the 'fix' may not produce sleep: in fact it may not do anything much but the person must have it. If drugs of the stimulant variety are used, obviously sleep is impossible except from exhaustion in the later stages.

8. *Physical state.* There is usually weight loss and the skin may lack lustre. If the forearms are examined there may be multiple scars, infected spots and inflammation of the veins (phlebitis) if the person uses the self injected method or 'main lining' in the addicts' terms. No care is taken over injections and water from lavatory pans may be used to dissolve tablets, hence the infection. It is not unusual for a blood-borne infection to occur (septicaemia) or a pneumonia caused by a variety of organisms. Such infections often require a number of antibiotics to control them. There may be tremors or convulsions during the withdrawal stages. Often there is nausea and vomiting.

14.42 Nursing care

Drug dependency is an urgent and an increasing social problem. Many addicts do not seek help until it is too late. Others agree to a period of treatment in order to build up physically and then return to their former habit.

Some who become dependent on drugs genuinely seek a cure. Motivation or the will to get better is vital if it is to be successful; it is no use compelling anyone to have treatment. There is much that can be done for those who want to break the habit. Withdrawal symptoms, even with a substitute drug, can be almost unbearable: there is psychological torture on the one hand and severe physical discomfort on the other. A skilled nurse can do much to make the burden more bearable. Continuous help, support and encouragement is needed, particularly in the early days. Skill is also required in arranging suitable occupational and recreational activities.

The crucial step comes when the person is on his feet again. He may need help to find his way in the world again having looked at it for so long through a drug induced fog. It may be possible to discover and develop talents and abilities which would make the person's life fuller and reduce the need to use drugs as a form of escape. Without the proper help and support the first few steps in society are also the first steps to renewed disaster.

As always, nurses' attitudes are important and if a nurse has strong personal feelings about drug abuse she should keep these to herself and adopt an objective outlook. Rapport is important and this is based on mutual trust and confidence. However there is need for a word of warning here. Addicts will go to any extremes to acquire drugs and some will co-operate in a treatment programme and continue to take large doses of the drug of addiction. The author remembers a case where the person appeared to be making good progress until it was discovered that he had a large quantity of morphine tablets hidden in a lavatory cistern; he was continuing to take about 300 mg of morphine daily as well as the substitute drug. Nurses must be alert for this possibility. Also keep a discreet check on all incoming packages—for hidden compartments, and on visitors who may pass on supplies.

14.43 Prevention

When one sees how the abuse of drugs can totally wreck young lives and even cause death among those in the bloom of youth, one wonders if all drugs should be dumped in the deepest ocean and further supplies be banned for ever. But of course this would be no solution. Drugs, including drugs of addiction, when properly used do much to relieve suffering. It is only when drugs are abused that they are so harmful. Efforts must therefore be made to prevent drug abuse. A start has already been made. The Drugs (Prevention of Misuse) Act 1964 has made it more difficult to get amphetamines. The Drugs Act 1965 and 1967, which requires doctors to report suspected addicts, helps to control the use of opiates. Such drugs can only be supplied by specially appointed doctors. More legislation is promised. The establishment of Treatment Centres and the registration of addicts helps in the control of the problem.

Legislation alone is not enough for there are always people who will break or find ways around the law. New attitudes are also needed and with this follows new values. Reasons must be sought for drug abuse and alternatives must be found. People must be helped to develop their resources and to stand on their feet without chemical props. Education would seem to have a lot to offer, but often education is a rat race. Is early selection, early streaming and early specialization possible, while at the same time developing other aspects of the personality? If the answer is 'no', then a more liberal element should be introduced into education.

Apart from legislative, general and educational measures to control the abuse of drugs, much research work needs to be carried out on the question of dependency, tolerance and associated problems.

14.14 Summary

Drug abuse is a serious problem particularly among young people. The causes of drug abuse are not fully known, but the effects which can be readily observed are serious and often tragic. Fit young people are turned into physical wrecks and are physically and psychologically dependent on chemicals. Social disintegration and social isolation soon follow and many die in wretched circumstances and in appalling conditions. Much is being done to control the problem, but there is room for much more effort.

15

Mental disorders with a physical basis

15.0 Introduction

There are a number of mental disorders with a definite physical basis and these can be divided into two categories. First there are those due to physical lesions in the brain and second there are those due to lesions elsewhere in the body. The first category will be the subject of the next chapter and in this chapter we shall consider the mental effects of lesions elsewhere in the body.

15.1 Endocrine disorders

There are two control systems in the body. The nervous provides the overall control and the endocrine system plays a significant part in the chemical control of the body. Disordered endocrine function means an upset in the body chemistry and many of these upsets have an effect upon the mind.

15.2 Cushing's syndrome

This syndrome is due to a new growth in the pituitary gland. The overactive gland causes over activity of the adrenal cortex. This results in obesity and women grow hair on the face. Frequently there is acne. The blood pressure is raised and bones are rarefied causing osteoporosis and readily break.

The mental symptoms may be irritability and depression, though it is possible for a schizophrenic-like illness to develop depending on the pre-morbid personality.

The treatment of such conditions calls for a double approach. First the mental symptoms must be controlled with antidepressants or tranquillizers as appropriate. Second the condition must be treated by surgical methods or deep X-rays or a combination of both.

15.3 Myxoedema

This is due to the thyroid gland producing too little thyroid hormone. Physically all bodily functions are slower than normal. The blood pressure and body temperature are much lower than normal. There is obesity, constipation, loss of appetite and a coarseness of the skin.

Depression is the common mental condition, but sometimes there is mental deterioration resembling dementia. Treatment is by replace-

11

ment of the missing thyroid hormone, though in the meantime mental symptoms may need to be controlled with antidepressants.

15.4 Thyrotoxicosis

This is the opposite of myxoedema and is due to too much thyroid hormone being produced and the symptoms are also of an opposite nature. Mentally there is restlessness, excitement, irritability and anxiety. On a more severe plane there may be mania or a schizo-phrenic-like reaction with delusions and hallucinations.

The treatment is to correct the underlying condition whilst at the same time controlling the mental symptoms.

15.5 Diabetes mellitus and insulin

Too little insulin, as occurs in diabetes mellitus, results in confusion, restlessness and coma. Too much insulin resulting in too little sugar circulating in the bloodstream (hypoglycaemia) causes a variety of mental symptoms ranging from confusion and forgetfulness (amnesia) to coma. The excessive insulin may be produced in the body by an islet cell tumour, or it may be given by injection for the treatment of diabetes mellitus or as modified insulin treatment.

The treatment is the treatment of the underlying cause.

15.6 Adrenal insufficiency

The adrenal glands produce hormones, the cortex produces a group of hormones called steroids and the medulla produces adrenaline. When the output of these hormones is inadequate (adrenal insuf-ficiency) a variety of symptoms occur such as loss of weight, loss of energy, lowered blood pressure and excessive loss of mineral salts (electrolytes) from the body. There is often depression which clears up when the hormone levels are restored to normal.

15.7 Infections

Infections can affect mental function in two ways. In the period before and in the early stages of an infection people often feel very well mentally and better than normal. At one stage this led to giving people with mental illness T.A.B. (typhoid vaccine), for there are usually general symptoms and a raised temperature associated with this. The practice has long been abandoned. In the later stages of some infections there may be mental symptoms. These are sometimes referred to as *toxic confusional states* and may be found in the later stages of pneumonia, for example. There may be delirium in typhoid fever or malaria. Influenza is often followed by depression.

15.8 Drugs and poisons

We have already considered the effects of alcohol and the drugs of addiction. Now we shall consider other drugs and a number of poisons which may affect mental function.

15.9 Steroids

These hormones are commonly used in treatment often because of their anti-inflammatory action. They may be used for chronic inflammation such as pulmonary tuberculosis, asthma, dermatitis or ulcerative colitis. As well as reducing the body's reaction to inflammatory agents, steroids also produce a sense of well-being (euphoria). In some people, particularly those with a history of mental instability, steroids can precipitate a mental illness such as schizophrenic or manic reactive. Very often small doses will trigger off such reactions. The author has met a case of a woman who was given a small dose of steroid for a troublesome eye infection and had a schizophrenic type illness requiring admission to hospital. A general hospital nurse is more likely to meet such reactions in the course of her work.

15.10 Lead

This is a commonly found metal and is sometimes used in children's toys, paints, car batteries and in glass blowing. People involved in lead paint spraying, battery manufacture or lead glass blowing run the risk of lead poisoning if adequate precautions are not taken.

Lead accumulates in the body and gives rise to a number of symptoms such as loss of appetite, abdominal discomfort, constipation and headaches. Later there may be abdominal cramps and anaemia. There is bleeding around the teeth and this is known as the 'lead line'.

The mental symptoms are those of confusion with delusions and hallucinations. There may be delirium and occasionally convulsions occur. Reactions to lead can sometimes be very distressing. The author remembers a fit muscular man, who had been lead painting in an oil refinery, being admitted accompanied by six harassed medical students and four equally harassed policemen. The man was overactive and aggressive and continually fought and spat at everyone in sight. An intravenous infusion was set up and *calcium disodium versenate* was given by this route. This drug has the effect of a *chelating agent* and converts the lead into soluble compounds which are then removed from the body by the kidneys. In this case the man showed improvement after three or four days and was completely better in two weeks.

Prevention is better than cure and wearing the prescribed protective clothing usually gives full protection. More care is now taken over lead toys and lead paint should not be used on places where children can scrape it off and eat it.

15.11 Mercury

This is not used as frequently as lead, but exposure to mercury can cause irritability and depression. It also causes tremors of the lips, the tongue and the hands.

Mercurial poisoning is treated by giving a drug called *dimercaprol* (B.A.L.) This is given by intramuscular injection at regular intervals.

15.12 Carbon monoxide

Oxygen which is essential for the life of all cells is transported in the haemoglobin of the red blood corpuscles; the haemoglobin has an affinity for oxygen. Haemoglobin has a stronger affinity for carbon monoxide so that it is taken up in preference to oxygen. When there is a high concentration of carbon monoxide in the atmosphere, this means that little or no oxygen reaches the cells of the body and permanent damage or death follows. This is particularly so in the case of brain cells for they have the greatest need for oxygen and confusion and unconsciousness readily follow if supplies are inadequate.

Carbon monoxide is produced by motor car exhausts, by incomplete combustion of carbon and household gas (this applies to town gas and not natural gas) contains up to 25 per cent of this gas. We have already mentioned gas in relation to suicide and saw that it is the most common method used. Few cases of carbon monoxide poisoning are accidental, most are suicidal. The majority of those who recover from carbon monoxide poisoning have few ill effects, but the intellect is sometimes blunted and some suffer from dementia.

The treatment is first to remove the person from the source of the gas and to replace the carbon monoxide in the blood with oxygen. This may be by mouth-to-mouth artificial respiration, by oxygen mask and in special cases hyperbaric (high pressure) oxygen.

15.13 Acidosis

Acidosis as its name suggests means an excess of acid and is generally used to mean an excess of acid in the blood. The degree of acidity or alkalinity of a solution is measured with reference to the pH scale. pH means the hydrogen in concentration. H is the chemical symbol for hydrogen and the small p is used to indicate that it is a log scale; this means that each point on the scale is 10 times stronger or weaker than the next one. The scale ranges from 0 to 14 and the neutral point is 7. Numbers from 7 down to 0 represent an increasing degree of acidity and those from 7 to 14 an increasing degree of alkalinity. The pH range of the blood is small and is between 7·0 and 7·70. Acidosis may be due to depression of the respiratory centre by drugs, disease or paralysis. The main mental symptoms are progressive drowsiness with blunting of the intellect, delusions and hallucinations. Prolonged acidosis can lead to dementia. The treatment is to correct the cause if possible. In the meantime mental symptoms may be controlled by the use of the appropriate drugs such as the phenothiazine group.

15.14 Alkalaemia

This is the opposite of acidosis and it means that the blood is excessively alkaline. Over breathing (hyperventilation) causes alkalosis by removing too much carbon dioxide (acidic) too quickly. This sometimes happens in the panic phases of fear and anxiety reactions. Alkalaemia may cause loss of consciousness and it can precipitate a fit in epileptic persons. Treatment consists of treating the underlying anxiety. Reassurance is needed during an attack and some form of diversion is also needed. It is sometimes helpful to make the person count four between breaths.

15.15 Uraemia

Protein is the only nutrient to contain nitrogen. When protein has been used in the body, the remaining nitrogen is excreted in the urine in the form of urea. When the kidneys are diseased or fail for some reason, urea and other end-products of metabolism accumulate in the blood, and give rise to uraemia and many symptoms.

The mental symptoms are restlessness, irritability, fatigue and confusion. The symptoms often develop slowly especially in chronic kidney disease. There may be fits and there is a gradual loss of consciousness.

Treatment is to correct the underlying cause of the kidney failure. As drugs are excreted by the kidneys, they are not prescribed in uraemia.

15.16 Surgical operations

These are stressful events. There may be anxiety about the outcome of the operation, pain, loss of function or employment prospects afterwards. As well as the stress there is often an imbalance of the mineral salts in the body (electrolytes). We saw earlier that the electrolyte composition of the blood is altered in depression; it follows then that if the electrolytes are upset by operation, similar mental reactions may follow. Then there are infections which can affect mental function.

The mental effects of surgical operations are due to two principal causes, infective and toxic/electrolytic. The main symptoms are delusions and hallucinations. The delusions are often of a persecutory nature and the hallucinations may be visual or tactile—the person feels insects or flies crawling all over his body. Occasionally there may be delirium.

Despite the fact that surgical operations are stressful events, that there is frequently electrolyte upset and there is sometimes infection, mental reactions requiring treatment only rarely arise. In fact the morale in surgical wards is often very high and no doubt this contributes to the mental well-being of all concerned.

15.17 Childbirth

This is an event which is normally associated with happiness and joy. There are instances however when this is not so. The mother may be unmarried and thus may have to part with her child as soon as it is born, or the mother may have a large family already and the new arrival adds to her burdens. Even when the child is wanted there are varying degrees of pain; drugs may be used and there may be dehydration and an upset of the electrolytes. A combination of these factors gives rise to mental disturbance and confusion. Following childbirth there may be mild depression with lots of tears, the so-called 'maternity blues', which last for 3 or 4 days. These are normal reactions, but sometimes there are more severe disturbances of mental function and these are given the term puerperal psychoses. (Puer, boy. Parere to bear). Puerperium relates to childbirth and the period during which the reproductive organs are returning to their normal condition following labour and lasts for six weeks.

15.18 Puerperal psychosis

Hippocrates (460–377 B.C.) was probably the first physician to describe a case of puerperal psychosis in 400 B.C. The condition has interested people since and today it is said to account for 2–9 per cent of all women's admissions to mental hospitals. A great number, up to 80 per cent, are admitted to hospital within three months of delivery, though in some cases the period between delivery and admission is longer.

Puerperal psychosis is not a separate disease in itself, the majority are affective-type reactions, mainly depression, and the remainder are mostly schizophrenic-like reactions. A puerperal psychosis is much more likely to develop in a person who has had a history of mental illness.

The early signs of a puerperal psychosis are restlessness and insomnia. This is accompanied by loss of interest in the husband and child. Later delusions develop. If it is an affective reaction the delusions are often those of guilt and if it is a schizophrenic reaction the delusions may be of a persecutory nature and there are also likely to be hallucinations. The mother, perhaps driven by the 'voices', may attempt to kill her baby (infanticide). This is a possibility which must always be borne in mind.

The treatment is to relieve the symptoms with antidepressants or tranquillizers as appropriate. Supportive psychotherapy is an essential part of the treatment. Protection of the child is important whilst allowing the mother as much contact as is practicable. This is best achieved in a mother-and-baby unit.

Prevention is difficult when puerperal psychosis occurs for the first time, but good ante-natal care can contribute much. If the condition has occurred on one or more occasions there might be a case for advising against having further children and offering sterilization. The question of sterilization must always be carefully considered in the light of individual circumstances.

15.19 Summary

There are many mental disorders with a physical basis. The reactions produced may be of an affective or a schizophrenic nature. There is a specific treatment in the majority of cases and the response is often dramatic. Some of these conditions can be prevented such as those caused by drugs and poisons. Those due to surgical operations and childbirth can largely be prevented by good health education and

good nursing care. There is a case for including a period of psychiatric experience in general nurse training and of course this now
happens in a great number of training schools.

16

Physical disorders of the nervous system

16.0 Introduction

In this chapter we shall consider some of the physical lesions found in the brain and we shall mention the mental reactions associated with them. *Neurology* is the term given to the study of these lesions. Neurological disorders and physical disorders generally, are due to congenital, infective, traumatic, metabolic, neoplastic, or degenerative influences and are considered here within that framework.

16.1 Congenital

A congenital condition is one which exists before birth or occurs at birth. Congenital conditions may be genetic in nature as in tuberous sclerosis or phenylketonuria, infective as in German measles or syphilis, or traumatic due to a forceps delivery for example. Some congenital conditions are due to developmental defects; spina bifida is an example.

16.2 Hydrocephalus

In hydrocephalus there is an excess of cerebrospinal fluid. This is due to a malformation which interferes with the free circulation of this fluid. Malformations may occur in several places, the cerebral aqueduct may be narrowed or absent, or there may be a blockage at the outlet of the fourth ventricle. The accumulation of fluid greatly increases the intracranial pressure.

The main sign of hydrocephalus is a great enlargement of the head. It may have reached such proportions before birth as to obstruct labour. The hydrocephalus in some cases may not be severe at birth but slowly develops in the first months of life. The head enlargement may be such that the diameter of the child's head may be 75 cm. (30 in.) or more.

Children with hydrocephalus of any severity are mentally subnormal. They are unable to move the enlarged head and are likely to have a spastic paralysis of the limbs.

Hydrocephalus can be corrected surgically by introducing valves to drain away the blocked fluid. In one such operation a *Spitz-Holten* valve is fixed so as to drain the fluid into a jugular vein.

16.3 Aneurysm (*G. aneurusmos*, a widening)

An aneurysm is a widening of an artery and the widening is usually accompanied by a weakening as well (Fig. 16.0). When an aneurysm occurs in an artery in the brain, it may lead to haemorrhage. Aneurysms give rise to two types of haemorrhage, subarachnoid, which is bleeding in the subarachnoid space and cerebral, which is bleeding in the brain and most commonly occurs at the internal capsule.

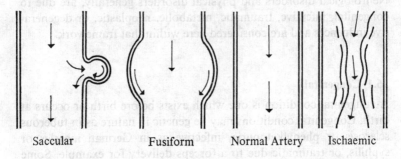

Saccular   Fusiform   Normal Artery   Ischaemic

Fig.16.0. Diagram to show types of aneurysm.

A haemorrhage in the brain in a young subject is frequently due to a congenital aneurysm and this is more likely to happen if the blood pressure is raised above normal. In an older subject haemorrhage is due to degenerative changes of the blood vessels—to be mentioned later—and raised blood pressure, though there may be a congenital weakness as well.

A subarachnoid haemorrhage due to an aneurysm often comes on without warning, though sometimes there may be a history of headache. A severe subarachnoid haemorrhage may produce a coma, shock and death within a few hours. A less severe one causes headache and vomiting. The person tends to want to be left alone and there is irritability, clouding of consciousness and confusion.

The following investigations help to confirm the diagnosis.

A. LUMBAR PUNCTURE. The pressure of the cerebrospinal fluid is raised and is blood stained.

B. X-RAY. A carotid angiography is very useful for it can show the site, the size and the shape of the aneurysm.

Apart from general medical care and nursing care, surgical operation is sometimes carried out provided the person is fit enough for an operation and provided the aneurysm appears to be amenable to surgery.

The outlook is variable; many die of the first haemorrhage, others survive only to have a further bleed. A number live a normal life-span without further inconvenience.

16.4 Epilepsy

This is an ancient disease. Hippocrates (460–377 B.C.) defined it as a chronic functional (having no organic base) disease, characterized by fits or attacks in which there is loss of consciousness with a succession of tonic (increased muscle tone) and clonic (involuntary muscular contractions) convulsions. This definition is as valid now as when it was first made.

16.5 Causes

A variety of physical disorders such as uraemia, drug withdrawal, injury and new growths give rise to convulsions and epilepsy due to any of these causes is called *symptomatic epilepsy*. No such physical basis can be found in the greatest proportion of epileptics and such epilepsy is known as *idiopathic epilepsy*.

Genetic factors are important in idiopathic epilepsy for it has been shown that the incidence of epilepsy is higher amongst the near relatives of epileptics than in the general population. Lennox (1951) and his co-workers did electroencephalographic studies on the parents of epileptics and found that they had abnormal brain waves more frequently than a control group.

16.6 Incidence

The incidence of epilepsy in Britain is about 1 in every 200 of the population, giving a total figure of up to 200,000. About 80 per cent of these live normal lives with a minimum of inconvenience. The others require varying degrees of supervision and help. Some may need psychiatric help for though epilepsy in itself is not a psychiatric condition, a psychiatric problem may occur in someone with epilepsy.

16.7 Physiology of a fit

The brain has a continuous spontaneous electrical activity and this electrical activity is recorded by the E.E.G. (electroencephalograph). When an epileptic fit occurs there is an excessive amount of electrical activity and this can readily be seen on the E.E.G. if the person is connected to the machine whilst having a fit. The extra electrical activity is said to originate in the cells of the cerebral cortex. It is sometimes described as an 'electrical storm' in the brain. The 'electrical storm' has two effects; it causes a loss of consciousness and the skeletal muscles are so over-stimulated that they contract involuntarily and give rise to convulsions.

16.8 Types of fit

There are two types of epileptic fit:

A. PETIT MAL. A petit mal as the name suggests is a small type of fit. There may be loss of consciousness for a few moments and there is no convulsion. Neither is there an aura (warning) and sometimes the subject may be unaware of the attack. The person may become pale, may stop talking or drop an object which is held. A school child may go 'glassy-eyed' and appear to be inattentive for a few moments. Sometimes there may be slight twitching of the facial muscles. Petit mal fits commonly occur in childhood and adolescence and are rare in adults. These fits, which may occur frequently, cause lack of attention or even confusion which may last for several hours. This can have serious effects on a child's education.

Petit mal fits give rise to a typical spike-and-wave E.E.G. pattern.

B. GRAND MAL. There are four stages in a grand mal fit:

1. The aura. This is a sensory warning and is peculiar to the individual. It may take the form of lights before the eyes, ringing in the ears, unusual skin sensations or peculiar tastes or smells. The amount of advance warning given also varies with the individual; some have time to lie on the ground. Others fall down almost immediately and lose consciousness. There may be a cry as the person falls and injury may be caused.
2. The tonic stage. This stage lasts from 10 to 30 seconds and during it there is a tonic spasm of all the skeletal muscles of the body. Breathing stops during this stage because the tonic muscles keep the glottis closed, the result is cyanosis (blue colour).
3. The clonic stage. The clonic stage may last for 3 or 4 minutes and consists of clonic jerking of the muscles. The tongue or lips may be bitten, froth may appear at the mouth due to the

air forced out of the lungs causing the saliva in the mouth to bubble. Urine and faeces may be passed during this stage.
4. The coma stage. When the convulsion stops the person remains unconscious, in a coma, for a varying length of time, but usually not more than an hour.

Following recovery from the fit the person is usually bewildered and confused and may complain of headache and fatigue. In some people the coma is followed by a stage automatism. During this stage the person may wander off in an undressed state and may commit violent acts.

Sometimes a person may have one grand mal fit after another and this is called status epilepticus. This is a serious threat to life and calls for skilled management. It involves caring for the unconscious person as well as treatment measures to control the convulsions.

16.9 Management of a fit

The important thing about petit mal fits is to recognize them for what they are and to seek treatment. This is in the province of parents and teachers rather than nurses. Parents should seek advice about complaints of inattention and poor concentration, especially if it is associated with a poor or a deteriorating school performance.

The maintenance of respiration is the most important thing when a grand mal fit occurs. This is done by maintaining a clear airway and holding the head to one side to allow for drainage of the saliva. It is important to prevent damage during the fall if this is possible. Some injuries are inevitable and it is a good idea to have suturing materials already prepared. It is a good idea to put something such as a padded spoon handle in the mouth to prevent the lips and tongue being bitten, but this is not always possible. There is no point in restraining the person during a fit as the site or origin of the fit, the brain, is beyond restraint. Only enough restraint to prevent injury should be used. The passage of urine or faeces during the fit is a cause of embarrassment and should be attended to as soon as possible. When consciousness is regained it is important to have someone at hand who is known to the person, then the bewilderment tends to be less.

16.10 Varieties of epilepsy

There are many varieties of epilepsy as follows:

A. PSYCHOMOTOR SEIZURES. These seizures are sometimes known as 'psychic equivalents' or epileptic equivalents. In psychomotor seizures there are disturbances, but not loss, of consciousness and there is usually no convulsion. The clouding of consciousness may last for hours, though occasionally it may last for days and during this time automatic acts may take place.

B. TEMPORAL LOBE EPILEPSY. In this type of epilepsy the 'electrical storm' comes from the temporal lobe area only. The person experiences hallucinations involving the senses of smell and taste, or musical tunes may be heard. The person becomes dazed and does not respond when addressed and may engage in automatic acts. Aggressive behaviour is a feature of temporal lobe epilepsy.

C. JACKSONIAN EPILEPSY. In 1888 John Hughlings Jackson (1835–1911) first described a convulsion which originated in the precentral area of the motor cortex. It begins with clonic movements of a small part of the opposite side of the body. The thumbs or the big toe may be involved, but often the whole limb is involved. If the convulsion is a big one there may be loss of consciousness.

D. MYOCLONIC EPILEPSY. Sometimes people with idiopathic epilepsy may suffer from repeated jerks which occur early in the morning. Such jerks may stop of their own account or may be followed by a grand mal fit.

E. NARCOLEPSY. In this condition consciousness is lost, but convulsive movements are absent. Unlike ordinary epilepsy the person can be aroused and is normal when aroused.

F. CATAPLEXY. This condition is related to narcolepsy and the two conditions may occur at the same time. In cataplexy voluntary power is lost and the person sinks helplessly to the ground. Consciousness is not lost though the person may be unable to speak.

G. EPILEPTIC PERSONALITY. The majority of epileptic persons are quite normal and have no recognizable personality traits. Some however do show personality traits, especially those confined to institutions of any kind. These sometimes take the form of quarrelling, fighting and violent behaviour. Others adopt a different line, become very religious and walk around with a Bible under one arm. Despite a self-professed love for the Bible and all that is good, such people carry tales to the doctors and administrators, they antagonize opposite shifts and generally create unpleasantness.

H. HYSTERO-EPILEPSY. Sometimes a person with hysteria may also present with epilepsy. It is important from the point of treatment to know the true nature of the epilepsy. Nurses are sometimes asked for detailed observations in order to provide information for the formulation of a diagnosis. The main point about hysterical convulsions is that they occur only in the presence of an audience. Their onset is gradual and consciousness is not completely lost. The movements are not clonic in nature, but can be seen to be carried out voluntarily. The movements increase if any attempt is made at restraint, whilst in a grand mal convulsion restraint makes no difference. In hysterical convulsions the tongue is not bitten and incontinence of urine or faeces does not occur.

16.11 Diagnosis of epilepsy

Epilepsy is diagnosed by taking a careful history and by carrying out a full neurological examination. The diagnosis is confirmed or excluded by an E.E.G. recording. In Chapter 5 we have already considered the neurological examination and the E.E.G. investigation.

16.12 Principles of treatment

Drugs form the principal part of the treatment of epilepsy. Phenobarbitone (Luminal) was the first anticonvulsant and is still commonly used for that purpose. Other drugs used are phenytoin sodium (Epanutin), methoin (Mesantoin), primidone (Mysoline), phenacemide (Phenurone) and troxidine (Tridione). A full list of anticonvulsants including the dosage, the indications and the side effects is given in Appendix 2 at the end of the book.

If there is a psychiatric problem at the same time, then the appropriate drugs are needed to control the symptoms and psychotherapy may be needed. Occupational therapy is an essential feature of treatment. In some forms of epilepsy there may be a lesion amenable to surgery but this occurs very infrequently.

16.13 Social problems of epilepsy

These are many. First epilepsy may upset a child's schooling and in some cases the child may need to go to a special school. In higher education epileptic students are restricted from taking engineering courses, or handling chemicals, electricity or radioactive materials. Epileptics are not accepted to study medicine or nursing. There are a number of jobs, which are unsuitable for epileptic workers such as any job which involves climbing and heights, jobs involving machines and driving. Under the Road Traffic Act, 1930, an applicant for a driving licençe must state whether he suffers from epilepsy and the Motor Vehicle (Driving Licences) Regulation, 1950 was designed to prevent epileptics from taking the driving test. Epilepsy presents problems in relation to marriage. Should an epileptic get married and have children? With the development of Genetic Counselling it is possible to forecast with considerable accuracy the likelihood of a child of an epileptic parent, becoming an epileptic. Even with this advice available, marriage is likely to present the epileptic with a dilemma.

There are other problems for the epileptic. At one time epilepsy was associated with the presence of evil spirits. There are still many people who do not understand epilepsy and thus have an attitude of suspicion and ignorance. Such attitudes depress some epileptics who tend to consider themselves as people apart rather than as integral members of society.

16.14 Nursing care

The majority of epileptics need no nursing care and are quite able to manage their own affairs. For those who do, there are two aspects to the nursing care. First there is the management of the fit and we have already discussed this. Second there is the general nursing care. This involves knowing the person and establishing rapport with him. This is important when he is recovering from a fit and is confused and bewildered, and should have a familiar face and a familiar voice around. Knowing the person and his pattern of epilepsy can also be helpful. A variety of factors such as changes of routine, constipation and emotional upsets can bring on a fit. With skilful management the number of fits can be kept small and in some cases it is possible to know when a fit is likely to occur and therefore be prepared.

A good occupational and recreational programme is essential for boredom and idleness have an adverse effect. As we mentioned, a small number of epileptics have an epileptic personality and the nurse should be aware of this and the disruptive influence such a person can have.

16.15 Infections

A large number of organisms may invade the nervous system or its membranes causing encephalitis or meningitis. Organisms which produce pus (*pyogenic*) cause meningitis or brain abscess. Any organism invading the brain may cause encephalitis, but this term is generally reserved for virus infections.

16.16 Encephalitis

This is due to a virus infection of the brain and its coverings and is characterized by a raised body temperature, headache, drowsiness and in severe cases confusion or coma. Convulsions may occur in children and there may be paralysis. The pressure of the cerebrospinal fluid is increased and laboratory examination reveals an increased cell count. The protein content is likely to be raised, but the sugar and chloride levels are normal.

There are several types of encephalitis:

A. ENCEPHALITIS LETHARGICA. The main feature of this type of encephalitis is the upset of the normal sleep pattern. It is sometimes called sleeping sickness because sufferers fall asleep during the day and become alert and awake at night. A late feature of encephalitis lethargica is the development of a form of Parkinson's disease.

B. INCLUSION ENCEPHALITIS. This is a form of encephalitis which occurs in children in the first decade of life. There may be mood changes at first and later intelligence is affected and involuntary movements occur. This form of encephalitis is often fatal.

C. HERPES SIMPLEX ENCEPHALITIS. Herpes simplex is a common virus infection involving the peripheral nervous system and gives rise to lesions in the skin. Sometimes the brain is involved giving rise to encephalitis.

There is no specific treatment for encephalitis as there are no antiviral drugs available. Treatment consists of relieving symptoms such as headache and general nursing care. Noise is very disturbing for people with encephalitis and they are best nursed in a quiet side ward.

16.17 Poliomyelitis

This is a virus infection of the nervous system which affects the anterior horns of the grey matter of the spinal cord and the motor nuclei of the brain stem. The cells involved are destroyed and paralysis results.

Poliomyelitis is described in two stages:

A. THE PRE-PARALYTIC STAGE. The symptoms during this stage are a raised temperature, headache, sleeplessness, flushing and stomach upsets. The symptoms may ease in 48 hours, but sometimes they become more intense and there may be delirium. There may be neck rigidity and if one of the person's legs is moved so that it is at right angles to the trunk, the person is unable to straighten his leg at the knee joint. This is due to spasm of the big hamstring muscles at the back of the leg and is known as a positive *Kernig's sign*.

B. THE PARALYTIC STAGE. The paralytic stage follows quickly on the pre-paralytic stage and is accompanied by pain in the limbs and tenderness of the muscles. The paralysis may be localized or it may be widespread. Sometimes the respiratory muscles are involved giving rise to respiratory paralysis. When the cells of the brain stem are affected the function of swallowing is impaired or impossible. Apart from being unable to eat, saliva and other secretions are in danger of being sucked into the lungs and causing asphyxia. This is called bulbar paralysis. Sometimes there is a combination of respiratory and bulbar paralysis and this presents a serious threat to life.

When the nerve cells supplying the muscles of the limbs are involved, the paralysis which results is complete and is known as a flaccid (L. flaccus, flabby) paralysis. The motor cells of the cerebral cortex are known as upper motor neurones and the motor cells of the spinal cords are known as lower motor neurones. The flaccid paralysis which is part of a paralytic poliomyelitis infection is sometimes called a lower motor neurone lesion. In such lesions the affected limbs become wasted, most or all function is lost and the reflexes are sluggish or absent.

There is no specific treatment for poliomyelitis. If there is respiratory paralysis it may be necessary to use an artificial respirator. The nursing management includes making the person as comfortable as possible and making the most use of whatever muscle function remains.

16.18 Meningitis

This is an infection which involves the pia mater and arachnoid mater covering the brain. As the subarachnoid space, containing the cerebrospinal fluid, is between the pia and arachnoid mater it means that the cerebrospinal fluid is involved. There are three varieties of meningitis according to the type of organism involved.

A. PYOGENIC MENINGITIS. This is caused by pus-producing organisms such as the Neisseria meningitidis, Diplococcus pneumoniae, Haemophilus influenza, Streptococcus and the Staphylococcus.

B. TUBERCULOUS MENINGITIS. This is caused by the Mycobacterium tuberculosis organism and is secondary to an infection elsewhere in the body. It may occur at any age, but children are most frequently affected.

C. ASEPTIC MENINGITIS. This is the term given to meningitis caused by non-pyogenic organisms, usually viruses. This type of meningitis is similar in many respects to other types, the main point of difference being that it is not possible to isolate the organism from the cerebrospinal fluid, hence the term aseptic.

16.19 Symptoms of meningitis

There are some features which are common to all types of meningitis. Headache is often the first symptom and the body temperature is raised to 39 °C (102 °F) and sometimes even higher. The pulse rate is slow in the early stages but later on it may become rapid and feeble. There is frequently nausea and vomiting convulsions occur particularly in children.

The signs which may be observed are neck rigidity and in severe cases this causes head retraction and Kernig's sign (already mentioned) may be positive. The meningeal irritation may cause children to make high pitched noises which are referred to as the *meningeal cry*. There is frequently delirium in the early stages which later gives place to drowsiness or coma.

Meningitis is diagnosed by considering the history, the symptoms and the physical signs. The diagnosis is confirmed by examination of the cerebrospinal fluid which is obtained by a lumbar puncture.

16.20 Treatment and nursing care

Drugs are the main form of medical treatment. Antibiotics according to the sensitivity of the organism are given in pyogenic meningitis, penicillin or tetracycline may be used. Tuberculous meningitis is treated with Streptomycin which is given by lumbar puncture (intrathecally). There are no specific drugs for aseptic meningitis. Drugs may be used to relieve symptoms such as headache, but care must be exercised in using these because of their effects on an already disordered nervous system.

The nursing care consists of providing absolute quiet. This is best achieved in a single room. The curtains should be drawn for such people cannot tolerate light (photophobia). Nursing care should be carried out as quietly as possible for even the rustle of a nurse's apron or sheets is extremely irritating for people with meningitis. The diet should be light and drugs should be given as prescribed. Temperature, pulse and respiration observations should be recorded four hourly, though it may sometimes be necessary to carry out these observations more frequently. A record of the fluid intake and output is also essential to ensure an adequate intake and as a check that the kidneys are functioning. Bowel actions should be recorded to make sure that regular emptying takes place.

If the person is unconscious then continuous nursing observation is necessary for unconsciousness poses a serious threat to life. There should be a suction apparatus available to remove the secretions from the air passages and thus maintain respiration. In addition to the above observations, it is necessary to observe the level of consciousness. This usually consists of testing the subject's ability to respond to questions. The person may be asked how he is able to move his limbs and so on. Next the pupils of the eyes are examined for their ability to respond to light (a torch), for size and for equality of size. The response to stimuli is then assessed. This may be done by gently pinching the person or by using a pin. A person who is deeply unconscious will not respond to questions, his eyes will not respond to light and the pupil size may be unequal, and there will be no response to painful stimuli.

To avoid the eyes becoming too dry and the delicate corners becoming injured, liquid paraffin drops are put in the eyes which are then kept closed using Sellotape. The unconscious person needs to be fed artificially using a Ryles tube which is introduced into the stomach. Milk forms the basis of such a diet and Complan is frequently used. The diet should meet the calorie and the nutrient requirements of the person. The mouth should be cleaned after each feed.

In unconsciousness, urine may be passed involuntarily (incontinence) and a catheter may be introduced and left in the bladder.

The catheter drains into a bottle or a bag which should be emptied at regular intervals and the amount measured and recorded.

Care of the skin is very important and the person should be given a daily bed bath. The person's position in bed should be changed at two-hourly intervals and the pressure areas should be massaged at the same time.

16.21 Syphilis

This infection is caused by the Treponema pallidum. It looks like a corkscrew in appearance and such organisms are called spirochaetes. The infection is passed from one person to another at sexual intercourse, though it is sometimes passed from mother to child (congenital syphilis).

Syphilis does not always affect the nervous system, but when it does it does so in two ways:

A. It affects the brain by causing inflammation and degeneration of neurones, that is, encephalitis. Mental function is affected giving rise to General Paralysis of the Insane (G.P.I.) which is characterized by impairment of intellectual efficiency, poor concentration and memory defects. We considered this condition as a cause of presenile dementia in Chapter 9.

B. It damages the sensory pathways of the spinal cord with the result that the person develops a stamping walk (ataxic gait) and easily becomes unbalanced. This condition is called *tabes dorsalis*. Sometimes G.P.I. and tabes dorsalis occur together in the same person and the combination is called *tabo paresis*.

Syphilis quickly responds to antibiotics such as penicillin and as people come readily for treatment, it is likely the incidence of G.P.I. will be less in the future.

16.22 Cerebral abscess

This is usually an extension of a pyogenic infection to the brain from the nasal sinuses, the middle ear or the mastoid process.

The symptoms of a cerebral abscess are headache, delerium and in severe cases coma.

The diagnosis is made on the history and by physical examination and may be confirmed by lumbar puncture. The pressure of the cerebrospinal fluid is increased and the protein content is also increased. An E.E.G. can be helpful in pinpointing the site of the abscess.

The treatment is a combination of surgery and antibiotics. The abscess may be removed at operation or its contents may be aspirated, followed by the injection of the appropriate antibiotic into the site of the abscess.

16.23 Trauma

Each of us is given one set of nerve cells and if we abuse or ill-use these cells they cannot be replaced. The brain and spinal cord are encased within protective bony structures and are cushioned in fluid. Such an arrangement provides a good deal of protection, but despite this the nervous system is frequently injured. These injuries are most commonly associated with injury to the head.

16.24 Head injury

Road traffic accidents and industrial accidents are the most common causes of head injury and the estimated number is 100,000 a year.

A head injury can have three effects. It may cause:

A. CONCUSSION (*L. Concussio* from concutere, to shake). Concussion has been defined as a condition of widespread paralysis of the functions of the brain which comes on as an immediate consequence of a blow on the head, has a strong tendency to spontaneous recovery, and is not necessarily associated with any gross organic change in the brain substance. People who 'pass out' following a fall from a bicycle or a similar accident usually come to quickly and appear or may describe themselves as a 'bit shaken', have had concussion.

There is a loss of memory associated with concussion. Events which occurred immediately before the accident are forgotten (retrograde amnesia). Similarly there is a loss of memory for a period after consciousness is regained and this is known as post-traumatic amnesia. The degree of amnesia is dependent on the severity of the injury.

B. CEREBRAL CONTUSION (*Contusion L. contusio*, from contundere, to bruise). A cerebral contusion is a widespread disturbance of the brain following head injury and is characterized by oedema and capillary haemorrhages. Contusion may occur without concussion, but usually consciousness is lost and frequently the unconsciousness is deep. Sometimes a cerebral contusion is fatal, but there may be recovery, though there may also be residual damage.

C. SUBDURAL HAEMATOMA. A haematoma is a swelling filled with blood. Bleeding into the subdural space may result from a head injury. Blood cannot escape from this space and symptoms follow.

The symptoms of a subdural haematoma may appear immediately or may take some time to develop. These are headache, drowsiness and sometimes confusion and there may be localized paralysis depending on the site.

The treatment is surgical removal of the clot.

Many people with head injuries are completely cured. Others are not so fortunate and after-effects may include perpetual headaches, dizziness, poor concentration, paralysis of varying degrees of severity and epilepsy (post traumatic epilepsy). In other cases the damage may be so great as to cause presenile dementia. If the frontal lobe of the brain is damaged and other parts are relatively intact, severe behaviour disorder is likely to occur. Such people have little or no emotional control and fly into a rage on the slightest provocation; they present a difficult psychiatric problem. As we mentioned in Chapter 9, a severe head injury can result in complete apathy and inactivity.

16.25 Metabolic

The neurones have nutritional needs similar to other cells in the body and they also have specific needs. They particularly need an adequate intake of the vitamin B group of vitamins. Deficiency of vitamin B gives rise to a number of syndromes.

A. WERNICKE'S ENCEPHALOPATHY. This has already been mentioned in relation to alcoholism.

B. KORSAKOFF'S SYNDROME. This has also been mentioned in relation to presenile dementia and alcoholism.

C. VITAMIN B_{12} (Subacute combined degeneration of the spinal cord). Vitamin B_{12} has two functions in the body, it is necessary for the formation of healthy red blood corpuscles—a deficiency results in pernicious anaemia—and for the nutrition of the nervous system. The effects of deficiency of vitamin B_{12} on the nervous system are tingling and numbness of the extremities, and sensory disorders such as inability to appreciate hot and cold stimuli. In severe cases the gait may be ataxic and this is a feature of subacute combined degeneration of the spinal cord. If the pernicious anaemia is effectively treated, neurological signs do not appear.

D. HEPATO-LENTICULAR DEGENERATION (WILSON'S DISEASE). This disease is due to a disturbance of copper metabolism in the body. It mainly affects the basal ganglia and gives rise to symptoms and signs similar to those found in Parkinson's disease. This condition has been mentioned in Chapter 9.

E. PORPHYRIA. This is a metabolic disorder in which porphyrins are retained in the tissues giving a higher than normal concentration in the blood and in the urine. Porphyrius (*G. porphyria*, purple dye) normally occur in protoplasm and they form the basis of the respiratory pigments.

Porphyria has two effects in the body. It causes demyelinization of peripheral nerves and it produces mental changes which may be those of depression or fear and anxiety reactions.

The disease, which is said to be due to a Mendelian dominant genetic defect, produces symptoms intermittently. These symptoms are controlled usually by antidepressants or tranquillizers as appropriate. Other varieties of the disease are due to Mendelian recessive genetic defects.

If you are interested in the historical aspects of this condition you should read the book by McAlpine and Hunter (1966). These authors have come to the conclusion that the recurrent insanity George III (1738–1820) was due to acute intermittent porphyria. George III was King from 1760 to 1820 and had serious mental disturbances for the last ten years of his reign.

16.26 Neoplastic

The term neoplastic means new growths. These growths may be benign and innocent or malignant and cancerous. We briefly mentioned brain tumours in Chapter 9 and we shall now consider them in a little more detail.

16.27 Glioma

This type of cerebral neoplasm involves the cells which form the glia, the supporting tissue of the nervous system. There are several varieties of glioma and the majority are malignant. This means that they infiltrate areas away from the primary site and thus often make surgical treatment impossible.

16.28 Meningioma

This type of tumour arises in the cells of the arachnoid villi. They are thus most commonly found in the intracranial sinuses since the arachnoid villi returns the cerebrospinal fluid to the circulation by draining it into these sinuses. Sometimes the bones of the skull overlying the tumour are affected.

16.29 Angioma

An angioma is a congenital malformation of blood vessels. We have already mentioned a particular variety of this condition in Chapter 9 which causes mental subnormality (see haemangiomatosis and Sturge-Weber Syndrome).

16.30 Secondary (metastatic) tumours

A proportion of all brain tumours are due to secondary infiltration from primary tumours elsewhere in the body. These primary sites may be in the lung, breast, stomach, prostate gland, thyroid gland or the kidneys.

Some brain tumours develop quickly and others take some time. The tumour occupies space which would normally be occupied by brain tissue and is thus called a space occupying lesion. The effect of occupying such a space is that the intracranial pressure is increased and this is characterized by headaches, vomiting and eye changes called papilloedema. Depending on its site, a tumour may cause epileptic fits, paralysis, visual defects, deafness or haemorrhage.

Sometimes mental changes may be the first to appear and may include vagueness, forgetfulness and poor concentration. Brain tumours, as mentioned in Chapter 9, are a cause of presenile dementia. A brain tumour may also cause a progressive clouding of consciousness and coma.

16.31 Diagnosis and treatment

Brain tumours are diagnosed by considering the history and by physical examination. The diagnosis may be confirmed by the following investigations:

A. X-rays.
B. Lumbar puncture.
C. E.E.G.
D. Psychological tests are sometimes helpful. The various tests are discussed in Chapter 5.

If it is possible the best form of treatment is surgery but often the tumour is not accessible or it may be so widespread as to make removal impracticable. Radiotherapy is occasionally, but not generally, used. Other forms of treatment aim at lowering intracranial pressure and include giving hypertonic saline to cause dehydration.

16.32 Degenerative conditions

Degeneration (*L. degenerare*, to depart from) in this context means a deterioration in quality or function. In some conditions the neurones degenerate and impaired function follows. In other conditions the quality and function of the blood vessels deteriorate and indirectly affect mental function. We shall now consider degeneration of the blood vessels.

16.33 Atheroma (*G. athare*, porridge)

In atheroma there is a fatty degeneration of the inner layer of the arteries. This fatty degeneration causes a narrowing of the arteries involved which means there is greater resistance to the flow of blood, that is, raised blood pressure. It also means that volume of blood supplied to the distant organ is less than normal. Degeneration of the blood vessels is a normal part of the ageing process, though many things have been blamed for it, including too high an intake of fatty food. In diabetes mellitus, degenerative changes in the blood vessels occur frequently. Small reductions in the blood supply can be tolerated without serious impairment of function, but severe reductions giving rise to ischaemia seriously affect function.

16.34 Cerebral ischaemia (*G. iskhein*, to hold back; *haima*, blood)

This may be generalized due to the narrowing of the arteries supplying an organ or it may be localized due to the narrowing of one artery. We shall now consider the effect of generalized ischaemia on the brain and the localized effects will be considered under thrombosis and embolism.

Mental symptoms are common in generalized ischaemia of the brain with impairment of intellectual function, memory defects and emotional liability. Confusion occurs and this is made worse by an upset in routine, such as admission to hospital.

The intellectual deterioration may be so great as to give rise to dementia (See Chapter 9). Epileptiform fits are another feature of ischaemia of the brain and aphasia and agnosia may also be present. Cerebral haemorrhage is also likely to occur (strokes).

16.35 Cerebral thrombosis (*G. thrombos,* clot)

A thrombus is a clot of blood in a blood vessel and is usually caused by a sluggish circulation or by changes in the walls of blood vessels (degeneration). A thrombus in an artery prevents the blood from passing beyond that point and there is ischaemia. Complete and prolonged ischaemia results in the area supplied by that artery dying. When this happens necrosis is said to occur. The disruption of brain function depends on the size of the artery blocked. A small thrombosis may produce transient or no symptoms whilst thrombosis of a major vessel may produce unconsciousness.

Thrombosis may also occur in veins and in the case of the brain the intracranial sinuses may be involved. The cavernous, the transverse and the superior sagittal sinuses may be involved. The main effect of a thrombus in a sinus or a vein, is that the area drained becomes congested and oedematous. This gives rise to increased intracranial pressure with headache, vomiting and papilloedema. Convulsions and paralysis may occur.

There are anticoagulants such as phenindione (Dindevan) available for the treatment of thrombosis, but it is not always possible to use them in thrombosis of the brain's blood vessels for they may cause bleeding from an infected area.

16.36 Cerebral embolism (*G. en,* in; *ballein,* to throw)

An emboli is a particle, usually a blood clot, though it may be of any material, fat being an example, which is detached from its site of origin and is transported in the bloodstream until it becomes stuck in a blood vessel too small to allow it to pass.

The effect is similar to the effect of a thrombus, but the symptoms come on much more quickly. The person suddenly becomes confused, has a headache and may have a fit. Consciousness may be lost if a big vessel such as the internal carotid artery is blocked.

People with an embolism are nursed at complete rest to prevent further emboli from getting into the circulation. Anticoagulants are also used in order to prevent blood clots from forming.

16.37 Cerebral haemorrhage ('stroke')

The most common cause of cerebral haemorrhage is raised blood pressure (hypertension) and the associated degenerative changes in the arteries. Cerebral haemorrhage occurs most commonly in the area of the internal capsule, though it may occur in the cerebellum or in the pons. The subjects are usually in their fifth or sixth decades or older, for it takes some time for degenerative changes to have effect.

The onset of a cerebral haemorrhage is sudden and the rupture of the blood vessel may be brought on by excitement or physical effort, though it may occur during rest or sleep. The person becomes dazed and in the majority of cases quickly loses consciousness.

As we mentioned in Chapter 2, the body is controlled by the opposite side of the brain. A 'stroke' produces paralysis of one side of the body (*hemiplegia*). The nerve tracts from the neurones in the cerebral cortex (upper motor neurones) are affected in the area of the internal capsule and though the main nerve supply to the muscles is cut off, the muscles still have a nerve supply from the extrapyramidal tract and the reflexes are intact. This means that some muscular movement, though coarse and unco-ordinated, is possible. For this reason the paralysis is called a spastic paralysis and the reflexes are exaggerated.

The main treatment of people with cerebral haemorrhage is skilled nursing care and this can be divided into two phases.

During the unconscious phase the nursing care is as outlined earlier for meningitis. The airway must be kept free and a suction apparatus is necessary to do this. Artificial feeding must be given and so must an adequate fluid intake. The person may need assistance to empty his bowels and suppositories are sometimes necessary. There is frequently incontinence of urine so that it may be necessary to have a catheter in position. A careful fluid record is essential. Because of the paralysis there is a considerably increased risk of bedsores so that the pressure areas need particular attention to prevent this. The position should be changed two-hourly for it is much better and easier to prevent bed sores than to cure them once they have occurred. Passive movements of the limbs should be part of the two-hour attention. These will prevent stiffening of the joints and contractures, and may be given by the physiotherapy staff or nurses. The best results are obtained when there is close co-operation between the nurses and the physiotherapists.

When consciousness is regained there should be an active rehabilitation programme for there are many difficulties to be overcome. People who suffer from strokes are often very active and are angry when their activity is reduced. Not being able to do things for themselves causes intense anger and frustration. Others are overwhelmed by their incapacity and become apathetic. The most important thing is to make the person accept his incapacity whilst at the same time making the most of the remaining potential.

Communication is often a big problem for the person with a stroke. This is particularly so in the case of right sided hemiplegias, for the speech centre (Broca's Centre) is in the left side of the frontal lobe of the brain in right handed people. A haemorrhage in the left side of the brain may damage the speech centre. There are two main speech problems. The use of the wrong words to express what is meant (*dysphasia*) or the inability to convert words into sounds that can be understood (*dysarthria*).

The long-term correction of these speech difficulties are the concern of a qualified speech therapist. In the meantime nurses should develop a system such as using a slate and chalk or a system of printed cards containing questions and a choice of answers. For example, do you want to go to the lavatory? yes/no. Such an arrangement can add to the person's security and spare the nurse's time.

Eating presents another difficulty. One side of the face is likely to be paralysed and the mouth is likely to drop at one side so that chewing may not be possible on the affected side and food may accumulate or dribble out. A right-sided hemiplegia in a person who is right handed may mean that he is unusually awkward when compelled to use his left hand. If cutlery is modified, for example a long-handled spoon may be used, this may help with such a difficulty. Encouragement is very important, for such people can easily give up on the grounds that it is all too much.

Walking is often a major obstacle. First there is the muscular weakness due to the paralysis and second there is the psychological problem of lost confidence. It is important that there should be plenty of physical and psychological support particularly when the person takes those first few steps. Walking frames and walking sticks may be necessary at first. The person should be encouraged to get on his feet as soon as possible for there is no doubt that the longer it is left the more difficult it becomes. Some modification of the shoes may be necessary as there is a tendency to drag the feet.

Once the person is mobile, an appropriate form of occupational therapy should be used to maintain muscle function. It is good for morale to be able to do something constructive.

A stroke is a common form of illness and it often affects people who are active and energetic. In such people such an illness causes great frustration. For an insight into how such a person feels, every nurse should read the book by the late Douglas Ritchie, details will be given at the end of this book.

16.38 Disseminated sclerosis (multiple sclerosis)

This is a common neurological disorder and it is due to degeneration of the myelin sheaths of the axons. Following the degeneration of those sheaths, an excess of glia is produced and forms a sclerotic plaque over the nerve or nerves. This sclerotic plaque interferes with the transmission of nerve impulses and disorders of function result.

The precise cause of the condition is not known but a number of observations have been made. It has been noted that disseminated sclerosis is more common in the northern hemisphere and the incidence is high in northern countries such as Sweden and Norway. The incidence is low in countries with a tropical climate and in the southern hemisphere. The incidence is low in Australia. The condition tends to run in families, for about 5 per cent of cases have a family history. There are a number of precipitating factors such as infections, trauma and fatigue.

For a diagnosis of disseminated sclerosis to be made the symptoms must be disseminated in both time and place. That is there must be a symptom-free period following the onset of the symptoms and there must be neurological symptoms arising from different sites in the body.

The symptoms may include numbness of some part of the body, double vision, weakness of a limb or difficulty in passing urine. A combination of any two of these may be present.

Disseminated sclerosis frequently affects young people in their twenties and thirties. It is not unusual for a young person to become blind, paralysed, completely helpless and bedridden. The person may recover completely from the first episode, lead a full and active life, play games and participate in sports. After a period, and the length of time varies, the symptoms return. The combination is usually different on the second and subsequent occasions. Eventually the symptoms are present all the time so that the person is permanently disabled. The average duration of life from the onset of the symptoms is 20 years. Death occurs from chest or urinary infections which are inevitable when there is a combination of paralysis and inactivity.

One would expect young and previously fit people to be very depressed with their plight, but in the majority of cases this is not so, for many have an unfounded sense of well being. The author remembers one man in his early forties who had some service with the

R.A.F. as a non-commissioned officer, who continually made plans to take up gliding. He did this despite the fact that he was blind, had both feet paralysed, was doubly incontinent and had limited use of his hands. He would vividly describe the imagined pleasures of gliding in an enthusiastic and exciting way. He was convinced that it would only be a week or two before he was in the air. Such unfounded well-being and optimism is called euphoria.

There is no specific treatment for disseminated sclerosis. Steroids are sometimes used in the acute stages of the condition, though they are unlikely to have any effect in the long term.

The nursing care varies from very little in the early stages to doing everything for the person in the later stages. Incontinence is often a major problem and from this two further problems arise; those of urinary infection and irritation and breakdown of the skin from constant contact with urine. For these reasons it is often necessary to keep a catheter in the bladder all the time. In addition to irritation from urine the skin is at risk when paralysis is present. Frequent attention to the skin is essential if pressure sores are to be avoided. If the person is bedridden his position should be changed two-hourly and the pressure points should be massaged.

16.39 Parkinson's disease

We have already mentioned Parkinsonism in relation to some tranquillizing drugs and also as a sequel to sleeping sickness (encephalitis lethargica). We shall now mention Parkinsonism arising from a degenerative process.

Parkinson's disease or paralysis agitans was first described in 1817 by James Parkinson (1755–1824). It is due to degeneration of neurones in the basal ganglia. It affects people from middle life onwards and occurs more commonly in men than in women.

The effects of degeneration of the basal ganglia are many. What strikes one first is the facial appearance. The face appears immobile and the eyes tend to stare. Such people are unable to show emotion and may appear to be permanently depressed.

The basal ganglia co-ordinate muscular movement and when this control is lost, tremors follow. The thumb assumes a position over the other fingers and the involuntary movement and tremor is referred to as 'pill rolling'. There is unusual rigidity of the limbs. For example, if an arm is flexed, this cannot be done smoothly—the action is jerky like that of a cogwheel. The rigidity is called 'cogwheel' rigidity.

Movement is very slow and the gait is characteristic. The person is bent forward and though he has difficulty in getting started he shuffles along gaining momentum all the time. The result is that after a little while the person may be running.

Parkinson's disease in the majority of cases does not shorten life and most are ambulant until near the end of their lives.

There are two forms of treatment available.

A. DRUGS. The drugs most commonly used are:

   a. Benzhexol (Artane) up to 8 mg. daily in divided doses.
   b. Ethopropazine (Lysivane), up to 200 mg. daily.
   c. Orphenadrine (Disipal), up to 20 mg. daily.
   d. L. Dopa, this is a new drug and much is expected of it, but it has not been in general use for long enough to have proved its worth.

B. SURGERY. Destruction of the affected cells in the basal ganglia by surgical methods often brings about a dramatic improvement of the symptoms. Techniques have been developed whereby an instrument may be inserted through small openings in the skull to destroy the appropriate area and thus avoid the necessity of opening the skull and exposing large areas of the brain. This type of surgery is called *stereo tactic surgery.*

16.40 Huntington's chorea

This chronic degenerative, hereditary type of chorea was first described in 1872 by George Huntington (1850–1916). It is due to a dominant genetic defect and causes wasting (atrophy) of the brain, particularly in the frontal area. There is also degeneration of the basal ganglia and the result is very unco-ordinated movements.

We have already mentioned this disease in Chapter 9 as one of the conditions which gives rise to presenile dementia.

16.41 Other

The field of neurology is a big one and large volumes have been written on the subject. In this book many conditions have been mentioned very briefly, others have been left out altogether. There are however a few conditions which should be included and which do not conveniently fit into any of the groups already mentioned.

16.42 Headache

This is a very common symptom and may be caused in many ways, for we mention headache as a symptom in encephalitis, poliomyelitis, meningitis, cerebral abscess, head injury, neoplasms, thrombosis and increased intracranial pressure. Although there are many causes there are two principal ways in which pain can be produced. First the blood vessels of the brain are pain sensitive and many headaches are due to the affect of disease processes on them. Raised blood pressure is an example. The increased pressure causes increased tension within the vessel and this in turn causes pain and is felt as headache. Second the sensory nerve roots may give rise to headache because of neuritis or neuralgia. Pain from such sites as the eyes, the sinuses and the teeth may be referred to the head and cause headache. Pain from the frontal sinus gives rise to an unpleasant form of headache known as a 'vacuum' headache. Some headaches are a response to stresses and strains and are said to have a psychosomatic origin. Such headaches are often described as causing 'pressure' on the head'

Many headaches respond to a mild analgesic and give no further trouble. Persistent or recurring headaches should always be investigated to exclude the possibility of a serious underlying condition.

16.43 Temporal arteritis

This is a condition found mainly in the elderly and causes a severe headache. As its name suggests there is inflammation of the temporal artery which may cause it to stand out and be clearly seen. The eye of the affected side may be involved and blindness can result. Temporal arteritis responds to steroid treatment.

16.44 Migraine

This is a headache, usually one-sided, which occurs at irregular intervals and may be accompanied by visual disturbances and vomiting. It is a common condition and it is said that up to 5 per cent of the population have suffered from migraine sometime in their lives. Migraine occurs more commonly in women than in men.

Migraine is due to dilatation of the branches of the external carotid artery. It is not known how the changes in these blood vessels are produced, but it is known that attacks may be brought on by the intake of certain foods, alcohol or by an emotional upset. Eyestrain may also cause an attack. People who suffer from migraine tend to be conscientious, hardworking people who set themselves high standards and who drive themselves hard to attain these standards. There is usually a strong obsessional trait in the personality.

Migraine produces a blinding headache and eye disturbances are frequently the first thing that is noticed. These distortions of vision may be dangerous in the case of motorists suffering from this condition. The person is unable to see in part of his field of vision where everything appears misty. Sometimes coloured haloes appear around lights. The headache begins as the visual disturbances get better and this may take a half an hour or more. The pain associated with the headache is often described as if a hole were being drilled in the head. The temple of the affected side is the most common site for the pain, but it may spread over the whole of the affected side of the head. Nausea may be present and vomiting may occur during an attack. The length of an attack varies from a few hours to several days.

There are a number of drugs available for the treatment of migraine:

A. Aspirin or codeine are sometimes, but not always, sufficient to relieve the headache.
B. Ergotamine tartrate may by subcutaneous injection relieve an attack of migraine or it may be given by mouth when the need is less urgent. The dose by injection is 0.25 mg. and the dose by mouth 2 mg.
C. Methysergide (Deseril). This is useful in preventing attacks of migraine, but its regular use is not recommended because of side-effects.
D. Amylobarbitone (Amytal) or phenobarbitone are sedatives which may help to prevent attacks.

Migraine cannot be prevented until the true nature of the condition is known, but those measures which can be taken, reduce the number of attacks. Fatty foods, eggs, chocolate and fruit are examples of foods associated with attacks. Often in individual cases, one or one group of foods are involved and should be avoided. Alcohol should be taken in small quantities.

The main points in the nursing care of a person with migraine are to provide absolute quiet for noise is very irritating. In addition to quietness the room should be darkened for such people have a dislike of light.

16.45 Summary

A consideration of physical disorders of the nervous system reveals the many functions of that system and how these functions may be affected. A variety of things can cause a clouding or a complete loss of consciousness with the serious threat to life which it presents. Convulsions may be caused by an equally variable number of factors. Muscle action is affected in many ways. An infection such as polio-myelitis causes flaccid paralysis when no muscle movement is possible. A 'stroke' causes a spastic paralysis, unco-ordinated movement and loss of power. The degeneration of Parkinson's disease causes tremors and a characteristic gait and the degeneration of Huntington's chorea causes wildly unco-ordinated movements.

Congenital, infective, traumatic, metabolic and neoplastic conditions of the brain, can cause mental subnormality in children if of a severe nature and if not adequately treated. In the adult, conditions of similar nature give rise to disturbances of mental function ranging from minor to severe dementia.

17

Legal aspects

17.0 Introduction

The legal aspects of mental illness no longer occupy as prominent a position as previously, for 80 to 85 per cent of those needing help are now admitted to hospital informally. There is, however, still a need for legislation to deal with the minority. It is needed because a person may be a danger to himself or to society. If a person is so disturbed that he has to be removed from society against his will, then it is important that this is done within a legal framework. It is also important that there should be legal machinery available to allow for appeal against such removal, and the person's property and affairs should be safeguarded. This is what the Mental Health Act, 1959 is about.

As a nurse you will need a working knowledge of the Mental Health Act and you should have access to a copy of the Act. In this chapter we shall make a synopsis of the Act and we shall give some detail of sections of particular interest to you.

17.1 The Mental Health Act, 1959

This document is presented in 9 parts and there are over 150 sections:

PART 1. PRELIMINARY. This part of the Act deals with the repeal of previous legislation and the definition and classification of mental disorder.
Section

1. *Section 1* repealed the Lunacy Act, 1890, the Mental Treatment Act, 1930 and the Mental Deficiency Acts of 1913 and 1938.

2. *Section 2* dissolved the Board of Control. This body, as its name implies, had legal control over those admitted to mental hospitals.

3. *Section 3* made provision for the establishment of Mental Health Review Tribunals (M.H.R.T.'s). These tribunals have taken over the functions of the Board of Control. Unlike the Board of Control, which was sited in London, the M.H.R.T.'s are sited regionally and there is one in every Regional Hospital Board area in England and Wales.

The members of M.H.R.T.'s are appointed by the Lord Chancellor and include:

13

a. Legal members (legal members provide Chairman).
b. Medical persons.
c. Lay people. Such people come from the fields of administration or the social services or have similar relevant experience.

M.H.R.T's have the power to discharge any patient from hospital and applications may be made in three ways:

a. By a patient (in writing).
b. By a relative.
c. By a person authorized to act, for example a Guardian.

Hearings are normally conducted in private and the applicant may be represented.

The onus is on the patient to make an application and to present it in the best light. Because of this the National Association for Mental Health and the National Council for Civil Liberties have experimental schemes where volunteers help patients prepare their case.

4. *Section 4* defines and classifies mental disorder as follows:

a. In this Act 'mental disorder' means mental illness, arrested or incomplete development of mind, psychopathic disorder, and any other disorder or disability of mind; and 'mentally disordered' shall be construed accordingly.

b. In this Act 'severe subnormality' means a state of arrested or incomplete development of mind which includes subnormality of intelligence and is of such a nature or degree that the patient is incapable of living an independent life or of guarding himself against serious exploitation, or will be so incapable when of an age to do so.

c. In this Act 'subnormality' means a state of arrested or incomplete development of mind (not amounting to severe subnormality) which includes subnormality of intelligence and is of the nature or degree which requires or is susceptible to medical treatment or other special care or training of the patient.

d. In this Act 'psychopathic disorder' means a persistent disorder or disability of mind (whether or not including subnormality of intelligence) which results in abnormally aggressive or seriously irresponsible conduct on the part of the patient, and requires or is susceptible to medical treatment.

e. Nothing in this section shall be construed as implying that a person may be dealt with under this Act as suffering from mental disorder, or from any form of mental disorder described in this section, by reason only of promiscuity or other immoral conduct.

5. *Section 5* deals with the informal admission of patients. It should be pointed out that patients are not admitted under the terms of the section in the ordinary sense. Section 5, through repeal of previous legislation, makes informal admission possible.

PART II. LOCAL AUTHORITY SERVICES. This part of the Act deals with the functions of the local authorities in relation to mental illness. Welfare functions, the Children's Act, 1948 (now the Children and Young Persons Act, 1969), the Education Act, 1944 and training centres are considered.

PART III. MENTAL NURSING HOMES, RESIDENTIAL HOMES. Part III is concerned with the registration and conduct of mental nursing homes.

PART IV. COMPULSORY ADMISSION TO HOSPITAL AND GUARDIANSHIP.

Section 25. Admission for observation. An application may be made in respect of a patient on the grounds:

a. that he is suffering from mental disorder of a nature or degree which warrants the detention of the patient in a hospital under observation (with or without other medical treatment) for at least a limited period; and

b. that he ought to be so detained in the interests of his own health or safety or with a view to the protection of other persons.

The main features of section 25 can be set out as follows:

Type of Admission	*Observation*
Persons authorized to make application:	Nearest relative, Mental Welfare Officer or person authorized under section 52.
Medical recommendations:	2 medical recommendations.
Forms:	Application and medical recommendation forms.
Duration:	28 days.

Section 26. Admission for treatment. An application for admission for treatment may be made in respect of a patient on the grounds:

  a. that he is suffering from mental disorder, being

    (i) in the case of a patient of any age, mental illness or severe subnormality;

    (ii) In the case of a patient under the age of twenty-one years, psychopathic disorder or subnormality; and that the said disorder is of a nature or degree which warrants the detention of the patient in hospital for medical treatment under this section;

and

  b. that it is necessary in the interests of the patient's health or safety or for the protection of other persons that the person should be so detained.

Section 26

Type of Admission	Treatment
Persons authorized to make application:	Nearest relative, Mental Welfare Officer, Person authorized under section 52.
Medical recommendations:	2 Medical recommendations.
Forms:	Application and medical recommendation forms.
Duration:	One year.

Section 29. Admission for observation in case of emergency.

Type of Admission	Emergency
Persons authorized to make application:	Nearest relative, Mental Welfare Officer.
Medical recommendation:	1 Medical recommendation.
Forms:	Application and one medical recommendation form.
Duration:	72 hours.

Section 30. Applications in respect of patients already in hospital.

The terms of this section apply when a person who has been admitted to hospital informally wishes to discharge himself and is not well enough to go home.

Section 30

Type of Admission	*Already in hospital*
Person authorized to make application:	Consultant in charge of person.
Medical recommendation:	1 medical recommendation from consultant in charge.
Forms:	1 Section 30 form.
Duration:	3 days.

Section 36. Correspondence to patients. Any letter or parcel addressed to the patient can be withheld from him if, in the opinion of the medical officer, the receipt of it would interfere with the treatment of the patient or cause him unnecessary distress. Such packets shall be opened, and if the sender's name and address can be discovered, must be returned to him by post.

Letters or postal packets sent by the patient may be withheld from the Post Office if:

a. The person to whom they are addressed has written to the hospital asking that any communication addressed to him by the patient be withheld.

b. The medical officer considers that the contents would be unreasonably offensive to the recipient, if it is defamatory of other persons (except people on the staff of the hospital) or would be likely to prejudice the interests of the patient.

Letters written to anyone on the following list must be posted, for such people play a part in safeguarding the patient's interests:

1. The Secretary of State for Health and Social Services.
2. Any member of the House of Commons.
3. The Master or Deputy Master or other officer of the Court of Protection.
4. The managers of the hospital.
5. To any other authority or person having power to discharge the patients.
6. At any time when the patient is entitled to apply to a Mental Health Review Tribunal.
7. A solicitor acting for the patient.

PART V. ADMISSION OF PATIENTS CONCERNED IN CRIMINAL PROCEEDINGS AND TRANSFER OF PATIENTS UNDER SENTENCE

Section 60. Powers of courts to order hospital admission or guardian-

ship. Section 60 enables the court to order the admission of a person to hospital and his detention there.

Section 60

Type of Admission	Hospital order
Person authorized to make application:	Magistrates Court Assize Court Quarter Sessions Court.
Medical recommendations:	Written or oral evidence of two medical practitioners.
Forms:	Hospital order forms.
Duration:	As specified in order.

Section 65. Powers of higher courts to restrict discharge from hospital. When a patient is admitted to hospital under section 60 above, the court may also apply the terms of section 65 which means that the person cannot be discharged from hospital whilst this is in force.

Section 71. Persons ordered to be kept in custody during Her Majesty's Pleasure. When a person guilty of a criminal act is also found insane, such a person is transferred to a special hospital such as Broadmoor or Rampton and is detained during Her Majesty's Pleasure, that is, without limit of time.

Section 72. Removal to hospital of persons serving sentences of imprisonment. The Secretary of State, on the evidence of at least two medical practitioners, may direct that a person serving a prison sentence may be removed to and detained in a hospital.

PART VI. REMOVAL AND RETURN OF PATIENTS WITHIN UNITED KINGDOM. This part of the Act deals with the transfer of patients within the United Kingdom, the removal of alien patients to their own country, and for the return of patients who are absent without leave.

PART VII. SPECIAL HOSPITALS. This part of the Act deals with the provision of institutions for treatment under conditions of special security.

PART VIII. MANAGEMENT OF PROPERTY AND AFFAIRS OF PATIENTS.

Section 100. Judicial authorities and Court of Protection. Sections

100 to 107 deal with aspects of the functioning of the Court of Protection.

Section 108. Lord Chancellor's Visitors.

Section 109. Functions of Lord Chancellor's Visitors. The remaining sections of this part of the Act deal with further aspects of the Court of Protection.

PART IX. MISCELLANEOUS AND GENERAL. This part of the Act contains a number of general regulations.

Sections 122 to *124* deal with the proceedings of Mental Health Review Tribunals.

Section 125 deals with forgery and false statements by relatives, guardians, doctors, nurses and welfare workers.

Section 126 is concerned with the ill-treatment of patients.

Sections 127 and *128* deal with the Sexual Offenders Act, 1956 and with the question of sexual intercourse with patients.

Section 129 with the assisting of patients to absent themselves without leave.

Section 133. This section deals with the provision of pocket money for in-patients in hospital.

Section 136. Mentally disordered persons found in public places.

If a policeman finds a person in a public place who appears to be suffering mental disorder and in need of care or control, the policeman may remove the person to a place of safety. A person admitted to hospital in this way may be detained for 72 hours. At the end of this period the person may be discharged. If, however, further treatment is needed, the person may agree to remain in hospital informally, or it might be necessary to make an order under one of the sections of the Act.

Section 147. This section gives a list of definitions as applied to the Act.

The Mental Health Act, 1959 is an improvement on the previous legislation relating to the mentally ill. The Mental Health Review Tribunals, organized on a regional basis, are better placed to deal with local problems than a centrally based and thus a remote Board of Control in London. Provision is made for closer liaison with local authorities and thus the way is open for better community care.

17.2 The McNaughton Rules

The first of the McNaughton Rules states: 'To establish a defence on the ground of insanity it must be clearly proved that, at the time of committing the act, the party accused was labouring under such a defect of reason, from disease of the mind, as not to know the nature and quality of the act he was doing, or if he did know it, he did not know he was doing what was wrong'. In 1843, Daniel McNaughton was tried for the murder of Edward Drummond, the private secretary to Sir Robert Peel. During the trial it emerged that Mr. McNaughton had had delusions of persecution for many years and that the murder was a direct result of these delusions. Mr. McNaughton was one of the first patients to be admitted to the then newly built Criminal Lunatic Asylum at Broadmoor (now designated a Special Hospital). The McNaughton Rules were drawn up by 15 judges as a result of questions in the House of Lords in relation to the case and they have provided a framework for dealing with other similar cases.

17.3 The Criminal Justice Act, 1948

The main provision of this Act, as far as hospital work is concerned, is that it provides the court with power to order psychiatric treatment as well as punishment. At the level of the magistrates court it often means that a convicted person is required to submit himself for out-patient treatment as a condition of probation.

17.4 The Homicide Act, 1957

This Act provides for a verdict of manslaughter instead of murder where it is shown that the accused was suffering from such abnormality of the mind as substantially impaired his mental responsibility for his acts or omissions in doing or being party to the killing.

17.5 The Suicide Act, 1961

From 1845 until 1961 suicide was a criminal offence in England, though for a long time people believed that such people were in need of treatment rather than punishment. The 1961 Act means that suicide is no longer an offence.

17.6 Drug legislation

Nurses handle drugs every day in the course of duty and it is therefore important to have a working knowledge of the legal aspects. Three is no need to be overawed by these for the regulations are based on common sense and are of a sort which nurses put forward themselves if asked to do so. There are three Acts of Parliament relating to drugs which are of concern to nurses.

A. DANGEROUS DRUGS ACT, 1920; REGULATIONS, 1964 AND THE DANGEROUS DRUGS ACT, 1965

1. *Provisions.* These Acts are designed to control those drugs which cause people to become dependent (addicted). There are provisions to control the production, manufacture, distribution and administration of these substances.

2. *Examples of drugs controlled by the Dangerous Drugs Acts (D.D.A.s).* Examples of D.D.A.s are opiates, such as morphine, diamorphine (Heroin), papaveretum (Omnopon), cocaine, cannabis, physeptone, pethidine and pethilorfan.

It is an offence to possess such drugs without authority. These drugs must be kept locked and the key is kept by an authorized person such as a registered nurse who is a staff nurse, ward sister or charge nurse.

3. *Ordering.* The ward Dangerous Drugs book should be used in conjunction with individual prescription sheets. Book number 90–500 is the one commonly used.

4. *Storage.* These drugs should be kept in a locked cupboard marked D.D.A. and the key kept by a registered nurse, that is, the sister or charge nurse.

5. *Administration.* The word Dangerous Drug Record Book (No. 90–501) should be used and the following information should be recorded:

Date	Time	Patient's name	Amount given	Given by (Signature)	Witnessed by (Signature)	Stock balance

The entry should be made in the book at the time of giving the drug as accuracy is essential One of the nurses must be a registered nurse and the dose of the drug must be checked with the patient's prescription sheet. Both nurses should go to the bedside; it is not sufficient to check the drug in the clinical room, the actual giving of the drug to the right person must be witnessed. The principle of giving the right dose of the right drug by the right route to the right patient at the right time applies to D.D.A. drugs as it does to all drugs.

B. THE PHARMACY AND POISONS ACT, 1933, THE POISON RULES, 1964, 1965.

1. *Provisions.* This Act is designed to control drugs, not included in the D.D.A., which are poisons and for which legislative control is desirable.

2. *Examples of such poisons.* Drugs which are controlled by this Act are the barbiturates, some amphetamines (*See below), sulphonamides, anti-histamines, digitalis, atropine, Mersalyl and tranquillizers such as Fentazin, Largactil, Sparine, Melleril, Moditen Librium, Miltown and Stelazine. Other drugs include ephedrine, arsenic and strychnine.

3. *Schedules.* This Act has several schedules but only 1 and 4 are of concern to nurses. Schedule 1 preparations in the form of weedkillers or rodent killers may be purchased from a chemist provided the buyer is known to the chemist, states how the substance is to be used and signs the Poisons Register. Schedule 4 preparations are obtainable only on a doctor's prescription. In practice it is usual to refer to all these drugs as Schedule 1 (S1) whether Schedule 4 (S4) applies or not. The pharmacist has the authority to label preparations as he thinks is warranted, 'Store as Schedule 1'; this is useful for new unclassified drugs.

4. *Ordering.* S1 and S4 drugs must be prescribed by a registered medical practitioner. They are then ordered in the ward order book. Individual prescriptions are usually dispensed, but in certain cases 'Stock' bottles may be issued. Records must be kept for two years.

5. *Storage.* S1 and S4 preparations should be stored in a locked cupboard clearly marked 'Poisons Cupboard.'

6. *Administration.* S1 and S4 drugs should be checked by a registered nurse. It is not mandatory to keep a record as for D.D.A. preparations, but some hospitals have a local system.

C. THE THERAPEUTIC SUBSTANCES ACT, 1956 (T.S.A.)

1. *Provisions.* The Therapeutic Substances Act, 1956 controls the

---

*Amphetamines such as Drinamyl (Purple Hearts, 'French Blues'), Durophet ('Black Bombers'), Dexedrine, Methedrine and L.S.D. are controlled by The Drugs (Prevention of Misuse) Act, 1964. The main provision of this Act is that possession of these drugs without authority is an offence.

sale, supply, dispensing, and administration of penicillin, other anti-biotics and the corticosteroids.

2. *Examples.* The antibiotics covered by the Act are aureomycin, chloramphenicol, erythromycin, neomycin, streptomycin, viomycin and of course penicillin.

Corticosteroids covered by the Act include hydrocortisone, prednisone and prednisolone.

3. *Ordering.* T.S.A. preparations are obtainable only on a pre-scription.

4. *Storage.* T.S.A. preparations should be stored in a non-schedule cupboard which is kept locked.

5. *Administration.* There are no special administration require-ments except an application of the principles which apply to the administration of all drugs. Gloves should be worn when administer-ing antibiotics.

D. STORAGE OF DRUGS. There should be separate cupboards, or more usually in practice, separate compartments with a single cupboard for the following groups of drugs and chemicals.

1. *D.D.A.s.* These should be stored in a locked cupboard and clearly marked 'D.D.A.' The key should be be kept by a registered nurse.

2. *Schedule Poisons.* S1 and S4 poisons should be stored in a locked cupboard clearly marked 'Poisons Cupboard'. The key should be kept by a registered nurse.

3. *Non-Schedule medicines* such as T.S.A.s, aperients, antacids and vitamins. These should be kept locked and the keys should be kept in a convenient place such as sister's office.

4. *Reagents.* These include chemicals used in the testing of urine.

5. *Disinfectants.* These should be kept in distinctive bottles to avoid the danger of confusion. The keys for the reagent and disin-fectant cupboards should be kept in a convenient place which is safe and readily accessible.

E. ADMINISTRATION OF DRUGS. There are a number of general points which should be observed in relation to the administration of drugs:

1. Drugs in any shape or form must be prescribed by a medical practitioner.
2. Abbreviations are generally best avoided as their use sometimes results in tragic mistakes.
3. All drugs should be checked at the time of administration and not at any other time.
4. The person's individual treatment sheet should be taken to the bedside. Medicine lists of any sort should not be used.
5. It is not enough for the nurse to give a drug, she must also see that it is taken by the patient.
6. When giving antibiotics and similar materials by injection gloves should be worn as a means of protecting against skin reactions.

F. DRUGS (NOTIFICATION OF ADDICTS) REGULATIONS, 1968. This is another piece of legislation relating to drugs and its title is self explanatory.

17.7 Summary

People have mixed feelings about the law. Most people will agree a system of law is essential in order to achieve a regulated society and that such laws should be based on common sense. Yet the same people will admit that they are frequently baffled by the complexity of the law, this is despite the fact that legal draughtsmen take great trouble to make their meaning clear.

It must be remembered that ignorance is never accepted as a defence in law. It is therefore important that nurses should be familiar with the general terms of the law as it affects them. A nurse who maintains a high level of professional conduct need not have anything to fear. Nevertheless it is a wise precaution to belong to a professional organization or trade union for such organizations provide legal aid for members in need.

APPENDIX I

Examples of Drugs Used in the Treatment of Mental Illness

A. TRANQUILLIZERS OF THE PHENOTHIAZINE GROUP

Approved name	Other name(s)	Dose	Indications	Contra-indications	Main side effects	Antidote
a. CHLORPROMAZINE	LARGACTIL	75–600 mg. daily	States of excitement and extreme agitation as seen in schizophrenia for example	Liver disease Other drugs (The action of alcohol and barbiturates is potentiated)	Jaundice Extrapyramidal symptoms (Parkinsonism) Dermatitis Hypotension Hypothermia	1. Hypotension. This is a dangerous complication as the blood pressure may fall to a dangerously low level *a.* Lay person flat with head lower than legs *b.* Noradrenaline by intravenous drip
b. PROMAZINE	SPARINE	75–600 mg. daily				
c. TRIFLUOPERAZINE	STELAZINE	2–30 mg. daily				2. Parkinsonism *a.* Anti-Parkinson drug
d. PROCHLORPERAZINE	STEMETIL	25–100 mg. daily				
e. PERPHENAZINE	FENTAZIN TRILOFON	10–30 mg. daily				
f. ACEPROMAZINE	NOTENSIL	30–90 mg. daily				
g. THIORIDAZINE	MELLERIL	30–600 mg. daily				
h. FLUPHENAZINE	MODITEN	1–5 mg. daily				
	MODITEN	1 ml. injection of 25 mg. Controls symptoms for 14–21 days				
	MODECATE	As above but effects last up to 28 days				

B. TRANQUILLIZERS OF THE BUTYROPHENE GROUP

Approved name	Other name(s)	Dose	Indications	Contra-indications	Main side effects	Antidote
a. HALOPERIDOL	SERENACE	0·75–6 mg. daily	Mania Schizophrenia Agitation	Parkinson's disease and other basal ganglia lesions Spastic conditions Arteriosclerosis	Parkinsonism Drowsiness Increased salivation Muscular spasm Skin reactions	1. Chlorpromazine for muscular spasms 2. Anti-Parkinson drugs
b. TRIFLUPERIDOL	TRIPERIDOL	1–5 mg. daily				
c. FLUANISONE HALOANISONE	SEDALANDE	40–400 mg. daily				

C. TRANQUILLIZERS OF THE BENZODIAZEPINE GROUP

Approved name	Other name(s)	Dose	Indications	Contra-indications	Main side effects	Antidote
a. CHLORDIAZEPOXIDE	LIBRIUM	30–100 mg. daily	Anxiety tension and delirium tremens Behaviour disorders in children	—	Ataxia, skin rashes Drowsiness Potentiates the effects of barbiturates and alcohol	—
b. DIAZEPAM	VALIUM	2–10 mg. daily				

D. ANTIDEPRESSANTS OF THE MONOAMINE OXIDASE INHIBITOR GROUP

Approved name	Other name(s)	Dose	Indications	Contra-indications	Main side effects	Antidote
a. NIALAMIDE	NIAMID	75–150 mg. daily	All forms of depression	Impaired liver function. History of heart disease as these drugs mask anginal pain Should not be in conjunction with morphine, pethidine, adrenaline or anti hypotensive drugs	Headaches Dizziness Hypotension Dry mouth Blurred vision Restlessness	1. Avoid mixing with other drugs or alcohol 2. Avoid certain foods such as cheese, beans and Marmite
b. PHENELZINE	NARDIL	15–45 mg. daily				
c. TRANYLCYPROMINE	PARNATE	10–60 mg. daily				
d. ISOCARBOXAZID	MARPLAN	10–30 mg. daily				
e. MEBANAZINE	ACTOMOL	15–30 mg. daily				

E. ANTIDEPRESSANTS OF THE TRICYCLIC VARIETY

Approved name	Other name(s)	Dose	Indications	Contra-indications	Main side effects	Antidote
a. IMIPRAMINE	TOFRANIL	75–200 mg. daily	Endogenous and involutional depression	Epilepsy and cardiac failure Should not be used in conjunction with mono amine oxidase inhibitors	Dry mouth Tachycardia Visual disturbances Tremors Skin reactions Excitement Insomnia Hypotension	No specific antidote 1. Restore blood pressure if there is hypotension 2. Discontinue drug
b. DESIPRAMINE	NORPRAMIN PETROFAN	50–200 mg. daily				
c. TRIMIPRAMINE	SURMONTIL	75–200 mg. daily				
d. AMITRIPTYLINE	HORIZON SAROTEN TRYPTANIL TRYPTIZOL	75–200 mg. daily				
e. NORTRIPTYLINE	ALLEGRON AVENTYL	20–100 mg. daily				
f. OPIPRAMOL	INSIDON ENSIDON	100–150 mg. daily				

APPENDIX II

Examples of Anticonvulsants

Group		Approved name	Other name(s)	Approximate total daily dose	Indications	Contra-indications	Main side effects
1. Barbiturates	a	PHENOBARBITONE	LUMINAL	100–300 mg.	Grand mal	Petit mal (made worse)	Occasional rashes Dependency
	b	PRIMIDONE	MYSOLINE	250–200 mg.	Grand mal Psychomotor		Sleepiness Nausea, ataxia which disappear after a few doses
	c	METHYLPHENO-BARBITONE	PHEMITONE PROMINAL	250–1000 mg.	Grand mal		
2. Hydantoins	a	PHENYTOIN SODIUM	EPANUTIN DILANTIN	300–600 mg.	Grand mal Psychomotor	Best avoided in children	Hyperplasia of gums (especially in children). Ataxia, headache, tremors, rashes, blood disorders. Hirsutes
	b	METHOIN	MESONTOIN	300–600 mg.	Grand mal Psychomotor		
	c	ETHOIN	PEGANOME	2000–3000 mg.			
3. Oxazoldine-diones	a	TROXIDONE	TRIDIONE	600–1200 mg.	Petit mal	Grand mal (made worse)	Photophobia, day blindness and dazzle Nephrotic syndrome Blood disorders Rashes
	b	PARAMETHADIONE	PARADIONE	900–1800 mg.	Petit mal		
4. Succinimides	a	ETHOSUXIMIDE	ZARONTIN	500–1500 mg.	Petit mal Psychomotor		Sleepiness, dizziness Vomiting Leucopenia
	b	PHENSUXIMIDE	MILONTIN	1000–3000 mg.	Petit mal		Nausea, dizziness Drowsiness Occasional rashes

Group		Approved name	Other name(s) daily dose	Approximate total	Indications	Contra-indications	Main side effects
5. Phenglacty lureas	a	PHENACEMIDE	PHENURONE	500–1500 mg.		Very toxic used only as a last resort	Personality change Liver and bone marrow damage
	b	PHENTURIDE	BENURIDE	200–400 mg.			
6. Others	a	BECLAMIDE	BENZCHLORPROPANIDE NYRDRANE HIBICON	2000–3000 mg.	Grand mal	Petit mal	Said to be non-toxic
	b	SULTHIAME	OSPOLOT	200–600 mg.	Grand mal Psychomotor	Petit mal	Nausea, headache Dizziness Paraesthesia
	c	MEHPHENESIN	MYANESIN TOLSERAM	1–6 g. 1–6 g.	Myoclonic	Petit mal Grand mal Psychomotor	Drowsiness Ataxia, nausea
	d	CARBAMEZEPINE	TEGRETOL	600–1000 mg.	Grand mal Temporal lobe	Petit mal	Dizziness Drowsiness Dry mouth Tight sensitive Dermatitis Aplastic anaemia

APPENDIX III

Examples of Barbiturates

A. ULTRA QUICK ACTING (ANAESTHETICS)

Approved name	Other name(s)	Dose	Indications	Contra-indications	Main side effects	Antidote
a. HEXOBARBITONE	CYCLONAL EVIPAN	The drugs in this group are used as anaesthetics				
b. THIOPENTONE	PENTOTHAL INTRAVAL					
c. METHEXITONE SODIUM	BRIETAL SODIUM					

B. SHORT ACTING (HYPNOTICS)

Approved name	Other name(s)	Dose	Indications	Contra-indications	Main side effects	Antidote
a. PENTOBARBITONE	NEMBUTAL	100–200 mg.	Inability to get to sleep type of insomnia	Barbiturate sensitivity Impaired kidney or liver function	Rashes Dependency	1. BEMEGRIDE 2. AMPHETAMINES 3. MANNITOL for use in forced diuresis
b. QUINALBARBITONE	SECONAL	100–200 mg.				

C. INTERMEDIATE ACTING (HYPNOTICS)

Approved name	Other name(s)	Dose	Indications	Contra-indications	Main side effects	Antidote
a. AMYLOBARBITONE	AMYTAL	100–200 mg.	As for short acting barbiturates	Respiratory depression		
b. BUTOBARBITONE	BUTISOL SONERYL	100–200 mg.	Effect lasts longer			
c. CYCLOBARBITONE	PHANODORM	200–400 mg.				
d. AMYLOBARBITONE SODIUM	SODIUM AMYTAL	100–200 mg.				

D. LONG ACTING (SEDATIVES)

Approved name	Other name(s)	Dose	Indications	Contra-indications	Main side effects	Antidote
a. BARBITONE	VERONAL MEDINAL	300–600 mg.	Anxiety	See Anticonvulsants		
b. METHYLPHENO BARBITONE	PHEMITONE PROMINAL		Epilepsy } Epilepsy			
c. PHENOBARBITONE	LUMINAL	100–300 mg.				

APPENDIX IV

The Collection of Specimens for Laboratory Investigations

Attention to accurate details on request forms is *essential*. The patient's name (in block letters), age, ward, diagnosis (relevant information), and tests required must be entered and signed by Doctor.

1. CHEMICAL INVESTIGATIONS

Substance	Sample Required	Type of Container	Remarks (Use appropriate form.)
Glucose	Blood or Plasma	Fluoride/ Oxalate	Yellow bottle, 2 ml. required. Fluoride inhibits glycolysis.
Acid or Alkaline phosphates	Serum (or) Plasma	Universal container Heparin tube	Haemolysis interferes with result so: minimum constriction of arm, clean puncture, dry tubes, no shaking after collection—gentle mixing of heparin only. Sample must be separated and frozen as soon as possible, don't delay in transit.
Barbiturate	Blood	Heparin	A large volume of blood is needed for this test (10–20 ml.).
Bicarbonate	Plasma	Heparin Universal container	Bicarbonate (as CO_2) is rapidly lost to or absorbed by the air. CO_2 combining power gives almost the same information as bicarbonate estimation. Plasma for this test must be separated as soon as possible.
Bilirubin	Serum (or) Plasma·	Universal container Heparin tube	Haemolysis interferes with the result. Bright light destroys bilrubin so protect from light.
Calcium	Serum	Universal container	Collect blood *without venous stasis*. Estimation must be performed as soon as possible.
Chloride	Plasma	Heparin Universal Container	
Cholesterol	Serum (or) Plasma	Universal container Heparin tube	
Transaminase:			Haemolysis interferes with result.
S.G.O.T.			Separate Serum and
S.G.P.T. and Lactic de-hydrogenase	Serum	Universal container	Store at low temperature (4 °C.) until estimation can be performed.

Substance	Sample Required	Type of Container	Remarks (Use appropriate form.)
Iron	Serum	Universal container	Large volume required. Take 20 ml. blood. Avoid contamination with iron. Plastic disposable containers supplied by the laboratory are suitable. Glass containers, unless treated, are out. Plastic syringes should be used.
Phosphate		Universal container	The first part of the analysis must be performed immediately. Don't delay in transit. Avoid haemolysis.
Potassium	Plasma Serum	Heparin Universal container	Be most careful to avoid haemolysis. Blood cells contain far more potassium than plasma and haemolysis liberates this potassium into the plasma giving erroneously high results.
Protein	Serum	Universal container	Plasma can be used but fibrinogen is a nuisance in this estimation.
Pyruvate	Blood		Special collection needed; arrange with laboratory.
Salicylate	Serum (or) Blood	Plain tube	
Sodium	Plasma Serum	Heparin Universal container	
Urea	Blood (or) Serum	Universal container or sequestrene or heparin	Do not use fluoride (Yellow label) or double oxalate (white label).
Uric Acid	Serum (or) Plasma	Universal container Heparin tube	
Zinc & Thymol turbidity	Serum	Universal container	
Vit. B_{12}	Serum	Universal container	10ml. required.

Gastric Analysis (test meals), Sugar Tolerance, Urea Clearance or Concentration Tests, Ascorbic Acid Saturation Tests, 17 Ketosteroids and Congo Red Tests are performed by arrangement with the laboratory: Find out what is the local practice.

COLOUR CODE FOR ANTICOAGULANTS

In most cases, the stopper as well as the label is coloured.

Di-potassium sequestrene	Pink
Fluoride/Oxalate	Yellow
Lithium heparin	Orange (this is the heparin tube referred to above)
Universal container	White

2. URINE ANALYSIS

Routine chemical investigations   ordinary fresh specimens.

Urea Clearance ⎱
Ascorbic Acid ⎰ See separate instructions above.

3. FAECES ANALYSIS

Occult Blood—small specimen in container with spoon.

4. HAEMATOLOGY—use appropriate form.

Haemoglobin ⎫
Total R.B.C. and W.B.C. ⎪
Sedimentation Rate ⎬ Sequestrene bottle—2–5 ml.
Packed Cell Volume ⎪
Spectroscopy—by arrangement ⎭
Fragility—clotted blood—plain tube
Other investigations carried out by   Sterile screw capped bottle
Laboratory Staff at bedside. Cells in   containing oxalate. Immediate
Puncture Fluids (other than C.S.F.)   examination important.

5. SEROLOGY—use appropriate form.

Wasserman and Kahn Reaction ⎫
Gonococcal Fixation Test ⎪
Widal Reaction and Weil Felix Reaction ⎪
Agglutination against Br. abortus and ⎬ 5 ml. of blood collected in
  melitensis   plain sterile bottle.
Blood grouping (including Rh.) and ⎪
  cross-matching. ⎪
A.S.O. Titre ⎪
Paul Bunnell ⎭
Cold Agglutinins   Fresh specimen sent direct to
                     laboratory.

6. BACTERIOLOGY—use appropriate form.

   a. *Blood Culture*—10 ml. of blood divided into two blood culture bottles, both containing glucose broth. Collect aseptically.
   b. *Antibiotic Levels* —5 ml. of blood in plain bottle.
   c. *Sputum*   —For acid fast bacilli—screw capped carton or bottle. For organisms, fungi and cells—screw capped *sterile* bottle.
   (Immediate examination essential, therefore, no delay in transit).

d. *Faeces*   —For pathogenic organisms—screw capped carton or plastic bottle or rectal swab.
(N.B. A throat swab dipped in faeces is also suitable). For amoebae or parasites—freshly passed specimen to be sent to laboratory immediately.
Thread worm ova—Cellophane swab from perianal skin (obtainable from laboratory on request) Sellotape, sticky side, satisfactory.

e. *Urine*   —For organisms—*Clean* specimen from males and females

f. *C.S.F.*   —Sterile screw capped bottle.

g. *Puncture Fluid*—Sterile bottle containing oxalate.

h. *Pus*   —Sterile screw capped bottle (or swab if this can be sent to laboratory without delay).

i. *Antibiotic content of Blood or Body Fluids*—Fresh specimen in sterile container.

j. *Vaginal Discharge*—Swab (transport to laboratory at once). Trichomonas rapidly loses its motility.

k. *Pregnancy Test*—Clean early morning specimen.

The date of the last menstrual period should be given whenever possible. Six weeks should elapse from L.M.P. (last menstrual period).

If information is not available in the ward about obtaining specimens from patients for other tests, or if you are in any doubt, you should ask the laboratory staff.

BIBLIOGRAPHY

Suitable texts for a more detailed study once the principles outlined in the text have been mastered.

CHAPTER 1

BENNION, F. (1969). *Professional Ethics: the Consultant Professions and their Code.* Charles Knight.
EWING, A. C. (1962). *Teach Yourself Ethics.* English University Press.
LILLIE, W. (1957). *An Introduction to Ethics.* Methuen.
STRINGER, P. (1970). *Ethics and Judgement in Surgery and Medicine.* Heineman.
The Problems of Euthanasia (1971). British Medical Association.

CHAPTER 2

BEARD, R. (1969). *An Outline of Piagets Developmental Psychology.* Routledge & Kegan Paul.
CALDER, N. (1970). *The Mind of Man.* British Broadcasting Corporation.
CARTER, C. O. (1962). *Human Heredity.* Penguin.
COHEN, J. (1968). *Psychology—an Outline for the Intending Student.* Routledge & Kegan Paul.
COX, DAVID (1963). *How the Mind Works. Teach Yourself Books.* English Universities Press.
DAVIES, D. V. (Editor) (1967). *Gray's Anatomy.* 34th Edition. Longmans.
FLAVEL, J. H. (1963). *The Developmental Psychology of Jean Piaget.* Von Nostrand.
FRASER ROBERTS, J. A. (1970). *An Introduction to Medical Genetics* (4th Edition). Oxford Medical Publications.
HAMILTON, W. J., BOYD, J. D. AND MOSSMAN, H. W. (1962). *Human Embryology.* (3rd Edition). W. Heffer & Sons, Cambridge.
JAHODA, M. AND WARREN, N. (1966). *Attitudes.* Penguin.
JAMES, D. E. (1970). *Introduction to Psychology for Teachers, Nurses and Other Social Workers.* (2nd Edition). Constable.
KAHN, J. H. (1965). *Human Growth and the Development of Personality.* Pergamon.
LOVELL, K. (1969). *An Introduction to Human Development.* Macmillan.
MARSHALL, W. A. (1968). *Development of the Brain.* Oliver & Boyd.
McDOUGALL, W. (1912). (Reprinted 1952). *Psychology.* Oxford University Press.
The mind (1965). *Life Science Library. Time Life International* by John Wilson and Editors of *Life.*
THOULESS, R. H. (1958). *General and Social Psychology.* University Tutorial Press.
WALTER, W. G. (1953). *The Living Brain.* Penguin.
WILSON, HARRIETT. (1962). *Delinquency and Child Neglect.* Allen & Unwin.

CHAPTER 3

GILLIS, L. AND BIESHEUVAL, S. (1962). *Human Behaviour in Illness.* Faber and Faber.
HADFIELD, J. A. (1969). *Dreams and Nightmares.* Penguin.
Health Education. (1957). *Education Pamphlet 31.* H.M.S.O.
HOLLINS, T. H. B. (Editor). (1964). *The Aims of Education, A Philosophic View.* Manchester University Press.

MOLONEY, J. C. (1952). *The Battle for Mental Health.* Philosophical Library, New York.
ROBERTS, NESTA. (1967). *Mental Health and Mental Illness.* Routledge & Kegan Paul.
SKOTTOWE, I. (1957). *A Mental Health Handbook.* Arnold. London.
SODDY, K. AND AHRENFELDT, R. D. (Editors). (1965). *Mental Health in a Changing World.* Tavistock Publications.
TAYLOR, LORD AND CHAVE, S. (1964). *Mental Health and Environment.* Longmans, Green & Co.
WHEELER, O., PHILLIPS, W. AND SPILLANE, J. P. (1961). *Mental Health and Education.* University of London Press.
WILSON, J. (1968). *Education and the Concept of Mental Health.* Routledge & Kegan Paul.
WOOTTON, BARBARA, *et al.* (1959). *Social Science and Social Pathology.* Allen & Unwin.

CHAPTER 4

HOPKINS, P. AND WOLF, H. H. (1965). *Principles of Treatment of Psychosomatic Disorders.* Pergamon.
The Psychosomatic Disorders. Pamphlet No. 5. Mental Health Research Fund.
TREDGOLD, R. F. AND WOLF, H. H. (Editors). (1970). *U.C.H. Notes on Psychiatry.* Duckworth.
WOLF, S. G. AND WOLF, H. G. (1943). *Human Gastric Function.* Oxford University Press.

CHAPTER 5

CATTELL, R. B. (1965). *The Scientific Analysis of Personality.* Penguin.
HARE, R. (1967). *Bacteriology and Immunity for Nurses.* Longmans.
HILL, D. AND PARR, G. (Editors). (1963). *Electro-encephalography*—2nd Edition.
MILLS, J. W. (Editor). (1968). *Diagnostic Methods.* Butterworths.
VERNON, P. E. (1964). *Intelligence and Attainment Tests.* University of London Press.

CHAPTER 6

ATKIN, I. (1962). *Aspects of Psychotherapy.* Livingstone.
BALINT, M. AND E. (1961). *Psychotherapeutic Techniques in Medicine.* Tavistock.
BARTON, R. (1959). *Institutional Neurosis.* John Wright.
CAPLAN, G. (1969). *An Approach to Community Mental Health.* Tavistock.
CLARK, D. H. (1964). *Administrative Therapy.* Tavistock Publications.
CRAMMER, J. L. (1969). *Practical Treatment in Psychiatry.* Blackwell.
DANIEL, G. R. AND FREEMAN, H. L. (Editors). (1967). *The Treatment of Mental Disorders in the Community (Symposium).* Balliere, Tindall & Cassell.
HINTON, J. (1967). *Dying.* Penguin.
HOPKINS, S. J. (1968). *Drugs and Pharmacology for Nurses.* Livingstone.
FREUD, SIGMUND. (1914. Reprinted 1942). *Psychopathology of Everyday Life.* Penguin Books.
JONES, M. (1968). *Social Psychiatry in Practice.* Penguin
MARCUSE, F L. (1959). *Hypnosis: Fact and Fiction.* Penguin.
MARTIN, D. V. (1968). *Adventure in Psychiatry.* Faber & Faber.
OSWALD, I. (1968). *Sleep.* Penguin.
OTTAWAY, A. K. C. (1966). *Learning through Group Experience.* Routledge & Kegan Paul.

SARGANT, W. AND SLATER, E. (1963). *An Introduction to Physical Methods of Treatment*. (4th Edition). Livingstone.

SPENSER-PATTERSON, A. (1963). *Electrical and Drugs Treatments in Psychiatry*. Elsevier.

SPROTT, W. J. H. (1958). *Human Groups*. Penguin.

SPROTT, W. J. H. (1966). *Social Psychology*. Methuen.

CHAPTER 7

CARTWRIGHT, ANN. (1964). *Human Relations in Hospital*. Routledge & Kegan Paul.

CROW, L. D. AND CROW, ALICE. (1961). *Understanding Interrelations in Nursing*. Macmillan, New York.

HOLMES, M. J. AND WERNER, J. A. (1966). *Psychiatric Nursing in a Therapeutic Community*. Macmillan, New York.

MCGHEE, ANNE. (1961). *The Patient's Attitude to Nursing Care*. Livingstone.

MCGHIE, A. (1969). *Psychology as Applied to Nursing*. Livingstone.

ODLUM, D. M. (1952). *Psychology, the Nurse and the Patient*. Nursing Mirror Publication.

WEISS, OLGA. (1954). *Attitudes in Psychiatric Nursing Care*. G. P. Putnam's Sons, New York.

CHAPTER 8

MAGEE, B. (1968). *One in Twenty*. Secker & Warburg.

POMEROY, W. B. (1970). *Boys and Sex*. Penguin Books.

WEST, D. H. (1968). *Homosexuality*. Duckworth.

CHAPTER 9

Age is Opportunity. (1961). National Council of Social Service Incorporated.

A Glossary of Mental Disorders. (1968). H.M.S.O.

Arrangements for Old Age. (1969). Consumers Association.

FELSTEIN, I. *Later Life: Geriatrics Today and Tomorrow*. Penguin.

HALLAS, C. H. (1970). *The Care and Training of the Mentally Subnormal*. John Wright.

HEATON-WARD, W. A. (1967). *Mental Subnormality (3rd Edition)*. John Wright, Bristol.

IRVINE, R. E., BAGNALL, M. K. J. AND SMITH, B. J. (1970). *The Older Patient*. English Universities Press.

KIRMAN, B. H. (1968). *Mental Retardation*. Pergamon Press.

ROBERTS, NESTA. (1970). *Our Future Selves. Care of the Elderly*. Allen & Unwin.

STEPHEN ELSPETH. (Editor). (1970). *Residential Care for the Mentally Retarded*. Pergamon.

CHAPTER 10

EYSENCK, H. J. (1960). *Behaviour Therapy and the Neuroses*. Pergamon Press, Oxford.

LADER, M. H. (1969). *Studies of Anxiety. R.M.P.A.* Headley Brothers Ltd.

RYCROFT, C. (1968). *Anxiety and Neurosis*. Penguin.

CHAPTER 11

BARTLETT, F. C. (1958). *Thinking*. Allen & Unwin.

FISH, F. (1962). *Schizophrenia*. John Wright.

Royal Medico-Psychological Association Symposium (1967). *Recent Development in Schizophrenia*. Alec Coppen and Alexander Walk. (Editors). *R.M.P.A.*

WALLACE, CLARE MARC. (1965). *Portrait of a Schizophrenic Nurse*. Hammond, Hammond & Co., London.
WING, J. K. (1966). *Early Childhood Autism*. Pergamon Press, Oxford.

CHAPTER 12

ARNÓLD, A. B. (Editor). (1968). *The Nature of Emotion*. Penguin.
BURSTON, G. R. (1970). *Self-Poisoning*. Lloyd-Luke.
Royal Medico-Psychological Association Symposium (1968). *Recent Developments in Affective Disorders*. A. Coppen and A. Walk. (Editors). London.
STENGEL, E. (1964). *Suicide and Attempted Suicide*. Penguin.
VARAH, CHAD. (1965). *The Samaritans*. Constable.

CHAPTER 13

CRAFT, M. (1965). *Psychopathic Personality*. John Wright, Bristol.
LLOYD, R. AND WILLIAMSON, S. (1968). *Born to Trouble*. Cassirer.

CHAPTER 14

Alcohol Abuse. (1970). Office of Health Economics.
Drug Abuse—The Scope for Action. (1970). Association for the Prevention of Addiction.
GREENFIELD, SIR HARRY AND OTHERS. (1970). *Drug Dependence*. Institute for the Study and Treatment of Delinquency.
IMLAH, N. (1970). *Drugs in Modern Society*. Geoffrey Chapman.
KESSEL, N., AND WALTON, N. (1965). *Alcoholism*. Penguin.
PHILLIPSON, R. V. (Editor). (1970). *Modern Trends in Drug Dependence and Alcoholism*. Butterworth.
RITSON, B. AND HASSAL, C. (1970). *The Management of Alcoholism*. E. S. Livingstone.
Smoking and Health Now. (1971). *Report of the Royal College of Physicians*. Pitman Medical.

CHAPTER 15

TREDGOLD, R. F. AND WOLFF, H. H. (Editors). (1970). *U.C.H. Notes on Psychiatry*. Duckworth.

CHAPTER 16

BARHAM CARTER, A. (1968). *All About Strokes*. Nelson.
BICKERSTAFF, E. R. (1965). *Neurology for Nurses*. English Universities Press.
MARSHALL, J. (1956). *Neurological Nursing*. Blackwell Scientific Publications.
RITCHIE, D. (1965). *Stroke—A Diary to Recovery*. Faber & Faber.
SCOTT, D. F. (1969). *About Epilepsy*. Duckworth.
WILLIAMS, M. (1970). *Brain Damage and the Mind*. Penguin.

CHAPTER 17

KENYON, F. F. (1968). *Psychiatric Emergencies and the Law*. John Wright.
Mental Health Act, 1959. H.M.S.O.
SPELLER, S. R. (1970). *Law Notes for Nurses*. Royal College of Nursing and National Council of Nurses of the United Kingdom.

Index